D1807646

Therapy of Social Medicine

Byong-Hyon Han

Therapy of Social Medicine

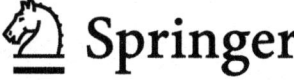 Springer

Byong-Hyon Han
Independent Scholar
Seoul, Korea (Republic of)

ISBN 978-981-287-747-5   ISBN 978-981-287-748-2   (eBook)
DOI 10.1007/978-981-287-748-2

Library of Congress Control Number: 2015956181

Springer Singapore Heidelberg New York Dordrecht London
Translation from the Korean language editions: 사회약료와보건의료체계 by Byong-Hyon Han,
© Seoul National University Press 2014. All rights reserved.
© Springer Science+Business Media Singapore 2016

This work is subject to copyright. All rights are reserved by the Publisher, whether the whole or part of
the material is concerned, specifically the rights of translation, reprinting, reuse of illustrations, recitation,
broadcasting, reproduction on microfilms or in any other physical way, and transmission or information
storage and retrieval, electronic adaptation, computer software, or by similar or dissimilar methodology
now known or hereafter developed.
The use of general descriptive names, registered names, trademarks, service marks, etc. in this publication
does not imply, even in the absence of a specific statement, that such names are exempt from the relevant
protective laws and regulations and therefore free for general use.
The publisher, the authors and the editors are safe to assume that the advice and information in this book
are believed to be true and accurate at the date of publication. Neither the publisher nor the authors or the
editors give a warranty, express or implied, with respect to the material contained herein or for any errors
or omissions that may have been made.

Printed on acid-free paper

Springer Science+Business Media Singapore Pte Ltd. is part of Springer Science+Business Media
(www.springer.com)

Preface

There is not only one right way to living a good life.
Just as there are many routes in climbing the top of Mt. Everest,
I wish to give hope to people with a "new route" in life,
which I will call "Social Medicine."

Many people in the pharmaceutical field are trying their best to discover and develop new drug products. However, what most people who take on the challenge don't know is that it takes more than a decade to create a new drug. In Aug. 22, 2013, there came good news. The research level and achievements of the College of Pharmacy at Seoul National University of Korea were evaluated as the world's best. I feel very proud that the news contributed to the increasing national standing of Korea. I know how hard the professors and students have worked to win this feat, and I dearly hope that they carry on the good tradition.

The world of drugs, based on new drug development, is a microscopic nano-world (10^{-9}). I hope new substances and drugs that can give hope to the humanity can be developed by our scientists, who are working at the frontiers of cutting-edge science technology.

The macroscopic world of "social medicine," however, is not something that can be seen with our eyes. It has been more than three decades that I made up my mind to develop social medicine. Finally, after the 30 painstaking years, social medicine started to beckon itself to me. As it turned out, social medicine has been in my everyday surroundings, and most importantly, it was in myself. So this is how the book made its way out into the world; I wanted to give hope to people.

Hope is like a road made on the ground,
it neither exists or not exists.
No road is there from the beginning,
but when many people walk the path,
it becomes a road.
- Lu Hsun (Hometown)

In this book, *Therapy of Social Medicine*, I focused on laying the theoretical foundation of social medicine and therapy of social medicine (or SM therapy):

First, social medicine is "everything that helps our health except drug products," which consists of two key elements originated from natural healing power (NHP) in Oriental medicine; homeostasis (natural healing strength (NHS)), and reciprocity (social healing strength (SHS)). As such, social medicine is woven by two strands of double healings rather than by two strands of double helix.

Second, twenty-first-century pharmacy should be a harmonious system by the conversion of traditional drug as a core part with the new social medicine as a remaining margin.

Third, theoretically, social medicine as a remaining margin can be screened and developed without limitation, but here I focused on daily life and complementary alternative medicine (CAM).

Fourth, on the eve of era for "healthy 100 years old," individuals should be health prosumers, which needs four major social medicines such as health diet, health exercise, health stressor, and beautiful laughter developed from our daily life.

Fifth, social medicine can be specialized into various SM therapies (i.e., aromatherapy, stone therapy, diet therapy, exercise therapy, light therapy, etc.) just as stem cell does.

Sixth, social medicine therapy can be defined as every event or activity including health behavior and illness behavior for health management and improvement or methodology derived from the theory of social medicine.

Seventh, although SM therapy is boundless, here I focus on "4+2 system." 4 means diet, body, stress, and facial image control and 2 refers to evacuation (–) and filling (+) methods originated from CAM.

Finally, "beautiful laughter" (BL) is newly introduced for pharmaco-gelotology, which includes enforced laughing for health.

Individuals, the society, and the nation all have their parts to play in promoting peoples' health. In the book, I concentrated on what individuals and the community can do and discussed social medicine, SM therapy, and pharmaco-gelotology from the general to the particular.

There is a saying that "A journey of a thousand miles begins with the first step." I do hope that my book can be the first step in our life's journey and ultimately give new hope to the readers around the world.

This book could not have been completed without the devoted assistance of translation by Mrs. Na Kyung-jin. I also thank my family (Young-joo, Sun-kyu, Chang-kyu, and wife Lee Yong-hae), mentor (Prof. B. A. Sorofman), colleagues, and friends including Chungwoohoe for their support, love, and especially their understanding as I completed this task.

Leopard of Kilimanjaro

A poem by Yang In-ja

Have you ever seen a hyena that wanders on the mountains to look for prey?
The hyena aims for the dead carcass of animals
But I wish to be a leopard, not a hyena
I want to be the leopard of Kilimanjaro,
which goes up to the mountain top and starve and freeze to death
I wake up to glory one day,
and to a battered life the other
And now I'm taking refuge at a dark corner of the world
I can't be found anywhere, by the splendor of city lights
Who cares if I'm left alone in the middle of this big city
There was even van Gogh, who was unknown in this life

I can't come like a wind
and leave like dew
I should leave a trace of me, like a column of smoke
Should I disappear without any piece of me,
I will burn up like the flames
Don't ask me why -
Why I wish to be raised to the top
Who cares if no one knows the fiery soul of a lonely man?

When it feels lonely and cold
the world has nothing in it to console such heart
but the only thing that makes the world beautiful
is love, is what they say
But they don't know how much love
can make the other love so lonely
they don't know they can get as lonely as love
You said you loved crickets
I love crickets, too
You said you loved lilacs
I love lilacs, too
You said you loved the night
I love the night, too
And I love again
Cheers to my youth,
my lonely youth, which seems full yet empty

Love is lonely, because you bet your life on it
You're lonely because you give everything to love
Love and ideals,
they all demand your everything
It's so lonely to bet with all the things you have
Love is a heartbreaking passion of goodbye
What is at the end of passion?
Love does not regret,

even if you lose everything
Then you can say you truly loved

Even in the deepest nights,
I will live on as a ray of light
Even in a barren land scorched with heat
I will live on as a stream of clear water
I will be a firmly grounded tree,
even if storms wither the trees and grass
I live on in this world,
because the 21st century called for me

Is it clouds or snow,
covering the mountain tops of Kilimanjaro?
I keep going forward in my journey
with a backpack on my back
Who cares if I shake hands with loneliness in the mountains
and become a mountain myself?

Seoul, Korea (Republic of)   Byong-Hyon Han
June, 2015

Contents

List of Figures

List of Tables

Chapter 1
Why Social Medicine?

1.1 The Rise of Social Medicine

On average, the pharmaceutical industry headed by visible drugs takes up about 1.5 % of overall industries in Korea. To put it another way, this means that the relative importance of the pharmaceutical industry among all industries in Korea stands at a meager 1.5 %. The small portion taken by the pharmaceutical industry tells us that medicine itself is not given much importance in the Korean society. Korea, already bearing the burden of being a divided nation, has been putting in much effort in achieving economic development. As a result, in a relatively short period of time after the establishment of the government of the Republic of Korea, it has accomplished both democratization and industrialization at the same time. Now, Korea should brace for the impacts of rising new waves of informatization, globalization, and an aging society. In this complex era, it seems that the pharmaceutical industry's importance in the society won't get much bigger in the short term, as Korea has another challenge of breaking the 40,000-dollar barrier in its per capita GDP.

Korean scientists have been taking on greater challenges in the pharmaceutical industry, however small its share may look in the overall Korean industry. As a result, professors in the College of Pharmacy at Seoul National University (SNU) have been formally acknowledged the best in their research level and achievements (p. A11, Chosun Ilbo, Aug. 22, 2013). Just as Samsung Electronics is topping the global market with its smartphones, with over 32.3 % of market share and accumulated sales volume of 319.8 million phones as of 2013, it is very hopeful that the research level of the College of Pharmacy at SNU is regarded the best around the world. However, what we should look back upon ourselves is that the scientists are only concentrating on the visible drugs in medical research. I know it is hard to point our fingers at them, because developing new drugs has been the norm in the field. Globally, pharmaceutical scientists have believed that the driving force of the history of medicine lies in the "productivity" of new drugs that creates "blockbusters." ("Blockbusters" refer to

© Springer Science+Business Media Singapore 2016
B.-H. Han, *Therapy of Social Medicine*, DOI 10.1007/978-981-287-748-2_1

innovative new drugs that can create more than 1 billion dollars' worth of sales each year.) Therefore, it's hard to deny the fact that research and development in the pharmaceutical world has been focused mostly on developing new, visible drugs, and it has been the mainstream discourse of the pharmaceutical industry to date.

In this book, I will introduce the concept of "social medicine" for the first time. I will argue that new drug development, the main discourse in the pharmaceutical community in the twenty-first century, is only one little part of the world of medicine, which is similar to only clinging to the "infrastructure" called productivity. Here, "infrastructure" refers to the sum of production means that form the basis of a society. I aim to reset the direction of the discourse by replacing "productivity" with "imagination." I believe that the world of medicine is made up of two parts: one, social medicine of the "superstructure," and the other, drug of the "infrastructure." "Superstructure" here means social institution, law, politics, religion, philosophy, and other forms of social rituals. With this in mind, I want to question the current dominant discourse that the productivity-based infrastructure defines the superstructure. As I mentioned, the world of drugs only takes up about 1.5 % of the entire industry in Korea. When the rest 98.5 %, which I believe is the legitimate share for social medicine, is discovered, it can give bigger hope to humanity as a whole.

As you can see, the world of social medicine is a very important new field, but it had been left untouched and therefore remained a virgin territory. Social medicine gives us greater promises as it can help us in fields such as treatment, disease prevention, antiaging, longevity, well-being, and happiness. Social medicine is an amorphous medicine that can be discovered and developed by using vitalizing energy, which is the origin of mankind.

For better understanding, I would like to explain social medicine by comparing it to arts. Social medicine is similar to atonal music created by Arnold Schoenberg. People believed that only the fixed scales of do, re, mi, fa, sol, la, ti, and do made up music. However, Schoenberg broke away from the tradition and norm and declared that all scales can be made into music, and he opened the world of modern music with his new idea. Social medicine also takes a similar stance, in that it views all things in the world to be used as medicine. In an artistic point of view, social medicine is a transformation from the classic representational painting, which focused on depicting the objects exactly, to cubist painting led by Pablo Picasso, who is the father of abstract painting that depicts objects in a free, modern way.

Therefore, the paradigm shift in the world of medicine is going from the traditional, visible drug to social medicine. It accompanies turning from the consumption of medical activities to the production of health or from lifesaving activity to vitalizing activity. The way we look at medicine will be taking a hopeful step forward.

The world of social medicine is a new system of medicine based on the so-called sociological imagination of C. Wright Mills. Sociological imagination calls us to look at our everyday surroundings with a new perspective. It makes us to look at ourselves out of our usual surroundings and contexts to be in a bigger picture. Through sociology, we get to learn that what was once thought of as natural, necessary, good, or true can be wrong. We understand that what we believed to be right can be influenced by historical incidents or social circumstances. Therefore, the world of social medicine is a new world that calls for new perspectives:

> Nowadays people often feel that their private lives are in a series of traps. They sense that within their everyday worlds, they cannot overcome their troubles, and in this feeling, they are often quite correct. What ordinary people are directly aware of and what they try to do are bounded by the private orbits in which they live; their visions and their powers are limited to the close-up scenes of job, family, neighborhood; in other milieu, they move vicariously and remain spectators. And the more aware they become, however vaguely, of ambitions and of threats which transcend their immediate locales, the more trapped they seem to feel.
>
> Underlying this sense of being trapped are seemingly impersonal changes in the very structure of continent-wide societies...
>
> Yet people do not usually define the troubles they endure in terms of historical change and institutional contradiction. The well-being they enjoy, they do not usually impute to the big ups and downs of the societies in which they live. Seldom aware of the intricate connection between the patterns of their own lives and the course of world history, ordinary people do not usually know what this connection means for the kinds of people they are becoming and for the kinds of 9/5/2015-making in which they might take part. They do not possess the quality of mind essential to grasp the interplay of individuals and society, of biography and history, of self and world. They cannot cope with their personal troubles in such ways as to control the structural transformations that usually lie behind them...
>
> It is not only information that they need – in this Age of Fact, information often dominates their attention and overwhelms their capacities to assimilate it. It is not only the skills of reason that they need – although their struggles to acquire these often exhaust their limited moral energy.
>
> What they need, and what they feel they need, is a quality of mind that will help them to use information and to develop reason in order to achieve lucid summations of what is going on in the world and of what may be happening within themselves. It is this quality, I am going to contend, that journalists and scholars, artists and publics, scientists and editors are coming to expect of what may be called the sociological imagination.
>
> The sociological imagination enables its possessor to understand the larger historical scene in terms of its meaning for the inner life and the external career of a variety of individuals. It enables him to take into account how individuals, in the welter of their daily experience, often become falsely conscious of their social positions. Within that welter, the framework of modern society is sought, and within that framework the psychologies of a variety of men and women are formulated. By such means the personal uneasiness of individuals is focused upon explicit troubles and the indifference of publics is transformed into involvement with public issues...
>
> The sociological imagination enables us to grasp history and biography and the relations between the two within society. That is its task and its promise. (Mills 1959)

When we look at humans and our history in societal sense, we can be assured that the world of social medicine is an "open world" that aims a healthier world. In the new, open, and uncertain world, the source of power lies not in productivity but in imagination. The world of social medicine can only be seen when we take a step backward from the real world. That is why people with "social navigation (an ability of reading the flow of the world by focusing on individuals, history, and society or wisdom of finding various correlations between variables)" can find their way through. It is a dynamic new world where "universal stream (i.e., an extreme state of vital energies collaborated among people based on humanism)" operates as well.

Auguste Comte said that to study the most complicated social institution in all of universal phenomena, one must start from the most simple and common field. With this, Comte announced the hierarchy of sciences, where he believed mathematics was the first step, the basis of positive philosophy, moving onto astronomy, physics, chemistry, and biology. After biology came the last step, which Comte announced is sociology. In my book, following in the footsteps of Comte, I will open a new world of social medicine by pointing out that medicine has been advancing and transforming in the following hierarchy based on drug development: natural products (herbal medicine, a part of nature or extracts including natural animal, plant, and mineral products), chemical products (compounds), biological products, and lastly, social medicine.

Professor T. Levitt of Harvard University emphasizes in his book *The Marketing Imagination* that imagination skills to come up with something new can "get you far more things at an instant than the scientific excellence, which had been put in time and money for a whole year, can give you" (Levitt 1983).

I would like to stress once again that there is not only one right way to cure disease and promote health. The readers of my book will find themselves in a place to decide whether they should stick to the so-called blockbuster drugs of the infrastructure or choose the universal stream that social medicine, based on the imagination of the superstructure, promotes.

I believe it will happen when the followings are understood by the public. First is the fact that they have the freedom to choose. Second is the fact that our life and health are made up of greater things than the economic values produced by traditional concept of "productivity" and that visible drugs are not perfect. Third is that to make life more meaningful for us and for those around us, we ultimately have to depend on social medicine, which can be helpful to the humanity. I want to add that a few months before Bobby Kennedy died in 1968, he said that people continually evaluate their life and society based on their standards. This still holds true today:

> It seems that we have forsaken the excellence and value of community in accumulating material things.
> …
> Simply put, GDP calculates everything except for the things that make our lives worthwhile. (Kennedy 1968)

1.2 Human Being: *Homo medicus*

In essence, humans are *Homo medicus*, which means people depend on medicine. The cycle of birth, aging, illness, and death is the natural cycle of life, but as we can't sit on our hands waiting to get old and sick, it is natural for people to make an effort to maintain a healthy life as long as they can. Life expectancy for a human has hit an all-time high of 100 years now. With this, health became the buzzword of our era, and medicine to promote health is gaining peoples' interest.

First, as the preamble to the UN Charter (1946) stipulates, health is not a simple condition of being free from disease or infirmity. It includes various aspects of being well in physical, mental, social, and spiritual sense:

> Health is a state of complete physical, mental, and social well-being and not merely the absence of disease or infirmity.

Interestingly, when the many aspects of health are summarized, it can be drawn into one single continuum that stems from absolute health to death. For an individual, health is a skill and ability. In this sense, being healthy includes having regenerative powers. A healthy person working to promote his health or coming back to a healthy condition from a temporary state of unease can be called to have increased his productive powers or been treated. Similarly, a person recovering from cancer or from an incurable disease is called being "regenerated." The fact that we have regenerative skills gives hope, although it isn't seen often in our daily lives. Norman Cousins who introduced "laughter therapy" said that he came to value regeneration skills very much after he recovered from ankylosing myelitis (Cousins 1992). Recently, humans have succeeded in regenerating hair cells, and it is giving hope to the development of medication for baldness, which remains yet to be solved. For individuals, health is not only a critical part of life but is also directly related to the freedom to choose what they want to do. That is why people say "when you lose health, you lose everything" (Grandjour 2008; Sen 2002). I believe that self-discipline is required in order to maintain one's health. Maintaining an individual's health is one of the prerequisites of the nation's duty in promoting human rights, and that is why each country is running health insurance policies that suit their circumstances. By doing so, nations aim to protect the members of the society from disease and the economic loss from it.

Health determines people's life and their quality of life, and disease is one of the main culprits that threaten health. As diseases take various forms, it is only natural that medicines to cure each disease are different. However, until now, only the drug from the "infrastructure" has been recognized and used as medicine. Therefore, at this point, I believe it is necessary to review several concepts of disease for better understanding.

First, it is the word "disease." It involves a special clinical symptom and refers to a medical point of view that includes a special pathogenesis of a condition. Disease is diagnosed and treated by doctors or medical experts. Disease also has with it the pathological change of the body, such as the flu, cancer, or heart disease. In short, the word "disease" emphasizes the objective aspect of a symptom.

Second, "illness" refers to the experience of being sick, in which individuals go through social and psychological changes in the physiological condition they are in. Illness refers to personal feelings and pains that come with changes in the body. The word "illness" stresses the subjective aspect of a symptom.

Third, "sickness" is a social term. People around the sick acknowledge the patient's condition and in this way, the sick person holds a special status or role in the society. The word "sickness" puts emphasis on the social aspect of a symptom.

As you can see, various concepts of disease not only include objective or subjective aspects but also a social one. Therefore, when an individual is sick, it is a matter that concerns people around him. There are certain social expectations for the sick, and when the sick doesn't follow what's regarded as required of him, he can be labeled abnormal.

Until the twentieth century, society saw individuals as medical consumers or patients in regard to maintaining health. This limited patients to be passive. Talcott Parsons was one of the theoretic leaders claiming the passivity of patients. He developed the "sick role" to describe the behavioral patterns of the sick. Parsons explained the concept in the following three aspects:

1. Patients are not personally responsible for being sick. Disease is considered as a result of physical elements that are beyond the reach of one's control. The onset of disease has nothing to do with the attitude or action of the patient.
2. The patient is given a right and privilege that includes the exemption from responsibility. As sick people don't take responsibility for their disease, they are exempt from duties and roles that they otherwise had to assume. Even impolite or thoughtless acts are forgiven. For instance, sick people are free from conventional duties from home, and they don't have to work, and they get the right to stay in bed.
3. Patients should consult a medical expert and agree on playing the role of a sick person and should strive to restore health. Sick role is a temporary and conditional role that should be assumed by the patient who wants to get healthy. The affirmation of disease by a medical expert prompts the others to believe that the patient is sick. The patient does what he can do according to the doctor's prescription, to restore health. Those who refuse to see the doctor or does not listen to the doctor's medical advice can't play the sick role (Parsons 1952).

However, Parsons' "sick role" theory became outdated as people's lifestyles and disease patterns changed. Now, individuals are eager to take the responsibility to fight off disease by themselves. The sick role theory, which was suitable for explaining acute bacterial diseases, doesn't work in the case of chronic diseases. As for chronic disease, we don't have a cure for now, and the best that the patients can do is to share with other patients how they carry on with the condition, maybe with the help of their family members, and to talk about their personal experiences. I believe all the aforementioned changes provide a fertile ground for social medicine to be the new vision and driving force for modern health system.

Prolonged life expectancy of humans shows that both the society and individuals have advanced. For instance, the life expectancy of Korean male and female during the 35 years from 1970 to 2005 rose by 16.4 and 16.3 years, respectively. The increased rate was the second fastest among 30 OECD (Organization for Economic Cooperation and Development) countries, trailing right behind Turkey (Hankookilbo, Dec. 11, 2011). Statistics Korea forecast that by 2060, the life expectancy for Korean male and female will rise up to 86.6 and 90.3 years, respectively (see Table 1.1). Then the level will be similar to that of Japan or Switzerland, which are well-known countries for longevity.

The new twenty-first century society where people are expected to live 100 years requires individuals to act as both consumers and producers. As *Homo medicus*, individuals will continue to play a passive role in the infrastructure, the role of a

Table 1.1 Comparison of life expectancy among Korea, Japan, and Switzerland

Life expectancy		2010	2020	2030	2040	2050	2060
Male	Japan	79.6	80.9	82.0	82.8	83.6	84.2
	Switzerland	80.3	82.4	83.9	84.6	85.3	86.0
	Korea	77.2	79.3	81.4	83.4	85.1	86.6
Female	Japan	86.4	87.7	88.7	89.6	90.3	90.9
	Switzerland	84.9	87.0	88.4	89.1	89.6	90.0
	Korea	84.1	85.6	87.0	88.2	89.3	90.3

Source: Press Release of National Statistical Office, Korea, 2013. 3. 28
*UN expects life expectancy in Korea to be 83 and 89.3 years for male and female, respectively, by 2060

patient or a medical consumer, and the government will bear most of the medical costs. At the same time, individuals will play the role of a health producer by using social medicine in the superstructure, thereby acting as a "health prosumer." Nowadays, people tend to put more value on disease prevention and health management before disease occurs. In everyday life, people practice disease prevention by rethinking their meal, exercise, work, relaxation, drinking, smoking, and sleeping habits. Stress mvanagement is also regarded as very important. One of social medicine's tools, various mass media programs related to health, is also a great boost to providing information for individuals to promote their health.

Originally, the word "prosumer" is a combination of the words "producer" and "consumer." It was first used by the futurist Alvin Toffler in 1980 in his book *The Third Wave*. He said that in the twenty-first century, individuals will play both the roles of a producer and a consumer. Prosumer directly engages in production and sales along with consumption and enjoys the rights of the consumer from the production stage to the distribution of products. Prosumers are not passive buyers who only get to exercise the right to choose items from the shelves but are active consumers who like to design their own products. Prosumers are making their appearance in literature, too, where readers don't limit their role to passive bystanders but act as producers of stories (Kim Ki-Ran and Choi Ki-Ho 2009).

As a health prosumer, individuals' role is no longer limited to a medical consumer, but he can take on a more active role of a health producer. He can use social medicine, which is easily accessible, to opt for productive choices, thereby improving health and quality of life. In the process, social medicine can become a catalyst and driver in creating a new health system in the superstructure. For instance, social medicine in the form of exercise, such as walking Dulle-gil, Olle-gil in Jeju Island, Korea, using bicycle roads and free public gyms are resources open to us whenever and wherever.

On the consumption side, individuals are showing a more active tendency to act as "sophisticated consumers." Consumer's right, which is gaining more ground socially nowadays, is the basis for the change. In the era of consumer's rights, consumer's selection is strengthened, which is giving power to self-help movements, where individuals are willing to take the responsibility for their own health. As these changes in trend show, medical consumers are taking great interest in complementary alternative medicine (Giddens 2013).

Then why the sudden rise of alternative medicine? First, traditional medicine is not 100 % reliable. Diseases such as cold (minor ailment), cancer (serious illness), and adult disease (chronic diseases such as diabetes, high blood pressure, and hyperlipidemia) are yet to be conquered, and there is no clear way to diminish stress following the conditions.

Second, the workings of modern medical system are another stumbling block. Long waiting hours, the inconvenience of visiting doctors, and high costs are some to name a few.

Third, there is anxiety over side effects of drugs and operations, which are the essence of traditional medicine. A glaring example is the "thalidomide incident." Thalidomide was a sedative and a sleeping pill invented in 1953 in West Germany and was distributed globally until 1961 throughout Europe. The USA was excluded due to import ban. Back then, thalidomide was approved by animal experiment, and it wasn't until later when people found out that it hindered the growth of blood vessels in the human body. Pregnant women used the drug to calm morning sickness, and it resulted in more than 12,000 victims of phocomelia, who had short arms and legs or none at all. Thousands more died due to the drug.

Fourth, the asymmetric power relations between the doctor and patient are burdensome. That is why some who want to take on a more proactive role of prosumer go through pains to go on "medical shopping" to look for nonauthoritarian doctors.

Fifth, some people object to the idea of dualism of the mind and body, which is the foundation of traditional medicine that sees the two as separate elements. To them, the idea is thought of as unacceptable in religious and philosophical senses.

Now, the five reasons mentioned above are why complementary alternative medicine, which aims to promote health and prevent disease, is gaining momentum. It is used along with the traditional medicine that is based on the biomedical model of health and disease, which appeared with the discovery of bacteria in the late nineteenth century. Social medicine includes all essential elements of alternative medicine but not visible drugs from the infrastructure.

In short, the fundamental problems related to health in the modern society are as follows. First, humans are not passive robots, and traditional medicine, equipped with cutting-edge science technology based on biomedical model, can't solve all diseases that people suffer from. Finally, it is hard to know what exactly "health" is through the biomedical model, as the model sees "health" as a state of absence of disease (Cho Byung-Hee 2010). Table 1.2 includes the presumptions and criticisms of the biomedical model.

Humans are social beings. Society is a community or a group where two individuals or more come together. In a society, various regulations and rules are established to satisfy people's social wants and needs. Society is a complex system of institutions where people are connected to each other in various social relations. People internalize social rules and act accordingly. Therefore, both human and

Table 1.2 Presumptions and criticisms of the biomedical model

Presumption	Criticism
Disease is the result of damage caused by a precise biological factor	Disease is labeled within the soc defined by "scientific" facts
Patients are passive beings who have a sick body and should be treated, and his mind should be separated from his body in treatment	Patients' opinions and experienc__ __ are essential in treatment. Patients are active, holistic beings and their overall welfare including physical health is important
Medical experts have "expertise" and only provide treatment to cure the patients' physical condition	Medical experts are not the only solution to promoting health and preventing disease. Alternative knowledge holds as much importance
Hospitals are home to cutting-edge medical technology and therefore they are where disease can be treated most effectively	Treatment can take place anywhere other than hospitals. Treatment composed of technology, visible drugs, and operation are not always superior

Source: *Sociology* (6th Edition), 2013, p. 368

society act as independent variables (main agents) but also as dependent variables (objects).

In a busy modern society, stress is an inevitable part of our lives, and it decreases peoples' quality of life, though we may not suffer from a specific disease. A healthy amount of stress can arouse challenging spirits in people, giving us the power to overcome barriers and increasing the potential and vitality in our everyday lives. However, negative stress results in negative reactions, giving rise to various physiological symptoms such as headache, stomach cramps, backache, rise of blood pressure, fatigue, and increased heartbeat. Stress is also the cause of behavioral disorders such as crying, car accidents, amnesia, screaming, criticizing, boasting, compulsive behaviors, and aggression. Emotional disorders resulting from stress vary from feeling concerned, blue, overly excited, anxious, angry, depressed, lonely, powerless, and worried (Jung Dong-Hwa 2010). The word "stress" comes from the Latin word "stringer," which means holding something tight. It has been used to explain happenings in not only natural science and engineering but also in human behavior and experience. Usually, when we say "stress," we refer to the negative meaning with the Latin root. The undesirable results from stress have a great impact on the health of an individual, causing the person to avoid the stressful situation and to get away from it.

In the twenty-first century, humans are still *Homo medicus*. However, people will move on from taking the role of a drug consumer to the role of a healthy prosumer, which encompasses healthier producer, reproducer, or sophisticated consumer who depends on social medicine. In this way, people will continue to pursue life beyond 100 years. Humans are not passive beings left behind in the "sick role behavior." When in a healthy state, people try to promote health and prevent disease by actively engaging in "healthy behavior." When people feel amiss or coming down with something, they would notice something is wrong and go to the doctor to be diagnosed and to look for proper treatment. They are all "illness behaviors," and I want oil-based extracts, how to boil with alcohol, and ways to pulverize, boil, filter, and disperse are introduced. According to research on 800 clay tablets that contain contents about drugs, among them is a clay tablet in the seventh century BC of King Ashurbanipal of Assyria. On it are written 250 types of plant drugs, 120 types of mineral drugs, and 180 types of drugs made with other miscellaneous ingredients.

In the Egyptian civilization, which is very similar to that of Mesopotamia's, one of the most meaningful relics can be the 11 medical papyrus. Among them, the Ebers Papyrus, which was written in 1500 BC, has more than 811 prescriptions and 700 drugs and specific ways to discern drugs. According to the papyrus, plant drugs such as colocynth, senna, and castor oil were used as relaxants. For animal drugs, pig's brain, the vagina of female dog, fly, and excretion of crocodiles were used. Alum, copper, and salt are listed as mineral drugs and they appear repeatedly in the papyrus.

In ancient Egypt, the system of managing drugs was established. The making of drugs, which is called "pastophor," and storage of drugs were separately performed under the supervision of doctors. Medical service was mostly provided through drugstores and there were helpers there who made drugs. There were also separate rooms to prepare drugs at temples and separate rooms to conduct experiments to store and test drugs at king's palaces. In these rooms, the collection and storage of drugs were conducted under the supervision of a special person in charge, and preparing drugs was the duty of the head of the drug preparation unit in the palace. His duty was to manage overall pharmaceutical procedures such as measuring, grinding, mixing, extracting, and boiling of drugs. What he prescribed was made into various dosage forms of medicine to be used, and the various types are as follows: medicine you keep in your mouth before cleansing with water, elements you mix with medicine to erase the bitter taste, smoking agent, inhalant, foam breaker, enema, suppositorium, medicine used as major element, salve, injection and instillations, etc. Just like in Mesopotamia, Egypt had its specific ways to manage drugs combined with its overall medical system.

In ancient China, herbal medicine that was orally handed down from Shen Nung, who is regarded as the father of medicine, was called "boncho (or original herb)." The written book of the oral tradition is called *Shen Nung Pharmacopeia*, which is the first book to read to know about "boncho," and there are 365 herbs listed in the book. Later, more drugs were added and Lee Si-Jin's *Boncho Classification Book* was published, where some 1000 herbs and 450 natural animal products were included to be used in 11,000 different cases. In ancient China, people believed that every disease has its own type of drug for treatment and that everything in nature can be used as medicine. In the sixth century, Dohonggyeong (AD 452–536), who was influenced by Buddhism and who was the father of Taoism, categorized herbs in the *Shen Nung Pharmacopeia* by yin and yang. He believed that drugs have an impact on the vitality and the harmony of living beings and thus categorized drugs in levels 1, 2, and 3. The 120 types of drugs in level 1 were called "gun" and 120 types of drugs in level 2 as "shin," which were tonic medicine. Lastly, level 3 drugs were called "gwasa" and there were 125 types. The drugs were prohibited from taking for a long period of time because of their venomous trait, and this shows the impact of Taoist hermit ideology on the drugs.

In ancient India, Ayurveda was the pharmacology of the Veda era, around 1500 BC. Plant drugs comprised most of Ayurveda, and more than 2000 types of drugs are mentioned in Charaka. For instance, drugs and spices that were popularly traded between the Indians and the Romans, such as white sandalwood, cinnamon, cardamom (a type of ginger), monkfish, ginger, pepper, Ranunculaceae, and licorice, are mentioned. Charaka not only had the list of drugs but also explained the effect of each drug. It gave instructions on the dosage of drugs and recommended ways to make drugs look, taste, and smell good in colors, flavors, and fragrance, respectively, by combining other substances. Later, around 500–1000 AD, Tantra medicine was integrated with Ayurveda and laid the foundation for chemical pharmacology. In 1400 AD of "Lasaratnasamukchaya" pharmacology, more than 5000 types of mercury medicine and medicine containing miscellaneous metals were listed. Until the fifteenth century, the collection of Ayurveda remained the answer to pharmacology.

1.3.2 The Greek and the Roman Period

1.3.2.1 The Greek Period

Minoan and Mycenaean civilizations, which flourished in the Greek islands, Crete, and other Asian regions since 3000 BC, were passed to Greece. That is how Greece was able to develop a unique hellenistic civilization, different from the Mesopotamian or Egyptian civilization, in the eastern Mediterranean from 600 to 300 BC. Hellenism is individualistic, cynical, and secular and emphasizes freedom and beauty. Greek medicine focused on nature, reason, and experience, which enabled it to treat disease, and on the cause of the condition by taking hints from nature, rather than resorting to superstition.

The theory of humoral pathology was taken as a golden rule in medical science, and it was originated from the four elements (air, water, heat, and earth) of Aristotle. The theory of humoral pathology became the theoretical basis in drug therapy, and for the last 2000 years, it remained unchallenged as the beginning of Western pharmacology and the study of medical effects. Drug therapy laid the foundation for allopathy by treating fever with drugs that can cool off heat and conditions related to dryness with drugs of humid traits. It was conducted according to the heterology of a particular body fluid of the patient.

The *Corpus Hippocraticum* doesn't contain pharmacology, but the followers of Hippocrates wrote about 200 types of plant drugs, 10 types of animal drugs, and 12 types of mineral drugs. Pedanius Dioscorides showed excellence in ancient Greek pharmacology, and his collection *Pharmacology* includes some 600 types of plants, 35 of animal drugs, and 90 of mineral drugs. With its massive coverage,

Pharmacology was widely used in the West for 16 centuries as one of the most prestigious books in medicine.

In the field of natural products, pharmacology, and pharmacotherapeutics, Greece was able to establish its name, but the management of drugstores remained only a part of the medical field. As drug therapy was rational, positive, and scientific, doctors consulted making drug prescription with experts.

1.3.2.2 The Roman Period

Medicine in Rome bloomed with the inflow of Greek doctors. Aulus Cornelius Celsus wasn't a doctor, but his book *De Medicina* was one of the most practical books at the time. His fifth book began with the categorization of medicine and became the first ancient pharmacopoeia. In his sixth book, Celsus talked about eye drops. The book was written in Latin and passed down Greek medicine. The book was able to come to light in the Renaissance period, when Pope Nicholas found and printed the book in 1478.

Gaius Plinius Secundus was also called "Pliny the Elder," and with his appetite for knowledge, he printed a large volume of *Natural History*. The book was printed in 1469, which contained some 20,000 records of observation by combining 2000 dissertations and books. From volume 18, Secundus started to mention medicine. Volume 20–27 contained contents about natural plant products, volume 28–32 about animal cures, and volume 33–37 about mineral drugs. However, his book was later criticized for carrying superstitious therapies without confirmation.

Claudius Galenus (AD 131–201) is the father of medicine, and his achievements exceed that of Pedanius Dioscorides. Galenus' book *Methodo Medendi* talks about single medicine, complexes for each ailing parts, and characteristics and mixes of complexes according to their forms. As his book categorized medicinal effect based on the theory of humoral pathology, his theory on drug therapy became somewhat doctrinaire. Galenus manufactured medicine by himself in Iatreion, which was where doctors manufactured drugs at the time, and stored drugs in Apotheca. He focused on the management of drugstores and drug therapy. His theory was widely spread in the West until Paracelsus challenged him in the sixteenth century.

In his book *Compositione Medicamentorum Liber* (AD 43), Scribonius Largus talked about various medication using 242 types of herbs, 36 natural mineral products, and 27 natural animal products. Based on pharmacology, Largus suggested the archetype of early pharmacy. In his preface to pharmaceutics, he stressed the importance of drugs in therapy and their effect and intensity. Oribasius, who was the palace doctor for Emperor Julian in the fourth century, summarized Galenus' achievements and therapies used in Greek medical institutions. His book *Collectorum Medicinalium* refers to 600 types of drugs from Dioscorides and Galenus. Oribasius had great knowledge in various medicines, and his works are meaningful in that they conserved, edited, and adapted the core theories of Galenus.

Roman doctors prescribed and manufactured drugs, just like Greek doctors, but they also had slaves manufacture and prepare special drugs. Roman doctors had people who prepared medicine, powdered medicine, and made salves and cosmetics work for them, and there were also drug sellers who went around towns to sell drugs. There were also drug peddlers who had their own shops. Fake doctors and spice traders existed as well. Although there were many people who worked in the pharmaceutical industry, professional pharmacists didn't come into being before the Roman Empire was on the road to collapse.

1.3.3   The Middle Ages

The 1300 years after the death of Galenus in the second century to the era of anatomist Vesalius in the sixteenth century is regarded as the Middle Ages of medicine. The cultural heritage of Greece and Rome was passed down to the Byzantine Empire of East Rome. After Byzantine lost its power, Arab medicine that combined the Eastern elements of the Saracens, Syrians, Persians, and Egyptians emerged.

1.3.3.1   History of Byzantine Medicine

The history of Byzantine medicine is the period from the third century up to 1453, when Byzantine was destroyed by Muhammad the 2nd of Turkey. Byzantine medicine inherited the tradition of the ancient Greek's rational medicine. Aetius (AD 502–575) lived in Amida near the Tigris River in the sixth century. He summarized Galen's theory and corrected some of Galen's categorization of medicine.

Alexander who lived in the same era as Aetius was evaluated as the best doctor in Byzantine. He focused more on treatment than theory and argued that the disease should be treated with any possible means. He accepted various medicines, and it included even having patients to have a talisman attached on their body. Paul was a surgeon in the seventh century and worked in Alexandria. His book was written in Arabic and was used as a tool for the Greek and Roman medicine to be spread to the Arab world.

1.3.3.2   History of Arab Medicine

The two important people in the history of Arab medicine are Al Razi (Rhazes) and Ibn Sina (Avicenna), who were both Persian doctors. Rhazes took the theory of Hippocrates and Galenus and wrote 237 medical books. The 14 books known as the *Liber Medicinalis* and *Continens Medicinae* are the most famous. He made mercurial ointment known to the Arab and the Western world. He was particularly interested in dosage forms and preferred pills, thinking it as the most suitable dosage form. In terms of treatment, he focused on maintaining physical health in the onset of disease and preferred not using medicine if diet was enough to cure the condition. He preferred single medicine and used complexes only when single medicine wasn't enough.

There was an event in Germany, which allowed running an apothecary as a special profession in the history of medicine in the Middle Ages. Emperor Frederick the 2nd announced an edict in 1240, which was similar to the Magna Carta of Medicine. It declared pharmacy as a professional field and regulated that opening and running of apothecary be checked by regional colleges of medicine. Pharmacists were given the duty to make drugs in the same way. There were three items in the edict, which had a great influence on the development of medicine in the later days: (1) separation of medicine and pharmacy, (2) institutionalized regulation on drugstore management, and (3) declaration of quality standard in the manufacture of drugs. It became the foundation of pharmacopoeia in the future.

Along with drugstores run by individuals, there were also public drugstores in the thirteenth century, and the two competed against each other. The drugstores stemmed from clinics in the abbey but were bought by private drugstores. In Basel, Switzerland, abbey drugstores and private drugstores coexisted for a long time, before the abbey drugstores disappeared after the Reformation of 1528. However, abbey drugstores continued to exist until the nineteenth century in Bavaria and Austria, where Catholicism ruled.

Pharmacognosy was greatly influenced by the overseas travels and trade by many merchants including Marco Polo (1254–1324). New medical herbs from overseas and spices were imported to Europe and expanded the scope of treatment.

1.3.3.6 Renaissance and Medicine

The advancement of art, literature, philosophy, education, religion, and science in the Renaissance era had their roots in the ancient world of Greece and Rome. However, the development was greater than the Greek and Roman influence. Observation by natural order, experiment, and reasoning was regarded as important in the medicine field, and it was a breakthrough for medical development.

In particular, Theophrastus Bombastus von Hohenheim (AD 1493–1541), who was known as Paracelsus, contributed much to the development of medicine by discovering new medicine that overturned the system of traditional medicine. He was born in Switzerland and was a bit wild. In June 24, 1527, he stomped on and burned the five books by Avicenna, which had been used as college textbooks in the era and declared a new theory of medicine. It was similar to Martin Luther, who undertook Reformation. Paracelsus also refused to use Latin in college lectures and used German. He saw the body as a chemical laboratory. In terms of chemical process, he called for "vital force" or "archeus" and "taking chemical substances" became the core of his theory and studies. In those days, the foundation of drug manufacturing was alchemists' skills. He argued that "the work of alchemy is not making gold or silver, but making drugs." By publishing *De Medicina*, he used alchemy in drug manufacturing and opened up the way for development of chemistry.

He stressed the three unmaterialistic elements of our body over the traditional four elements of Aristotle. Flammability was categorized as sulfur element, liquid and volatility as mercurial element, and safety and solidity as salt element. He used metallic compounds and had a new approach in drug therapy. He didn't simply depend on chemical drugs but saw that each disease had a corresponding cure and that similar drugs can cure similar conditions. His theory was in stark contrast with that of Galen's. His theory partly relates to "Oejing-ism," in that it uses oil from people's skulls in epilepsy.

He developed the distillation technique suitable for volatile elements and manufactured alcohol, wine, and essential substances. He also manufactured strong minerals and acetic acid. With the advancement of metallurgy, he was able to supply mercury, antimony, and lead. As production of arsenic, gold, bronze, cobalt, bismuth, and iron was made possible, new materials such as mercury substances prone to corrosion and calomel (mercury chloride) were able to be manufactured.

In 1608 Frankfurt, Oswald Croll published *Basilica Chymica*. As various other types of chemical books were published, people began to advocate Paracelsus. They also became more open to his "Oejing-ism." Until late sixteenth century, pharmacology became a foundation for a new document with the theory of Paracelsus, and he is evaluated as the one who left a glorious achievement in the history of medicine. In short, Hippocrates of Greece and Galenus of Rome were the ones who pioneered the first revolution of medicine, in the mythological, ancient medicine, based on natural products. Paracelsus used a chemical approach, taking one step further from the natural products, and made a second revolution in the field by allowing chemical substances to be used as medicine.

1.3.3.7 The Discovery of the New Continent and New Medicine

Since Columbus discovered America and the New World in 1492, many explorers discovered unknown lands. It opened up a new era of colonization for Europe. Rare herbs were imported from new continents to be used as new cures. The captain of the ships and pirates knew that the discovery of new drugs or the location of the existing herbs can be very profitable. In 1585, an English captain named Richard Hakluyt tried to make his voyage with 31 experts and wrote it in his plan. Among the 31 experts, "medicine experts" were the next in line after "mineral experts," and it shows the influence of medical experts and the importance of medicine in the era.

In those days, new types of medicine were rapidly discovered, as there was ample supply of exotic drugs such as camphor, ginger, and rhubarb, along with unknown medicines. The following were powerful new drugs introduced in the sixteenth century: guaiacum, introduced by the Spanish from West India; jalap and mechoacan, introduced by the Spanish in Mexico, which was exported to the West; capivi, introduced by the Portuguese in Brazil; Torun and Peruvian balsam introduced by Nicolas Monardes; winterian, introduced by the English in the Strait of Magellan; sassafras, known to be discovered by the Spanish and French; and sarsaparilla, introduced by the Monardes. Among the new drugs, sassafras was the most well known, and there was a "sassafras rush" to get the new drug. Walter Raleigh used to make great profits by monopolizing the bark and the tree. However, when it was revealed that the tree can be found almost anywhere, the price of the drug plummeted. Coca leaf was another new drug that was found in the new continent, and it wasn't used as a drug until the nineteenth century. In the nineteenth century, however, cocaine was extracted from the leaves, and it is a big social problem which destroys the society and humanity.

1.3.3.8   Pharmacopoeia and Books on Pharmacology

Since the Renaissance, pharmacopoeia (also called as dispensatorium or enchiridion) saw great advancement. Whether from an individual or a group, initial pharmacopoeia had the following goals: (1) the publishing authorities tried to set a standard of prescription, (2) and it was to set a prescription guideline to the pharmacists (3) and for the doctor to control the elements and intensity of the drug he prescribed and to supervise drug manufacturing.

The first formal pharmacopoeia was *Dispensatorium Pharmacopolarum*, acknowledged by the Nuremberg City government in 1546 in Germany. Later, pharmacopoeias were certified in Augsburg (1564), Koln (1565), Florence (1567), and Rome (1583).

The handbook of pharmacists became a third field in pharmacological document system. For instance, between the years of 1478 and 1488, Nicole Prevost published *Dispensarium ad Aromaticus* in Lyons, France. He described various single medicines and 575 types of complexes and included medical terms.

In Italy, pharmaceutical expertise was given an independent role, and Dr. Saladin di Ascoli wrote *Compendium Aromatariorum* in 1488 in Bologna. The book touched upon the differences between pharmacy and medicine in terms of science, practice, and institution. It became well known for its necessity as a great handbook and become the father of medical textbooks.

1.3.3.9   Education at College of Pharmacy

Pharmacology was an essential subject in the Middle Ages and at the college of medicine and pharmacy in the Renaissance era in Europe. Around 1540 in Padua and Pisa University, botanical gardens were established in the colleges for medical education. In 1536 in Paris, pharmacist trainers had to take at least two classes a week at the college of medicine. In 1588, those who wanted to obtain a master of medicine in Poitiers had to take a 1-year course at the liberal arts and science of college of pharmacy.

In 1558, pharmacists established a pharmaceutical course at Montpellier University with their own money. It was chair pharmacist Bernardin de Ranc who educated the course. He was the first pharmacist to be formally named as a faculty in Europe. In France, Henry the 4th made the department of surgery and pharmacy at Montpellier University in 1601. In 1675, Louis the 14th made a medicine manufacture major in Montpellier University. In the late sixteenth century, the documents issued by professors and college secretariat were taken as certifications that the person took courses at the college. The documents guaranteed the expertise of the people and distinguished them from nonprofessionals.

Such standards were set first in France than in colleges of pharmacy in Germany. Formal pharmaceutical education was established in late seventeenth century, and German pharmacists didn't have more than functional skills. Formal pharmaceutical education began in the eighteenth century.

In England, pharmacist licenses were given under the statutes by the Glasgow faculty, which was edicted by James the 4th in 1599. In 1657 Edinburgh, those who wished to open a drugstore in the city had to pass the qualification test. The training period and qualification test required for pharmacists are included in the statute, which was made by the London Pharmacist Association in December 6, 1617. It was the formal requirement credited by the government.

In Venice, Italy, the training period of students of college of pharmacy was set as 5 years. After graduation, they had to work for 3 years as a clerk and still had to pass a very hard qualification test. It was an example about the law regarding the education of pharmacists. It was due to the edict of the Pope back in 1429, where the guidelines for education training, place of the drugstore, and pharmacists were regulated, along with the separation of medicine and pharmacy long time ago. In Florence, doctors could employ pharmacists and vice versa. Therefore, doctors and pharmacists opened shops together and shared profit and this custom went on for several centuries.

1.3.3.10   Drugstores at Palaces

The selection of professional pharmacists who tended to kings and princes had existed since the Middle Ages. The operation of the Office of Royal Apothecary in England goes back to King John, who ruled from 1199 to 1216. In France, monarchs also designated palace pharmacists and they performed their duties, making rounds to royal family members. Palace pharmacists for German princes not only visited the royal families but also had to accompany monarchs when they went on trips or went to war. They palace pharmacists were given the title of "hof apotheker" or "reise apotheker."

Palace pharmacists manufactured drugs as well. In 1306, Richard de Montpellier was the pharmacist for Edward the 1st, and he made drugs that were prescribed by the king's doctor. The prescribed drugs included the following: 282 lb of electuary, 106 lb of powder salves, gum, fragrant oil, fat, turpentine medicine, ointment, alcohol used as medicine, ambergris, musk, pearl, precious jewelry, and salves that contained gold and silver.

The tasks of palace and royal pharmacists included dealing bread, fruits, and fragrant oil. They also applied preservative treatment to the dead body. There is a record that a wife of a pharmacist named John Rumbler brought with her four servants when she made her trip to France in 1624. This shows how rich and influential palace pharmacists were.

The pharmacology of the Renaissance era was expanded to two fields. One is a massive import of products already known and also massive import of new products from the East and the New World. Another was the introduction of new chemical drugs. Chemical drugs were distributed by pharmacists, and it broadened the knowledge of chemistry.

1.3.4 Modern Times

The foundation of Western science of today was established by the pioneers such as Bacon or Descartes in the seventeenth century. With rapid advancement of physics, chemistry, and biology, various theories that were promoted after the Middle Ages were denied. Galileo's telescope expanded the macroscopic visual scope we see with our eyes. Hans Lippershey and Zacharias Jansen of the Netherlands developed the microscope and opened a new way into the microscopic world. As the perspective was expanded, many presumptions were abolished or newly proven through experiments.

In most pharmacopoeias of the seventeenth through the eighteenth century, information about human skull medicine and medicine made from the wastes such as worm oil, ox bezoar, and stone or urinary calculus was included. However, German doctor Christian Paullini strongly criticized how ungrounded and unscientific they were, through his book *Dreckapotheke* in 1696. One of the biggest changes of the pharmaceutical world in the Enlightenment era was a strong desire for experiments. The desire was the starting ground for modern pharmacology. Fields related to poison and toxic agents were the most intriguing. In the eighteenth century, an Italian physiologist named Felice Fontana used 3000 poisonous snakes and 4000 animals to analyze 6000 types of poison from snakes.

The two people who had a great influence of the revision of the pharmacopoeia, with the advancement of science in the eighteenth century, were Linnaeus, who was a natural scientist of Sweden, and Antoine Lavoisier (1743–1794), a French chemist. In his books *System`a Naturae* (1753), *Species Plantarum* (1753), *Genera Plantarum* (1759), and *Philosophia Botanica* (1759), Linnaeus systematically categorized animals and plants of the nature. His categorization method was introduced in the pharmacopoeia, and the initial copies were double-checked with his categorization. In the process, the names that were written twice were erased, and an order was set in the categorization, which made the pharmacopoeia more scientific. As such, the chemical parts of the pharmacopoeia were helped by Lavoisier's book, *Traite Elementaire de Chimie*. A new system of naming chemical products was established. As a result, pharmacopoeia became more organized and its chemical parts more scientific.

In the late eighteenth century, C.W. Scheele separated various organic acids, but there wasn't enough knowledge and skill to analyze the natural products. However, in 1803, French pharmacist J.E. Deronse and his colleague Armand Seguin (1804) separated crystal from the opium. The chemical traits of the crystals were not revealed. Later, when Friedrich Wilhelm Adam Sertuerner (1783–1841), a German pharmacist, succeeded in separation in 1806, he named the element "sleep substance." The alkaline substance was a needle-crystal-like silk, and it was the first base that was extracted by plants. Later, Joseph Louis Gay-Lussac named the new substance, after "Morpheus (the god of sleeping)," as "morphine." It was found out later that morphine was a mere precursor and that many plants have various "alkalinity substances." The substances had organic base that contained nitrogen as active ingredients, and pharmacist Wilhelm Meissner called it "alkaloid."

After Sertuerner discovered morphine, many pharmacists focused on studies to extract and separate active ingredients from natural products. When glycoside, which was found in sugar form in plants, was successfully extracted, it became the second revolution of medicine. Until then, natural products were used in their original forms. With the extraction and separation of active ingredients from natural products, pure active ingredient was isolated. It led to the standardization and equalization of the active component, and the amounts could be controlled adequately. In the nineteenth century, there was a great breakthrough in pharmacology and chemistry, as private institutions run by one individual became popular and they all passionately pursued studies.

Pierre Joseph Pelletier and Francois Magendie separated emetine from ipecacuanha. Pierre Robiquet extracted narcotine from opium, and Claude-Adolphe Nativelle extracted digitoxin from digitalis.

1.3.4.1 Pharmacology in the Nineteenth Century

The 10 years in the late eighteenth century and another 10 years in early nineteenth century were hard times for medicine. The massive drug-based attack therapy was strongly criticized. There was belief that drugs and treatments don't work on sick organs and that the massive attack therapy didn't cure disease but was harmful to patients. Fortunately, German doctor Rudolf Virchow released "cytopathology," where he stressed that "Disease is related to cells, and not organs (1858)" and drugstores regained their reputation.

In those days, most medicines were plant products, and pharmacognosy remained as a branch of botany. However, pharmacognosy began to be regarded as an independent study with the release of *Histoire Naturelle des Drogues Simples* by Professor Nicholas J. B. G. Guibourt of the College of Pharmacy in Paris in 1820. The four representative pharmacognosists of the era are as follows: Jonathan Pereira (1804–1853), who translated the London pharmacopoeia into English and added scientific explanation, which became the foundation for Martindale and US Dispensatory; Daniel Hanbury (1825–1875) and F.A. Flueckiger (1828–1894), who completed the British pharmacographia together; and A.W.O. Tschirch (1856–1939), who emphasized that chemical elements of eatable plants are useful as medicine and who published *Handbuch der Pharmazie*.

Before the nineteenth century was over, physiologists revealed that the germ theory wasn't the only way to look for the cause of a disease and that lack of hormones can be one attributor. In the late nineteenth century, drug therapy was widely expanded due to the production of chemical products. To fight off disease, vaccine and antitoxins were added, and pharmacists began to treat the new drugs as products. This led to drugstores to be equipped with refrigerators, as biological products had to be stored away.

1.3.4.2 Pharmacopoeia of the Nineteenth Century

In the nineteenth century, nation-states and nationalism became the buzzword, and the quality of medical products had to be managed in national terms. Therefore, there was sensitivity toward the revision of pharmacopoeia or of its management. The 18th pharmacopoeia of Spain, Switzerland, Denmark, Portugal, and Prussia were used across the borders. In this trend, *Codex Medicamentarious Sive Pharmacopoeia Gallica* was nationally certified in France in 1818. In 1820, the *Pharmacopoeia of the United States of America* was made by doctors. With complexity of new products increasing, doctors participated to revise the book in 1882 and released *United States Pharmacopeia*, which became the foundation for pharmacopoeia of today. In 1888, the *U.S. Pharmacist* published the National Formulary (NF) and included medicines that were omitted from the *United States Pharmacopeia* and standards of handmade medicine. In 1906, the book was certified as official compendium along with the pharmacopoeia.

In 1864, the pharmacopoeia of London, Edinburgh, and Dublin were combined in England, and the *British Pharmacopoeia* was published. In England, the editor of the pharmacopoeia, as well as a pharmacist himself, William Martindale, released an attachment of the pharmacopoeia and developed it into *Martindale*. To date, the revised version of the book comes out periodically.

Bismarck founded a new unified country of Germany and published *Pharmacopoeia Germanica* in 1872, which promoted the spirit of a unified nation. Italy adopted *Farmacopea Ufficiale del Regno d'Italia* in 1892. In the case of Japan, the country published the *Japanese Pharmacopoeia* in 1886 after Western culture was introduced. As you can see, the pharmacopoeia established in each country did more than managing the quality of medicine. It was a source of national pride.

1.3.4.3 Pharmaceutical Industry of the Nineteenth Century

Industrial revolution had an impact on drugstores, and plant chemistry and synthesis chemistry created new derivatives of drugs in the past. New chemical products suitable for medical use were created by entrepreneurs, which were out of the reach of small, privately owned drugstores. Many pharmacists in France and Germany manufactured alkaloid products. Caventou and Pelletier, who were pioneers of alkaloid research, manufactured quinine. Heinrich Emanuel Merck discovered and produced papaverine. Until 1880, the Parke-Davis Company made 48 types of liquid extracts from plants that were collected from each branch. Medicines created and developed from drugstores were now produced by the pharmaceutical industry.

There were clinical tests on new materials in the 1880s. Let's look at the works of Hoechst on fever reducer. Wilhelm Filehne obtained the fever reducer kairin, which was synthesized for the first time, and it was tried on healthy people many times. It was tested on the patients to find the adequate amount before it was produced and sold. Before the twentieth century, drug companies couldn't conduct pharmacological or clinical studies.

With the development of a mechanical process, a new dosage form, tablet, was born (1884). Hard and soft capsules were developed as well. A capsule easily hid the taste of drugs and was easy to swallow and provided the accurate amount. At least 45 types of coating were used on pills and tablets. Medical advancement led to the creation of enteric-coated pills in the late nineteenth century. Mercury capsule and ampoule were introduced as well (1887).

The first patent on drugs was given to a magnesium sulfate manufacturer in 1698 in England. However, it was in the nineteenth century when the patent law had taken its modern form. Drugs with patents were very meaningful to the new industry, and the pharmaceutical industry was able to gain financial success with the patent law. The trademark system ultimately made the advertisement of medicine possible.

Modern pharmaceutical companies were mostly started by pharmacists in the nineteenth century. The following are the people and the companies they established: Heinrich Emanuel Merck established "E. Merck AG (1821)," and John K. Smith created "Smith Kline and French Lab" in 1830, which later became "SmithKline Beecham." Louis Dohme and Alpheus Phineas Sharp co-founded "Sharp and Dohme" in 1845, which later developed into "Merck Sharp and Dohme" in 1953. The drugstore of Schering became "Schering AG" in 1851, and Lilly founded "Eli Lilly" in 1876. Silas M. Burroughs and Henry S. Wellcome established "Burroughs Wellcome Co." in 1880. Doctor Edward R. Squibb made "E.R. Squibb."

Some of the most important modern pharmaceutical companies in Europe started from chemical, coloring, and dyeing industry. "Rhone-Poulenc" takes its roots from the chemical products factory (1858), and "Farbwerke Hoechst (1863)" also began as a chemical company. "Sandoz Chemical Company" started out as a coloring factory in 1886, and "J.R. Geigy (1758)" used to trade spices, dyes, and medicine. "F. Hoffmann-La Roche E Co." was created by Fritz Hoffmann-La Roche in 1896, but he only worked at a drug company in Belgium and didn't have any background education in drugstore or chemistry.

In the late nineteenth century, three revolutions opened up a new era for pharmacy. First, commercial production of diphtheria antitoxin helped the birth of a new treatment, such as biological products. Second, John Jacob Abel and Jokichi Takamine succeeded in separating and stabilizing adrenaline, which gave birth to an era of hormones. Third, Heinrich Dreser of the Pharmacological Institute of Bayer revealed the traditional effects of acetylsalicylic acid (the so-called aspirin) on neuralgia in 1899, and it became one of the most widely used chemical products in the modern times.

1.3.5 Twentieth Century and Medicine

The science technology of the twentieth century offered a wider perspective to medical research. Advancement of chemistry made structural formation of the chemical products possible, and various new products (chemical therapy) came flooding out. The continuous development of microbiology opened up way for antibiotics, and breakthroughs in immunology were accompanied by various vaccines, antitoxin, or immune serum. Physiological advancement and upgraded dietetics made the use of vitamins possible, and biochemistry development suggested new research branch of pharmacology and gave birth to pharmaceutical science. Nuclear physics brought about new changes in nuclear medicine, radiopharmacy, and radioisotope. Watson and Crick's discovery of the double helix structure of the DNA opened up new way of molecule biology and genetic engineering. It also gave rise to new production methods and the possibilities that gene revision could treat incurable diseases. Many scholars who received the Nobel Prize since 1901 contributed to the development of medicine both directly and indirectly.

1.3.5.1 Serum and Immune Therapy

The foundation of immune therapy was established by Jenner's vaccination therapy and Pasteur's research on rabies vaccine. After that, research to prevent various diseases such as infectious disease, the Black Death, measles, syphilis, and typhoid and paratyphoid fever was conducted. Serum therapy was the only way to cure particular infection before chemical therapy was generalized in the 1930s. The treatment serum antitoxin vaccine was rapidly developed in the early twentieth century and was used widely. One of the glaring examples is the polio vaccine. In 1955, Dr. Jonas E. Salk succeeded in inventing an injection-type vaccine, and since then, polio patients decreased by 1000 in 1961 (it was 6000 in 1959). When Dr. Albert B. Sabin developed the Sabin vaccine (oral vaccine) in 1961, polio was practically wiped off. Vaccines that work on pertussis, measles, rubella, and epidemic parotitis were introduced, and various combination vaccines are in use now. The examples are DPT (diphtheria, pertussis, and tetanus), DPT-polio, and MMR (measles, mumps, and rubella).

Vaccine to cure hepatitis B was manufactured from plasma in the early days. In 1987, they began to be produced and sold with the help of genetic engineering technology. As some of the vaccines and hematological products sometimes caused fatal problems, laws to control companies that manufacture biological products were established.

1.3.5.2 Endocrine and Hormone Products

With the development of biochemistry and endocrinology in the late nineteenth century, the workings of secretion were revealed in 1902. It was known to facilitate the secretion of bile and pancreatin. Three years later, it was named as "hormone" for the first time:

1. Thyroid hormone: When it was revealed that the thyroid is the endocrine gland (1844), the extraction of thyroid-stimulating materials succeeded, and it was named as "thyroxine" in 1914. Later, successful synthesis of thyroxine in 1927 led to its mass production in the Glaxo pharmaceutical company. Now it's widely used in thyroid hormone deficiency.
2. Parathyroid hormone: Parathyroid hormone was discovered in 1849 for the first time, and the lack of it was known to cause tetanus (1896). W.G. McCallum and Carl Voegtlin reported in 1909 that the parathyroid controls the calcium metabolism of bones. In 1925, James Bertram Collip extracted valid substances from the parathyroid and named it "parathormone."
3. Adrenal hormone: Epinephrine was separated from the adrenal medulla in 1895, and adrenaline was separated from the adrenal cortex in 1901. In 1904, Friedrich Stolz (1860–1936) successfully synthesized the hormone (adrenaline) artificially for the first time in history. Hans Selye (1907–1982) reported "stress theory" in 1946, and he argued that being under stress for a long time makes the adrenal cortex secrete hormone excessively in order to defend the body. He added that it ultimately gives rise to various diseases such as cardiac disease, rheumatoid arthritis, gastric ulcer, high blood pressure, and kidney disease, which are called as "general adaptation syndrome or GAS" against stress. The discovery, separation, artificial synthesis, and success of clinical adaptation of cortisone were a great breakthrough in pharmaceutical history. In September 21, 1948, 100 mg of cortisone was injected to a 13-year-old girl (acute rheumatism patient) through her muscle. In just 3 days, she miraculously recovered, and that's how the "miraculous medicine" was born. In 1950, doctors Kendall, Hench, and Reichstein received the Nobel Prize in Physiology or Medicine for their study on cortisone.
4. Sex hormone and oral contraceptive: Adolf Friedrich Johann Butenandt (1903–1995) of Germany isolated estrogen in 1929. Later, he isolated androsterone and progesterone which is the hormone related to pregnancy. He received the Nobel Prize (Chemistry) in 1939 when he proved that the hormones are steroids. In 1959, Searle & Company's norethynodrel medicine "Enovid" was approved by the FDA as oral contraceptive for the first time in the USA. Since then, various oral contraceptives came out, and social controversy related to open sex and the safety of the drugs was aroused. Treatment using hormonal contraceptives was widely used as abortion pill. "RU 486," produced by the company Mifepristone and Roussel, was found to be effective as oral medicine that can carry out abortion in the early stages of pregnancy. Despite opposition from religious groups,

China and France immediately approved the use of the medicine as it was easy to use, safe, and economic and was able to protect private life.

5. Pancreas insulin: In 1909, de Meyer named the active component secreted from the islet of Langerhans in the pancreas as "insulin." In January 11, 1922, a 13-year-old boy named Thomson, who was hospitalized at the Toronto General Hospital, was given refined insulin. He was able to be released from the hospital, and the news was spread around the world. Insulin came to save a lot of lives of patients who died from diabetes mellitus. In 1923, Frederick Grant Banting (1891–1941) and John James Rickard Macleod (1876–1935) received the Nobel Prize in Physiology or Medicine with their discovery of insulin.

1.3.5.3 Vitamin Products

Development of industries spurred population concentration in the city, and supplying food to a large number of people became a problem. Scholars were given a duty to scientifically find out nutrients in foods. In 1827, William Prout (1785–1850) promoted the "three nutrients theory" which included sugar, lipid, and protein. He argued that milk contains all three nutrients. The head of Japanese Navy hospital, Takaki Kanehiro (1849–1915), who came back from studying in England in 1880, improved the diet of soldiers. By adding more nutritious fish, vegetable, and meat to rice, he was able to cure beriberi. In 1912, Casimir Funk picked out beriberi, scurvy, and rickets as hypoalimentation and argued that lack of small portions of food supplementary factor caused such conditions, which he named "vitamines." Vitamine was a combination of the words "vita (related to life)" and "amine." Later, "e" was erased from the word:

1. Vitamins A and D: The growth boosting factor that is needed for the growth of mice is contained in butter. In 1913, Thomas Burr Osborne (1859–1929) and Lafayette Benedict Mendel (1872–1935) revealed that the factor is fat-soluble vitamin A (retinol). Almost at the same time, Elmer Verner McCollum and Marguerite Davis found out that it is also in the yolk of eggs and in cod-liver oil. In 1919, Kurt Huldschinsky reported that rickets can be cured by artificial sunlight therapy. Up to 1930, various experiments in England found out that rickets can be prevented and cured by cod-liver oil and sunlight. It was suggested that vitamin A in liver oil has elements that prevent and cure rickets and was called vitamin D. In 1931, Robert Benedict Bourdillon succeeded in separating calciferol. In particular, vitamin D is known not only to help the absorption of calcium but also to control the moisture balance of cells. That's why facial massage with egg yolk is highlighted as a method of skin treatment and wrinkle improvement.

2. Vitamin B: Elmer Verner McCollum and Marguerite Davis discovered not only a fat-soluble vitamin in milk but also a water-soluble vitamin. They named it vitamin B. In 1926, Morris Isidore Smith (1887–1951) and E. G. Hendrick reported that vitamin B is composed of two different substances. One is destroyed

easily by heat and has antineuritic traits. The other is a growth-facilitating factor and can withstand heat. The former was called B1 and the latter B2 in England. In the USA, the former was called "thiamine." Richard Kuhn extracted and separated various natural colorings in food and called it "riboflavin (B2)." Later, he succeeded its synthesis and received the Nobel Prize (Chemistry) in 1938. In 1948, E. L. Smith extracted and separated the antianemia factor from the liver and called it B12. It was also called "cyanocobalamin" as cobalt and cyanic acid were in the molecule.

3. Vitamin C: After Funk suggested the existence of vitamin C, many scholars did follow-up studies, and in 1932, W.A. Waugh and Charles Glen King extracted vitamin C from lemon. He found out that it is the same as hexuronic acid extracted from the adrenal and named it "ascorbic acid." In 1934, Walter Norman Haworth (1883–1949) succeeded in its synthesis and received 1937 Nobel Prize (Chemistry). Vitamin C contributed to the fighting of scurvy.

4. Vitamin E: In 1920, H. M. Evans found out that mice didn't recover fertility even when they were fed on sufficient milk. So in 1922, he and K. S. Bishop worked together and discovered a physiological effective substance for the first time and called it vitamin E. Later, vitamin E was also extracted from wheat and was called "tocopherol (fat soluble)."

5. Other vitamin B complexes: In 1930, vitamin B6 (pyridoxine, which helps the production of red blood cells) and, in 1937, vitamin B3 (known as nicotinic acid or niacin and induces pellagra when deficient) were separated and synthesized. By 1940, pantothenic acid, which is necessary when amino acid and fat turn into carbohydrate, was revealed. In 1943, biotin was uncovered, which plays an important role in the decomposition of amino acid.

1.3.5.4   Chemical Therapy Products

Paul Ehrlich (1854–1915) was the first person to introduce "chemotherapy," which treats disease with chemical substances. The chemical substances eradicate or repress the growth of infectious bacillus, without harming cells in our body. His co-researcher was Sahachiro Hata, and they tested the 606th chemical substance, arsphenamine (known as compound 606). It is the first medicine to be used in chemotherapy, and its effects were revealed 2 years later after its introduction in 1907. Ehrlich received the Nobel Prize in 1908 with his contribution to immunology. Later, the era of sulfas began after Gerhard Domagk (1932) discovered and extracted a chemical therapy product (sulfanilamide) from a synthetic dyestuff, prontosil. Arsphenamine was only effective on one germ, *Treponema pallidum*. However, sulfas was found to have effects on a variety of germs, from which many useful medicines were developed. Sulfapyridine, sulfadiazine, and sulfisoxazole are a few of the examples, and for the first time in history, diseases such as *Streptococcus* infection, puerperal fever, erysipelas, meningitis, coccal meningitis, *Shigella* dysentery bacillus, gonorrhea, and other diseases were fought. It didn't cure all infections but, in many cases, shortened the period of the illness and reduced multiple infections and death rate.

1.3.5.5 Antibiotics

In 10 years of time after sulfas was introduced, mankind discovered penicillin, a new type of medicine in the field of antibiotics. Antibiotics were taken from a live organism, and they repressed and killed other organisms. Antibiotics had the ability to attack infectious bacillus without harming the host. In 1928, Alexander Fleming (1811–1955) argued that lysozyme has a strong antibacterial effect and was studying it in St. Mary's Hospital in London. He discovered that when bacteria bouillons were left untended out in the air, *Penicillium notatum*, a type of fungus, killed other bacteria in the culture medium. He extracted the valid substance from the fungus and named it penicillin. He sensed that the fungus could be used as medicine but couldn't further his studies when he found out it couldn't be refined. When the Second World War broke out and the need for penicillin increased, a research team under Dr. Howard Florey was organized at Oxford University, under the support of the Rockefeller Foundation of the USA. They succeeded in getting pure penicillin that could be used on animal experiments. Through mice experiment, the team proved the effects of penicillin. They had difficulties in clinical tests due to lack of specimen but were able to publish their clinical report in 1941. The ten results reported were very promising, and there came a need for massive production, which was highlighted by the war. At first, a pharmaceutical company in England was to take part, but the war prevented it. So a pharmaceutical company in the USA took the first step in producing penicillin. By 1944, it was both in the USA and England that enough penicillin was produced to cure soldiers from both nations who were seriously wounded in war. Penicillin took over sulfas.

The next antibiotic discovered was "streptomycin" by Selman Waksman. It was obtained from actinomycetes and was the first medicine to be effective on tubercular bacillus. The development of streptomycin and isoniazid was a great step forward in fighting off "tuberculosis." Later, various aminoglycoside antibiotics were developed, and they are neomycin, kanamycin, gentamicin, tobramycin, sisomicin, and amikacin.

In 1947, a typhus epidemic spread out in Bolivia, and the miraculous antibiotic that cured all 22 severe patients was chloramphenicol. It was the first antibiotic to be used on so many people clinically. Nowadays, it's not used due to the side effects in blood-related diseases. However, it is still in use in treating incurable, severe conditions. Follow-up studies developed more generally used antibiotics similar to tetracycline. They are chlortetracycline (aureomycin), oxytetracycline, terramycin, and cephamycin.

Germs, bacteria, and fungus were tracked to develop new antibiotics. Along with this, a boom to develop derivatives by changing the chemical structure of penicillin (6-APA, 6-aminopenicillanic acid) aroused. In 1960, people developed antibiotics that worked on penicillin-resistant bacteria, which was called "methicillin ('semisynthetic' penicillin)." In 1961, the first-ever semisynthetic penicillin product called "ampicillin (penbritin)" was invented, which still had the effects on penicillin gram-positive bacterium but that could also cure the gram-negative bacterium. Later, cepha family antibiotics were developed and the following drugs were introduced: cephalothin and cephaloridine in the 1960s and cephapirin and cefazolin in the 1970s, followed by cefotaxim in the 1980s. Other drugs such as azamacrolide family, polypeptide family, antimycotics, and anticancer drug flooded out. From 1935 to 1970, death rate by influenza and pneumonia fell from 103.9 to 30.0 per 100,000. The numbers fell from 55.1 to 2.6 in tuberculosis, 14.1 to 1.3 in inflammation in the digestive system, and 91 to 2 for syphilis until 1970. The death rate by diphtheria toxoid, dysentery, pertussis, scarlatina, meningitis, and coccosis was near zero. As for polio, the rate of 37 per 100,000 people in 1952 fell to near zero in 1970.

1.3.5.6 Chemical Drugs

In the twentieth century, development of organic chemistry prompted researchers to find out the effects of valid substances from natural products. Moreover, efforts to use synthesized chemical substances in medicine were widely conducted. One of the glaring examples is aspirin. *Salix alba* were used as cure for gout, rheumatism, neuralgia, and toothache since the ancient times. In 1763, when it was reported that willow extracts have fever-reducing effects, Pagenstecher found out salicylaldehyde from a bridal wreath in 1838. Bridal wreath is a type of *Spiraea*, so it was called "spirsaeure" in Germany and thus the origin of the name of aspirin. In 1874, Kolbe and Lautemann synthesized salicylic acid and soda was preferred in treatment. Through Kolbe's method, it was synthesized and produced by the Heyden Chemical Co. In 1899, the head of pharmacological experiment at Bayer chemical research institute, Herman Dreser, reported that acetylsalicylic acid turns into salicylic acid and takes effect when absorbed in our body. He named it aspirin, and as it stimulated gastric mucosa less than salicylic acid soda, the Bayer Company took an astonishing step forward with the success of aspirin.

Barbital is a "soothing sleeping pill" derived from barbituric acid. Since its introduction in 1903, phenobarbital was developed in 1912, and more than 2500 types of the barbital family were synthesized since then. Among them, 50 are used clinically. Barbital products still have a value as a repressor in the central nervous system, but it's not widely used since the development of tranquilizer.

The first tranquilizer to be chemically synthesized was chlorpromazine (1954), and similar drugs (50 types) were developed for the next 20 years. Representative ones are meprobamate (Miltown, 1955), prochlorperazine (Compazine, 1956), chlordiazepoxide (Librium, 1960), and diazepam (Valium, 1963). They became very popular right after their launch, and it seems to reflect the craziness of human lifestyle in the modern days. With the introduction of tranquilizer, the number of patients hospitalized in mental institutions decreased significantly. After 1955, drug therapy replaced convulsion or operation therapy in mental disease treatment.

Cardiac medicine is one of the top three medicines that are sold well in the drug market in the USA. The most manufactured cardiac medicines before this century were digitalis, quinidine, and nitroglycerin. New discoveries in physiology such as alpha- and beta-receptor in the parts where adrenaline works (in the nervous system) opened up a new way for medicine to treat circulatory system conditions in the 1950s. Since the 1960s, doctors were able to choose from a variety of drugs, ranging from antihypertensive, antiarrhythmic drug, angina cure, coronary dilators, cholesterol-lowering agents, and lipid-lowering drugs to other drugs that work on our circulatory system. For instance, methyldopa (Aldomet) and clonidine hydrochloride (Catapres) were synthesized as antihypertensive from MSD (Merck Sharp & Dohme, 1962) and ICI (1969). The following are the drugs and the companies that discovered and introduced the drugs: vasodilator isoxsuprine hydrochloride (Vasodilan, 1959) was by Mead Johnson, lipid-lowering drug clofibrate (Android-S, 1963) was by ICI and fenofibrate (Lipanthyl, 1975) was by Fournier, and cholesterol-lowering agent cholestyramine (Questran, 1968) was by MSD, colestipol hydrochloride (Colestid, 1978) was by Upjohn, and lovastatin (Mevacor, 1988) was by MSD. Furthermore, a new approach to repress the angiotensin-converting enzyme was introduced by MSD, which led to the falling of death rate by 71 % from high blood pressure and cardiac disease in the 20 years from 1960 to 1981. For high pressure alone, the death rate fell by 39 %. Contributions of new chemical drugs are still ongoing. They changed peoples' diet and exercise habit and encouraged people to quit smoking. New ways of surgical operation also contributed to reduce the death rate by cardiovascular disease, which was one of the benefits of chemical drugs as well.

Drugs used in medical research in the past, which were needed for doctors' prescription and pharmacists' drug preparation, have increased in number and scale. It started from painkillers, anesthetics, diuretics, anticonvulsants, muscle relaxants, and anti-inflammatory drugs to be expanded to anticancer drugs and antivirus drugs. The development of antiviral agent is urgent not only to fight AIDS but also to conquer cancer. In particular, the HGP or Human Genome Project was completed in 2003, and new biological products (stem cell treatment medicine, therapeutic antibody drugs, vaccine, blood product, etc.) that came from the revolutions of biotechnology are giving us great hope. In the year of "Healthy 100 Years Old," the hope of increased life span and quality of living is just around the corner. As we have seen in the twentieth century, the phenomenal development of drug therapy in the twenty-first century will give us new hope for a new kind of medicine in the future.

Now, we looked through the history of medicine that was discovered, developed, and used by mankind. As you can see, people are dependent on medicine, meaning we are *Homo medicus*. In terms of form, medicine has developed from natural products in the nature to chemical drugs to compounds to biological medicine. The emergence of social medicine seems natural, in line with the flow of medical history. Furthermore, this shows that people are becoming more dependent on social medicine of the superstructure, from being reliant on drugs from the infrastructure. In essence, humans are *Homo medicus* and it's a fact that won't change. When we look at the history of mankind, we can predict that social medicine will be the perfection and the completion of all drugs.

References

Cho Byung-Hee (2010) Sociology of disease and medical care. Gypmoondang, Seoul, p 104

Cousins N (1992) Hope, laugh, and therapy (trans: Lee Jung-Shik). Bumyangsa Publishing Co, Ltd., Seoul

Giddens A (2013) Sociology (trans: Kim Mi-Suk, Kim Yong-Hak, Song Ho-Keun, Shin Kwang-Yung, Ryu Hong-Joon, Jung Seung-Ho), 6th edn. Eulyoo Publishing Co. Ltd., Seoul, pp 369–370

Grandjour A (2008) Mutual dependency between capabilities and functionings in Amartya Sen's capability approach. Soc Choice Welf 31(2):345–350

Jung Dong-Hwa (2010) Psycho-social stress. Korea Academy Information Co, Ltd., p 81

Kennedy RF (1968) John F. Kennedy Presidential Library & Museum. (n.d.). Quotations of Robert F. Kennedy. Retrieved 1 Sept 2009, from http://www.jfklibrary.org/Historical+Resources/Archives/Reference+Desk/Quotations+of+Robert+F.+Kennedy.htm. In Rath T, Harter J (trans: Sung Ki-Hong), Welbeing Finder, Winners Book, 2010, pp 199–200

Kim Ki-Ran, Choi Ki-Ho (2009) Dictionary of popular culture. Hyunsilmunhwa Research, Seoul, p 69

Lee Dong-Seok, Kim Shin-Keun (1997) The history of drug. SNU Press, Seoul

Levitt T (1983) The marketing imagination. The Free Press, New York/London. In: (Translation Saemirae Research Association), Marketing Imagination, 21c Books, 1994, p 5

Mills CW (1959) The sociological imagination. Oxford University Press, London. In Mills CW (trans: Kang Hee-Kyung, Lee Hae-Chan) The sociological imagination, Hong Sung Sa, 1978, pp 9–13

Parsons T (1952) The social system Tavistock, London. In Giddens A (trans: Kim Mi-Suk, Kim Yong-Hak, Song Ho-Keun, Shin Kwang-Yung, Ryu Hong-Joon, Jung Seong-Ho) Sociology, 6th edn. Eulyoo Publishing Co, Ltd., 2013, p 376

Sen A (2002) Why health equity? Health Econ 11(8):659–666

Chapter 2
What Is a Social Medicine?

2.1 The Concept of Social Medicine

In article 10 of the Constitution of the Republic of Korea, it is stipulated that "All citizens shall be assured of human worth and dignity and have the right to pursue happiness. It shall be the duty of the State to confirm and guarantee the fundamental and inviolable human rights of individuals." Health is the basic component that has always determined the happiness of people. Therefore, nations, along with individuals and the society, are working together to promote peoples' health. Drugs have contributed much to peoples' health, and the drugs from the infrastructure were the only drugs that were approved under the current medical health system.

When we look at the history where people depended on drugs, we know that drugs have gone through various developments and changes in each era. First, the discovery of the new continent made the entire world to be looked at as a treasure land with "resources." For drugs, it was a great achievement. Second, innovation derived from the advancement of science technology made people take a step ahead in various fields. Such development based on productivity is still ongoing. Finally, the era of social medicine is here for us. It makes people make use of all things, starting from the mind, body, nature, and surrounding environments to the society, culture and everything in the superstructure, coupled with "social navigation." Therefore, drugs have to be defined and categorized in a new and balanced way that is totally different from the Western perspective of the past.

2.1.1 The Remaining Margin

The remaining margin refers to an empty space. It is not a space that is left out, without power, but a world full of harmony and hope where vitalizing activity is in full action. Humans need energy in order to live. We eat, drink, breathe, and go to the bathroom every day to obtain energy (vital force). Along with vital principle, we

© Springer Science+Business Media Singapore 2016
B.-H. Han, *Therapy of Social Medicine*, DOI 10.1007/978-981-287-748-2_2

also have to think, see, listen, talk, and move to live. In order to live, we have to use the vital energy.

Let's think about this in plain science. Photosynthesis is taking energy from the sunlight to turn it into chemical compound. Organisms like humans can't photosynthesize, and we depend on the products of photosynthesis. That's why we take the products in the form of food and absorb energy through our bodily mechanism and the reaction of the metabolism that is facilitated by enzymes. The energy is later used efficiently for living.

Let's take one step further and look at the phenomenon and facts with a molecular-level perspective. The following explanation is an analysis of the two by modern Western medicine through biochemical mechanism. Our body is made up of about 100 trillion cells and there are mitochondria in the cell. They are the organs that produce vital energy and are similar to the engine of a car. Cars use petroleum or gas as fuel, but mitochondria use nutrients as fuel, such as glucose, fatty acid, and amino acid, which are obtained from decomposing food. The fatty acids, glucose, and amino acids are absorbed in the colon and travel around the body in the blood. They are absorbed into cells that need them, and ultimately make their home in the mitochondria in the cell. The nutrients go through several stages to be turned into acetyl-coenzyme A and power the Krebs cycle. In between the cycle, NADH comes out (they are reduced forms of acetyl-coenzyme A and nicotinamide-adenine dinucleotide or NAD) and the intermediary metabolites go through another stage (coenzyme Q10) to become ATP (adenosinetriphosphate, the form of vital energy) and is used in vital activities (Lee Yung-Keun and Choi Joon-Yung 2011a).

As we have seen, the essential concept of the remaining margin is based on the vitology of Oriental medicine. According to vitology, the movement of energy starts time and space, and the beginning of time sets the flow of energy in the space. The movement of energy is called "force." Generally, the force has five basic traits. First is dividing (the force to be separated from one another). Second is uniting (the force to be together). Third is gathering (the force to be collected). Fourth is scattering (the force to be dispersed). Last is organizing (the force to form a special functional frame).

When the basic forces come together to form a "conversion," various "hidden orders" of force are established, and when it's expressed as "displayed order," it then becomes "power" and "strength." In short, the trait of force appears, and "sex" refers to "power" and "quality" equals "strength." Expressions such as "authority" and "accent" (each word has the meaning "power" in Korean) are the same as "power" of the force. "Human power" and "muscle power" (each word has the meaning "strength" in Korean) equals the "strength" of force. For instance, there is a "hidden order" in our body that controls us. It is called gene, and the program (information) in the gene determines the "displayed order," which includes the height, physical structure, skin color, health, and life span. They are the components of our body. Ultimately, our body is made up of various combinations of vital force, and our body is the result of firmness and big and small traits expressed together (Jeon Se-Il 2004a).

Society is the place full of vitalizing activities, where vital force of each individual comes together to interact. Therefore, social medicine is a drug that centers on humans, originating from humans and founded on the basic force of vital energy. As a result, the innate characteristics of social medicine, the power and the strength, can be harmonized and converged to be sublimated to the "universal stream."

If we say that drugs are the essence of mechanical view of the world that originates from Western medicine and is materialistic in that it can't be developed any further without scientific research or experiment, social medicine is quite different. Social medicine is based on Oriental medicine, which has "the beauty of emptiness," full of vitalizing energy. It regards human experience based on vitalizing energy to be very important. In short, SM is effective whenever and wherever, using human mind, nature, environment, society, and culture. It is a formless medicine that has converging traits and can be discovered and developed in a creative and liberal way.

As a result, the remaining sector is the place where the vitalizing energy works. The important truth is, the vital force has the so-called, "natural healing power (NHP)" and can operate on its own. Moreover, the strength of the power is divided into two, known as natural healing strength (NHS) of the individuals and social healing strength (SHS) of the society. If the two can be peacefully united and sublimated, it can form "universal stream." Therefore, how we can discover and utilize the powers through "social medicine (SM)" is very important, as mankind's health and happiness depend on it.

2.1.2 Natural Healing Power (NHP)

Human beings are made up of mind and body, which is called "Sim-sin (mind-body)" in Korean. Just like every living being, human body has general trait of "homeostasis." The word was first made and used by Professor Walter Canon at the Harvard School of Medicine. He reported that the changes in homeostasis gives rise to "fight or flight" response. It means that we tend to respond in either ways, whether to fight or flight in case of danger. It is known that the over-secretion of catecholamine, a neurotransmitter in the sympathetic nervous system, is the cause (Byun Gwang-Ho and Chang Hyun-Gap 2012). In terms of vitology, homeostasis is the first innate instinct programmed in living organisms, as each of us strive to make the best possible environment in every moment to maintain our valuable life.

Nature is a large "system of order" where numerous livings coexist under harmony. Being healthy doesn't refer simply to a state of absence of disease. It is a state where the vitalizing energy flows and you have the enough capacity to do what you want. The organic condition to maintain a healthy life and to facilitate harmonious coexistence in the ecosystem is called "reciprocity." It is the second innate instinct that calls for the following three conditions (Lee Yung-Keun and Choi Joon-Yung 2011b):

First, living organisms have to communicate well. The buzzword of our society nowadays is "communication." As stagnant water rots, so does our body when blood circulation is not conducted well. The food we eat first meets the teeth, and the food is digested in our stomach and colon, and the absorbed nutrients are filtered through the liver to be sent to each organ and cells. Cells use nutrients that have penetrated the cell membrane and also use oxygen that came in through breathing to make energy and hormones. In this process, the waste undergoes detox process and is excreted out of the body through the colon or kidney. This is the healthy cycle of our body. The healthy flow and exchange of work between the liver and kidney, spleen and stomach, lung and kidney, and colon and small intestine makes our body full of energy, not to mention the organs.

Second, it should be regular and predictable. The human body is not a machine, but it is programmed to move in a regular and predictable way. Therefore, collapse of the "order of physiology" is the same as being unhealthy. For instance, being on one's period regularly each month and having a rhythmic pulse and blood pressure are all indicators of health. Metaphorically speaking, gears can be all different, and the numbers of cogwheels on the gears may differ. However, when gears rotate in a predictable way, it can move smoothly. Our body works in the same way. Health can be maintained when the workings of organs move in an expected way through everyday lifestyle and diet. In other words, eating and resting regularly will be useful in maintaining a healthy state. People nowadays often die from overworking, and it is a punishment from the nature for violating the "order of physiology."

Third, positive and active attitude on life is important. Health can be promoted when individuals and society can exchange opinions in an active way and when cells move in a regular, predictable way. For instance, stomach cancer cells are ordinary cells when our stomach is working well. However, when foods come in irregularly due to unhealthy eating habits, or when food is not digested well and stays in the stomach for a long time, the stomach notices that something is wrong. Then, stomach cells turn themselves into enterocytes, which are called, "intestinal metaplasia," referring to gastric mucous membrane cells' regeneration into intestinal mucosal cells. After some time, the cells turn into cancer cells and attacks ordinary cells. The balance in the body is erupted, and health is undermined.

In an ecosystem, the three conditions are very important. Unless the living organism is faced with a fatal danger or damage, the three conditions enable it to cure most injuries and illness on its own, and it's called "natural healing."

In short, NHP is the combination of NHS (it seeks to maintain homeostasis, which is the first innate instinct of human beings) and SHS (based on the reciprocity, which is the second innate instinct of human beings). It is a vital force with a broad meaning. Therefore, problems related to health and disease in the modern society can be fundamentally solved in the context of "loss and restoration of NHP."

2.1.2.1 Natural Healing Strength (NHS)

Living organisms are programmed to maintain homeostasis, which allows us to maintain our valuable life by making us keep the best condition. Let's take a deeper look based on vitology. Physiology is the program of life, and living energy is the vitalizing energy. Physiology and living energy work together for our mind and body to maintain a normal state. To that aim, a safety margin is set and it is controlled so that the mind-body status remains in the safety margin.

For instance, the examples of normal state are as follows: our body temperature has to be maintained at around 36.7 °C, the fasting blood sugar should be around 90–110 mg to be safe, and the systolic blood pressure should be around 100–140 mmHg. When our mind and body goes out of the safety margin to be in an abnormal state, due to stress or overwork, it is labeled as being unhealthy or suffering from illness. Making the body go back to normal state would be called "healing." The force to maintain the homeostasis, which we are inherently born with, is called "NHS or natural healing strength."

> Let's take an example of "Natural Healing Strength" with a clinical case. There is a patient suffering from a very high fever of 40 degrees Celsius. If the patient is given two pills of aspirin, which is most often used to reduce fever, the fever will go down a bit. Four hours later, he was still suffering from a fever of 39 degrees Celsius. The patient was given two more pills of aspirin, and the temperature decreased to 38 degrees Celsius. Repeated prescription of the pills in every 4~6 hours made his body temperature to go down to the normal range of 36.7 degrees Celsius.
>
> If he was repeatedly given the pills after restoring his normal state, would his body temperature continue to go down? To 35, 34, and 32 degrees Celsius? No, the temperature would go down when he had the fever, but after hitting the normal range, more pills wouldn't let his body temperature go down anymore. When the temperature was high, above the normal status, the strong natural healing strength would be aided by the aspirin to lower the temperature to reach normal levels. Once he reaches the normal temperature, however, the "power to decrease the temperature" stops working, and that's why the temperature doesn't go down. (Jeon Se-Il 2004b)

Based on the various natural healing processes in us, social medicine mobilizes various methods to participate in opportunities to maintain and contribute to life. That's because the healing process is made in our body with the help of NHS. In short, social medicine is just like medical experts medical doctors or therapists. It doesn't heal of itself, but it only works as an aid so that natural healing would occur and take effect, in terms of vitalizing energy.

2.1.2.2   Social Healing Strength (SHS)

Humans are social being, and we can't live alone. It is the social instinct of humans to recognize that we can't exist without other people. Later, we seek ways to cooperate with each other to benefit ourselves. The desire to interact with each other to maintain physical, mental, social, and economic health is what drives us to form a community. Here, community refers to a web of relations called ecosystem. Communities formed with various individuals coexist in our world, maintaining balance with each other and the individuals within (Drucker et al. 2001).

For instance, the World Cup games symbolize the soccer community. In the 2002 Korea-Japan World Cup, Koreans made the miraculous feat to enter the semifinal game. The incident made Korea to become a glorious community, to stand near the center of soccer world, from being on the margin. The skills of then national team coach Gus Hiddink and the soccer players were great, but the unified cheering phrase of "Dae~hanminguk (meaning "Korea" in Korean)" and the clapping sounds were the result of aspiration of all Koreans. It was one of those times when the vitalizing energy of our society was great, and it was the biggest festival that was such a joyous occasion for all Koreans. Throughout the month of games, the mind and body of Koreans were very healthy and happy. The soccer games in those days were a very good social medicine, which wiped Koreans of all worries in this world and replaced them with laughter and happiness. It was a good medicine that was better than any other drug. This shows how much power SHS, or social healing strength, coupled with vitalizing energy, can have. It will be remembered as one of the most representative "effective cases" of social medicine.

A successful society would consider future problems rather than clinging to the problems of today. Some sociologists have long argued that there is a strong correlation between crime and social exclusion in advanced societies. Crime rate can be a barometer of a gloomy reality of a society, where there are increasing numbers of people who feel that they are not valued in their society or community (Giddens 2013).

Therefore, when we see the global society with a perspective in which it should be a human community where people cooperate with each other in, we should "go beyond walls" of social exclusion. We should form a strong partnership with constructive, healing, and cooperating abilities so that we can make our children and families healthy. We have the calling to make our community a harmonious one where good schools, houses, and jobs are offered to promote human dignity. This is the dream of a social community. The community where its people cooperate to realize the dream is where hopeful leadership presides. There may be no preventative drug cure for cancer, cardiac disease, alcohol addiction, AIDS, violence, and other problems that arise from our society or community, related to the smoking of adolescents and the marginalized people. However, all of this can be prevented. So what we desperately need is social medicine from the superstructure, not drugs. The adults who are the main players of health promotion can offer strong social immunization, thereby strengthening SHS.

Laughter therapy, which emerged quite recently, is also based on social healing power. Laughter is a social medicine that has strong infection. Our society can become stronger with many laughter therapists working more actively in our society and with individuals who have a habit of laughing in their daily lives. The reason we have hope is that there are still people who sacrifice themselves and set an example in our world.

Teresa of Calcutta (1910–1997), a saint of the twentieth century, went to Loreto Convent at the age of 19 and devoted her entire life to the needy and sick in a poor village in Calcutta, India. She established "Missionaries of Charity" and is remembered as a person who used all her vitalizing energy to care for the health and lives of other people. As such, social medicine has innate SHS, whether it's by individuals or groups. Therefore, social medicine cures our society and turns it healthier.

The recent typhoon Haiyan (which hit the Philippines in Nov. 8, 2013, killed and wounded more than 12,000 people, displaced 10 million people, and caused more than 15 trillion Korean won worth of economic damage) can't let us down. It's because people have the universal stream (as the last stage of vitalizing energy, it refers to the most selfless "love and service" here), the noble social medicine. It gives us hope that we can cure ourselves on our own to restore the healthy state, without any coercion.

As you can see, the concept of the remaining margin has various basic beliefs. It believes that we can cure disease with the harmony of our body and mind, aided by social medicine. Moreover, our health can be maintained and promoted through it. We should take heed that the noblest social medicine we have to unearth and develop is the universal stream. Only transformed humans and communities can cure and change our society.

2.1.3 Composition of Medicine

I believe that medicine is composed of two parts, social medicine of the superstructure and drug of the infrastructure. Social medicine penetrates individuals, history, and social changes with social navigation. Social medicine is a formless medicine that can advance toward the universal stream with the convergence of active vital energy. Conventional drug exists in the infrastructure, which is the symbol of cutting-edge science technology and the essence of medical industry.

As I mentioned earlier, social medicine includes everything except for the visible drug. In this sense, society is a co-depending world where individuals, who are conscious beings that have determination and beliefs, reside in. It is well known that individuals' thoughts and actions are given impact by society or groups, and the idea has been researched in social psychology and group dynamics. When individuals are alone, they can think and act in any way they want, but as members of the society, their actions face various restrictions and limitations. That is why individuals tend to have a similar stance to that of the society and groups they are in, because those groups force the individuals to follow their regulations. It is called "social influence." "Conformity" is the result of social influence on individuals, and the conformity in turn has an effect on the group, giving birth to another social phenomenon (Lee Min-Joo 2001). Social medicine reflects history and sociality, so it is sensitive to social phenomenon and it develops in close relationship to how individuals think and feel.

Drug is composed of natural products, chemical products, and biological products according to its characteristics and developmental system.

The following (Fig. 2.1) shows how medicine can be composed of two parts: social medicine of the remaining margin and drug in the infrastructure that are based on medical history, social change, medical industry, and the ideology of capitalism.

If the newly established social medicine in Korea can be combined with the "drug-only" Western medicine and therefore settle down as a harmonious system, it will be a union of the idea of Eastern medicine and the history of Western medicine.

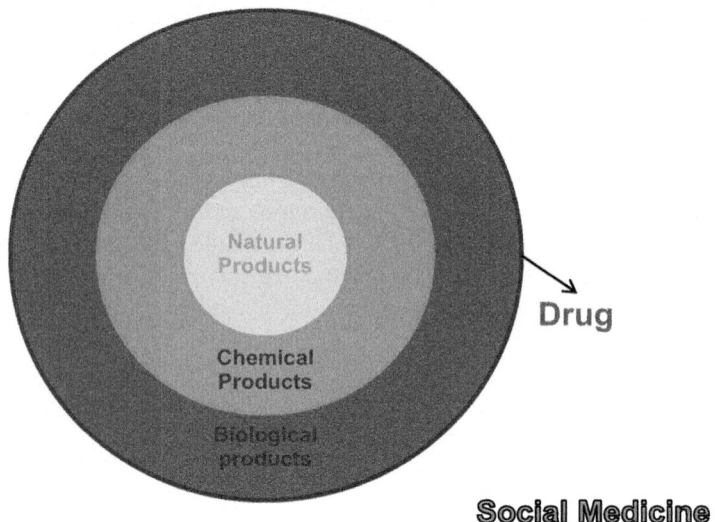

Fig. 2.1 The system of medicine

The integrated medicine will serve as the driving force for taking the 21st pharmacy to another level.

It is already known that humans are medicine dependent, or *Homo medicus*. Based on the fact that medicine is composed of the two parts, on the one hand, anyone who is healthy and wants to prevent disease and manage stress, promote antiaging and longevity, and pursue well-being and happiness can depend on social medicine. Patients, on the other hand, can depend on treatment-focused drugs and at the same time use social medicine as an alternative. When visible drugs alone can't cure, patients can look toward social medicine, which is based on the convergence of vital energies, and work for a better life. As such, social medicine has various resources and available resources, and it can advance toward metaphysical sector, which can't be attained by science. Therefore, social medicine and drug naturally have different developmental motives, processes, adaptation ranges, functions, and roles.

The best part of social medicine is that it can be easily found in our everyday surroundings and can be used right away. Let's say many people on the street spontaneously unfolded their umbrella because it suddenly rained. Umbrella is a part of people's everyday life, and it holds a symbolic value. In this way, the "ritual" that includes the action of unfolding umbrella can be more meaningful than just flipping open the umbrella to avoid the rain. This means that everyone on the street has the desire to avoid getting wet and suffer from a cold, and an umbrella can act as social medicine that prevents cold. How about stones or pebbles in the stream? When heated stone or pebble is put on the part of the body where muscles are knotted or where the digestive organs exist, it can also promote health, which is the popular "stone therapy" nowadays.

People say that we should watch out for what we ask for. When you praise a person and that comment stays on him, the person's thoughts can be provoked, and his body and mind can be healed. In this case, the praise acted as social medicine. As for people who suffer from not being able to find love, "love" can act as social medicine to cure their hearts.

In the modern society where much stress is aroused, people physically, mentally, and socially tend to feel various obstacles. However, most people just live on with it. But when they discover the existence of social medicine and its wonderful world, they can recognize then how social medicine has taken us this far in life by promoting health.

By improving NHS and SHS with vital force, which is the basis of humans, NHP can be used to promote health in many ways. In this respect, social medicine is a strong independent variable to health, and it is a social entity in material, physical, emotional, spiritual, human relational, and environmental respect that encompasses the promotion of not only individual health but also of social health.

2.1.4 Characteristics of Social Medicine

In the world of visible drugs, drugs only target patients with specific conditions, so it has to be selective and used under the supervision of medical experts. Therefore, drugs are subject to various limitations. However, social medicine can be anything other than visible drugs that are used to promote one's health, so the government has almost no say in it, and it works with the principles of free market capitalism or economy. Therefore, regulation is the key in the infrastructure, whereas free market is the representative trait in social medicine.

2.1.4.1 The Principle of Free Markets

A stark trait of the mobile media today is that it makes communication possible even when people are on the move. People can communicate whenever and wherever, and there is a sense of freedom from time or space-based restrictions. Social medicine is also separate from the regulations of traditional medicine of the infrastructure. As social medicine looks toward freedom, it is akin to mobile media.

According to Milton Friedman (1912–2006), liberalism stems from the following two words, "freedom" and "individual." In the late eighteenth century to early nineteenth century, the two words were recognized as "ultimate value" and "ultimate truth," respectively. In this context, too much government intervention in the individual's social and economic activities was met with fierce opposition, and there were demands that individual's freedom and the absolute value of private property be respected. However, after the late nineteenth century, in particular after the 1930s' Great Depression, individual's welfare and equality were put first, and active participation of the government to achieve this end was stressed. Some argue that it is why limitations on individual's freedom and right to private property were misinterpreted as liberalism. Friedman argued that the "real meaning of liberalism" should be restored.

In short, freedom is regarded as important, as freedom itself is the ultimate goal. Economic freedom is also a goal, as well as being an important tool to achieve political freedom. The history of the USA is both an economic and political miracle. The practice of the concept of "free market" promoted in *The Wealth of Nations* by Adam Smith (1723–1790) and the argument that "everyone has the right to pursue his own value system" written in the Declaration of Independence made it possible. Adam Smith said in his book that individual's freedom can be harmonized with others' in the cooperating process and in the market system, which is needed for economic activities. He added that outside pressure, coercion, and violating freedom are not necessary and that cooperation among individuals is possible, based on the fact that it is beneficial to all people. By the work of "invisible hands (it generally refers to market price and the selling and buying of services and goods through money)," we are guided to a goal that is not necessarily the same as his intention. Friedman reaffirms that Adam Smith expressed the power of "free market" in this way:

> Nor is it always the worse for the society that it was no part of it. By pursuing his own interest, he frequently promotes that of the society more effectually than when he really intends to promote it. I have never known much good done by those who affected to trade for the public good. (Smith 1776)

> The wisdom of Adam Smith is that price, which stems from the voluntary exchange from the seller and the buyer, simply put, the price of a free market, is understood as millions of people to cooperate with each other, as they purse their own interests, as well as working towards a more profitable way for everyone. The fact that the actions of pursuing one's own interest, without any pre-conceived intention, can give order to the economy, was a very surprising thought, and it still is today. (Friedman 2009)

However, the government is on the outskirts of market principles and competition, so it is mostly inefficient and far from democratic values. Civil servants want their group to become larger. The larger the size of the group, the more people and budget are gathered, ultimately increasing members' pride and authority. In short, it's not that there is much work calling for more people but rather more work needed for the increased number of people. New regulations are made to give them work, and new areas for intervention keeps adding up. When companies don't fare well in the market, they downsize by restructuring, but government bodies tend to increase their subgroups to solve problems when management is slack.

Friedman believed that the role of the government should be limited to the following areas: maintaining law and order and safety, guaranteeing private property, implementing duty of contract, promoting market competition, and maintaining currency and the protection of the elderly and the disabled. He argued that other government activities hinder efficiency of the market, weaken growth potential, and undermine free society that guarantees peoples' creativity. He maintained that government intervention in the market should be performed at the minimum level, adding that price theory and free market economy best explains the economic activities of people, and it most efficiently performs distribution of resources and capital. He measured and set a standard of the so-called Friedman ratio, the proportion of government spending to GNP or GDP. He proved that the higher the ratio, the lower the real economic growth rate becomes, thereby strongly arguing a "small government" and repressing government intervention.

The existence of a free market does not of course eliminate the need for government. On the contrary, government is essential both as a forum for determining the "rules of the game" and as an umpire to interpret and enforce the rules decided on. What the market does is to reduce greatly the range of issues that must be decided through political means, and thereby to minimize the extent to which government need participate directly in the game. The characteristic feature of action through political channels is that it tends to require or enforce substantial conformity. The great advantage of the market, on the other hand, is that it permits wide diversity. (Friedman 2007a)

In short, free market economy uses the following three functions of price to distribute resources in the most effective manner: first, by transferring information; second, by inducing to select the lowest cost production method so that available resources can be used for the most meaningful purpose; and third, by distributing income. For this reason, people who agree strong government intervention take "market failure" (where the price-setting body "market" can't function well) as an example so that the government should step in to raise effectiveness of resource distribution. However, opponents argue that it inevitably results in "government failure," which is more distorted and incurs high cost than the "market failure."

A liberal is fundamentally fearful of concentrated power. His objective is to preserve the maximum degree of freedom for each individual separately that is compatible with one man's freedom not interfering with other men's freedom. He believes that this objective requires that power be dispersed. He is suspicious of assigning to government any functions that can be performed through the market, both because this substitutes coercion for voluntary co-operation in the area in question and because, by giving government an increased role, it threatens freedom in other areas. (Friedman 2007b)

Let's look at how conventional drugs are being regulated in the real world. The role of drugs is to promote lifesaving activity, which has a direct bearing on people's lives, and that is why governments tend to put strict regulations on the safety of new drugs. After developing new drugs, the developer has to conduct various nonclinical and clinical tests that the government directs, before selling the products. After all the data and information are submitted to the Korean Food and Drug Administration (FDA, in the case of the USA) to get a sales approval. Later, when the products are out in the market, they are constantly under strict government supervision. In 2012, the Korean Food and Drug Administration, a subsidiary organization of the central government, was established to systematically manage cases of harmful medical products such as side effects of drugs in Korea. With the new body, drug supervision in Korea is being strengthened to promote people's health. The following is the essential regulations related to the new drug development in the scientific regulation aspect (Table 2.1).

Social medicine based on vital energy can be easily found in food, exercise, leisure activities, culture, arts, travel, rest, sleep, positive words, and laughter in our daily lives. Anyone can use social medicine without going through complicated developing process or GXPs, and its main role is "vitalizing activity," which is to aid people to live a healthier life. Because of its regulatory traits, drugs can only be developed by experts who are equipped with expertise and cutting-edge technology. After development, drug makers can enjoy exclusive rights over the products by placing patents in the market, and it can only be dealt by professions with licenses.

Table 2.1 Regulations on the process of new drug development

	Phase	Guideline contents
GLP	Analysis of various laboratories that are conducting nonclinical or clinical tests	Guidelines for various facilities in the laboratory, how they are operated, education of the experiment researchers, the system of information reporting
GCP	Clinical test phase	Guidelines for facilities where clinical tests are performed, how they are operated, education of the clinical test researchers, proper reporting to the patients or experiment participants
GMP	Production phase	Guidelines for facilities of the production base, how they are operated, quality control of raw materials, education of the production workers, quality management of products
GPMSP	Post-market entrance phase	Guidelines for reporting side effects after going on market, reexamination, reevaluation

GLP good laboratory practice, *GCP* good clinical practice, *GMP* good manufacturing practice, *GPMSP* good post-marketing surveillance practice

As for social medicine, anyone can have free access for its development, and it can be used at any time. However, drugs need more than 10 years of time and astronomical developing costs resulting from various regulations along the way, starting from research. Social medicine can be developed and used in a short period of time at little cost or is free of charge. It can be selected by people out in the market through free and fair competition.

The first principle needed for the discovery and success of social medicine is free market economy. Creativity, market trust, respect and protection of individual freedom and private property, and a small government are essential for the success of social medicine. We are living in a relatively very liberal society, and we tend to forget how we weren't in the past. Humans have "the right to pursue their wants" and "freedom to choose," so they should be able to choose social medicine freely for their health. Respecting individual's freedom and expanding economic freedom is the way for promoting successful health management through making the right choices.

2.1.4.2   Safety and Misuse/Abuse

Social medicine is also "medicine," so it has to be safe. The word "safe" here is related to having "no harm," and social medicine shouldn't be harmful to humans, as well as having risk-preventative functions. The main focus of social medicine is to promote safe health management. Social medicine is about utilizing NHS and SHS to engage in direct therapies on each disease. Furthermore, it is about increasing the quality of life by repressing misuse, abuse, or over-medicalization of drugs and by stress management. Social medicine seeks inclusive health management, protecting individuals and society from health risk factors, and engaging in disease prevention and treatment, patient's care, recovery, and health promotion. That is why health risk factors such as alcohol and cigarettes, which have been controversial in our society, can't be social medicine. Though the two are personal preferences and are used widely around the society, alcohol leads to alcohol addiction and smoking induces lung cancer. People should first consider the benefits and the risks of the two for their health and use them as social medicine when they believe the positive side overweighs.

People want health, not medicine. After the accident of thalidomide, drugs that followed underwent strengthened regulations and were made with more advanced pharmaceutical technology. However, though the safety of the drugs has been guaranteed, they should be the last resort for people. However good medicine it is, it can turn into poison when it is not used in an accurate way. In advanced medical systems, DUR (drug utilization review) is established to give drug safety-related information real time in drug prescription and preparation, so misuse of drug can be checked beforehand. When patients take several pills together or take it with food that interferes with the drug, unexpected side effects may arise. Therefore, it is not wise to rely on drugs whenever you feel even a little sick. If you can find social medicine that suits you and make yourself healthy with NHP, it will be a more desirable way.

Health-threatening, tolerant bacteria have risen by the misuse and abuse of antibiotics, which wasn't necessarily needed in drug therapy in the first place. Sometimes incidences of over-medicalization become a social issue, as accessibility and dependency on drugs increased due to development of health insurance and medical information. For instance, Ritalin, which is a cure for ADHD (attention-deficit/hyperactivity disorder), was misused as a "smart pill" to increase students' concentration skills. Safety of drugs and misuse/abuse of medicine need stricter management.

After going through the barrier of 20,000 dollars of per capita GDP, Korea has been enjoying a time of affluence, freed from poverty. There is a phrase that goes, "you would even drink detergent if they say it's good for health." It is used to describe the negative atmosphere of drug misuse in our society. Against this backdrop, the misuse/abuse problem of social medicine could become a bigger problem. Such phenomena are often found in food. Advertisement on natural products, health products, health functional food, organic food, natural food, vitamins, and enzymes lures customers, and even food aversion attracts people once they're said to boost power. Laughter is highlighted as "the best medicine" nowadays, but we've seen that it can be fatal to pregnant women. It shows that we should also think twice when considering safety and misuse/abuse of social medicine. Individuals have to be more cautious when choosing social medicine and a proper tool of social control on drugs is needed.

Societies can't work in harmony when the members don't follow social rules or when they don't play their roles. Therefore, social control is inevitable for the existence of a society. Here, social control means the mechanism used by the society to gather its members and to set regulations so that the members don't deviate (Kim Chae-Yoon et al. 2007). If one person is obsessed with the well-being of himself/

herself and breaks the rules of the society, he/she will be regulated or even punished. This provides a certain action plan to the other members of the society, regulates the person in question, and also works as a warning to potential deviator. In the same respect, a person who follows social rules will be acknowledged by other members of the society and will receive reward. In this sense, the government's recent setting of nonsmoking areas and strengthened social control on some social medicine that have safety issues or problems of misuse/abuse is desirable for both individuals and national health.

2.1.4.3   Freedom from Stigma

Everyone wants to be healthy as they live about their daily lives. The moment pills are taken, our social position changes from being a healthy person to a "patient." According to social constructivism, when a person gets on medicine due to illness, people around him gives "a new role (patient)" and the person himself also realizes his changed position. It becomes a type of "stigma" to him. It's social members (medical experts) who decide if the person has a disease and should take drugs. The patient's condition is determined by the "interpretation rules (of the condition)," which are shared through the cultural values and regulations of the society.

In structural functionalism, there is acknowledgement of the social system, which exists as an objective truth in macroscopic terms. In this case, illness is looked upon as a state of deviation in maintaining the social system. However, people who believe in social constructionism theory see social structure in microscopic terms, saying that it is formed by the relationships individuals have through interaction. They think people share a certain symbol of an action, which enables communication in the society, and it is the social order and social structure (Cho Byung-Hee 2010). Illness or medicine is regarded as "social reality," and the meaning is determined "in relative sense" in each situation. The new role of "patient" can become the life of the person I mentioned above, and it may be hard for him to get out of the "dishonor." It is similar to social exclusion and isolation.

The damaged identity due to illness may prompt the patient to stigmatize himself as a sick person. However light the illness is, for instance, a cold, it is hard for the person to think of himself as healthy in sociopsychological terms. Therefore, drugs stigmatize us as patients, rather than healthy people in the society, and it is the "paradox of drug." Of course, people are freed from the patient role once they get better with the help of medicine. However, the fact that he is on medication makes a healthy person into a patient in the society. That is why people tend to avoid drugs, and it is also true in the case of patients. Patients' "noncompliance" remains as the biggest hurdle of drug therapy.

Through social medicine of the superstructure, people can be freed from the stigma of being a patient or from the damaged identity, which is caused by drugs of the infrastructure. People can enjoy their social status as a healthy person and can continue to manage their health. This is important in that social medicine is added to the concept of drugs, which traditionally focused only on material drugs. Now the concept of drugs is enlarged to include not only the infrastructure but also the super-structure and the overall social system. It also shows the fundamental difference between drugs and social medicine. Both are effective as drugs (of course, the effects can differ), but whereas drugs make people "patients" in sociopsychological terms, social medicine allow people to remain as "healthy people." Social medicine is based on vitalizing energy and depends on NHS and SHS. Therefore, it prevents people from putting too much trust in drugs and represses over-medicalization that can arise from misuse or abuse of drugs.

2.1.5   Effects of Social Medicine (SM)

Then, can social medicine in the superstructure, based on vital energy, show effect in an objective clinical study apart from subjective effects on each individual?

Placebos are good examples which show social medicine can also work. Placebos refer to fake drugs that patients take as medication to get psychological relief. The word "placebo" is Latin, and it means "something suits oneself." It differs on the type of conditions, but it is widely believed that about 20–30 % of effect can be derived from placebos. In particular, placebos work well in cases such as pain, vomiting, asthma, and phobia, and 'New England Journal of Medicine' reports how placebos work:

> Researchers at Harvard College of Medicine studied some 40 patients with asthma to compare the effects of real drugs and placebos. The patients were subject to real inhalant (albuterol), fake inhalant (placebo), fake saliva treatment and how the patient felt about the treatment (subjective index) were measured before and after the treatment, along with pulmonary function test (objective index). As for objective, pulmonary function test, the results showed a 20 % increase when real inhalants were used. But when fake inhalant was used or fake saliva treatment was conducted, it only showed a 7 % increase. The results were not so surprising, but the following fact was noticeable. In terms of patients' subjective view, they felt about 50 % of increased vitality when real inhalant was used. In the case of fake inhalant or saliva treatment, a similar statistics were revealed, a 45 % of increased vitality. Whether the treatment was real or fake, there weren't many changes on the subjective view of the patients. (Wechsler et al. 2011)

In real life when clinical tests are carried out to develop new drugs or when treatment is being conducted, the use of placebos is not revealed to the patients. This is called blind manner. Many think that when patients take placebos knowing they are placebos, it will not be so effective. However, a study released in "PLoS One" in 2010 by another Harvard Medical research team shows that social medicine is effective:

> The research was conducted on 80 patients suffering from Irritable Bowel Syndrome. First, all patients were subject to a 15-minute presentation where the following four points were stressed.
>
> 1) The effect of placebos is great.
> 2) Human body automatically act to placebos just like to a conditioned reflex.
> 3) Positive attitude could help in treatment, but it is not necessary.

4) It is important to take placebos with trust.

Next, the group was divided into two, placebos-taking group and non-treatment group. Placebo-taking group was asked to take gelatin capsules regularly that are written "placebo" on them. No instructions were given to the non-treatment group. Three weeks later, those who took placebos fared better than those who didn't, and the level of improvement was similar to a new drug that was known to be effective in curing irritable bowel syndrome. (Kaptchuk et al. 2010)

Surprisingly enough, this shows that placebos work well even when patients know that they are fake drugs. It's similar to the case of "praise" mentioned earlier. Placebos are nothing essentially, but when it was taken with belief, the fake drugs produced good effect in the patients' body as real cure. This means that our mind and body react together. In other words, when something goes wrong in our body, it works to control physiological phenomenon so that recovery can be made on its own, which is the role of NHS. Placebos, as one part of social medicine, can be effective with its natural healing effect. However, follow-up studies are needed to distinguish the extent of the effects of real treatment and fake drugs.

To look deeper into the effects of social medicine, it seems that "mind-body medicine," which studies on the correlation between body and mind, can be of great help. It has already been proved in the Chinese traditional medicine and Ayurveda Indian treatment that mind in the superstructure is important in curing disease, and it has been the essence of the medicine for the last 2000 years. Hippocrates (B.C. 460–B.C. 377) believed that mind, environment, and natural treatment had to be considered in treating patients. A holistic approach of considering mind and body had been regarded important in traditional Eastern medicine. However, with the scientific advancement in the sixteenth to seventeenth century, the spiritual part and feelings were separately dealt from body in Western medicine. Later, the development of medical technology, such as the invention of microscope, stethoscope, and cutting technology in operations, widened the gap between body and mind. It also gave a correct and a more detailed insight into the microworld of tissues and cells.

Furthermore, development of drug therapy in the infrastructure nullified the mind, belief, will, and spiritual side of the superstructure, despite its impact on health. Defining and curing disease were thought to be in the area of objectivity, conducted by science and technology. In short, biomedical model in the Western medicine separated mind from body, and it was popularly believed that sufferings in the mind don't exist, as they aren't linked to physiology and biochemistry.

Nevertheless, with various studies on the interactions between mind and body after the 1960s, mind-body medicine appeared. Mind-body medicine focuses on the interactions among brain, mind, body, and human behavior, and it also concentrates on emotional, spiritual, social, and behavioral tools that can directly have a bearing on human health. As a result, more studies are pointing to the fact that neurotransmitting substances and hormones from the brain control the essence of human mind and feelings and that they cause physical conditions by physiological, chemical, and dynamic processes. Mind-body medicine focuses not only on the physical side but also on the mind, lifestyle, characteristics, and behavioral patterns in treatment. It relies on mediation therapy in the social medicine therapy, which is believed to promote health by relaxation, hypnosis, visual image, meditation, yoga, biofeedback, t'ai chi chuan, Qigong, cognitive behavior therapy, group support, autogenic training, and spirituality training. In particular, in mind-body medicine, disease is regarded as an opportunity for the individual to grow and transform. It is not regarded as a deviation or a stigma.

It is also a well-known fact that the reaction of a patient when he/she hears he/she has cancer during his general checkup impacts his future course of treatment, ranging from complete recovery to death.

2.2 Development of Social Medicine

In the modern society, individuals act as health prosumers. Among human instincts, the will to lead a long life is one of the strongest. Scholars agree that in the absence of special diseases or injuries, natural life span, or virtual life span, will be about 120 years. However, the problem is aging starts a disharmony in the homeostasis of the human body.

For instance, when people age more than 40, they react more sensitively to cold, which used to be a rare occurrence in their younger days. Catching a cold can be easier when the temperature gap gets wider between outdoors and indoors. Bone density tends to be the highest in 25-year-olds and calcium and minerals start to be lost from then on. It results in decreased muscles and lack of ability to absorb vitamins and minerals. Coupled with aging, due to the inactive metabolism in our body, it is harder to strike a balance between the production and consumption of vital energy.

A health prosumer who wants to age wisely should think about his/her lifestyle and stress management skills. I say this as aging is an "avoidable hurdle" in the aging society. Therefore, it is desirable that we discover and use social medicine for the occasion. The reason I want to discover and develop social medicine from our daily life is with a hope to avoid being drug dependent. By utilizing various resources around us, we can usher in NHS and SHS of our body to avoid drugs and to promote treatment, antiaging, and longevity in a healthier manner.

Complementary alternative medicine, or CAM, is gaining popularity around the world, and it is another important branch of social medicine. It relates well with social medicine as it seeks to manage health in various holistic ways.

Thinking that drugs in the infrastructure are derived from orthodox medicine or conventional medicine and that drug therapy also has its roots in them, it is very natural that complementary alternative medicine is included in social medicine. It also goes without saying that therapy or treatments by social medicine are regarded as SM therapy. However, we should be aware of the overcommercialization of social medicine by mass media, which can have a negative impact on the public.

2.2.1 Social Medicine from Daily Life

How we go about our everyday lives is the most important factor in determining health. People who wish to discover and take advantage of social medicine that suits them live the day with more enthusiasm and passion. They regard that the 24 h in a day is something very valuable. Those hours are specially looked on with a view to promoting health.

With more emphasis on lifestyle these days, food and exercise have become all the more important for people in preventing adult diseases and promoting well-being. To patients with chronic disease, doctors recommend regular exercise and diet along with drugs. Major adult diseases that are referred as "culture disease" stem from stress, overeating, and obesity. In many Western countries, excessive intake of animal fat and sugar has given rise to extreme obesity, arteriosclerosis, and ischemic heart diseases, making it a severe social problem.

In Korea, adult diseases are on the rise as well, as their dietary habit gets more Westernized. This shows that there is a close correlation between diet and adult disease. With the increasing average life span, it is everyone's dream to live longer in a healthier way. To do so, social medicine such as healthy diet and regular exercise should be used to counter the shortcomings in our daily lives. By doing so, people should not only focus on defending themselves from the threat of adult disease but also promoting their health at all times.

I would like to talk about two types of social medicine that stemmed from our daily lives. One social medicine is about our lifestyle that encompasses diet and exercise. The other is about stress management.

2.2.1.1 Lifestyle Habit-Based Social Medicine

Health Diet

The Economics Nobel Prize winner, Thomas Schelling, referred to gluttony as the following: "We act like two different people. One wants a slim body, and the other one wants to eat dessert (Schelling 1978)." Gluttony, which results in obesity, is an original instinct that is hard to be controlled on our own. It is also one of the representative causes that produce unhealthy lifestyle. Let's take smoking for example. People already know the correlation between smoking and lung cancer. However, many people still find it hard to cut smoking and are immersed in unhealthy lifestyle. It is a burden not only on the smokers but also on their families. In order to have a healthy lifestyle, knowing what type of food is unhealthy for us is not enough; we need a stronger incentive that can make us change our lifestyle.

Therefore, social medicine to cure our "lifestyle disease," which is a hurdle as we eat, drink, move, sleep, and rest, should come from food culture. By using social navigation of diet improvement, we can better understand the correlation between disease and food. It is the basic foundation on which people can get away from the

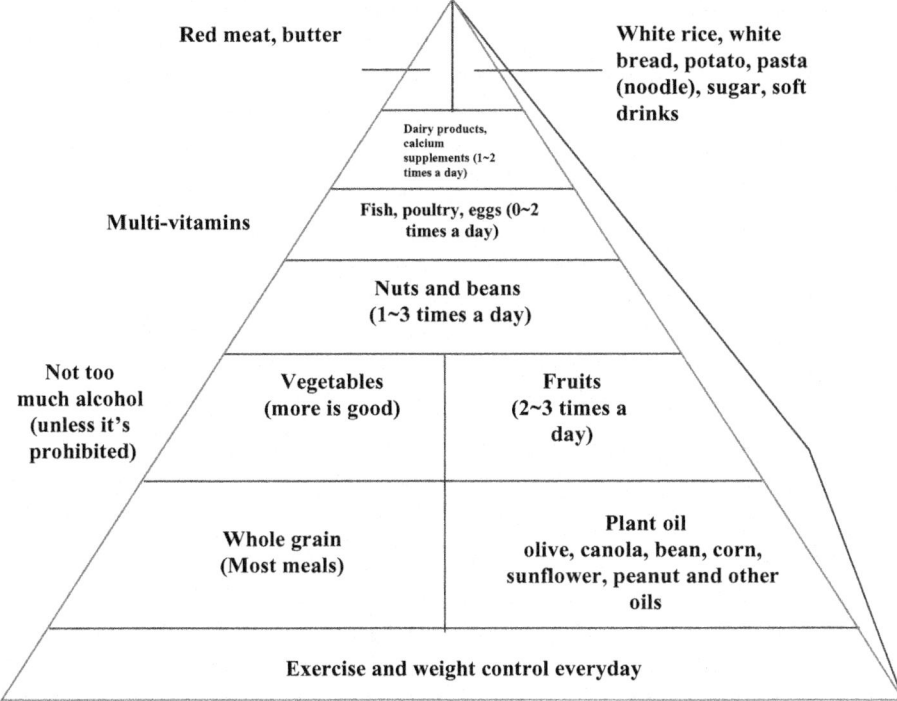

Fig. 2.2 Health diet pyramid (Source: "Eat, Drink, and Be Healthy: The Harvard Medical School Guide to Healthy Eating," 2009, p. 16)

threat of disease and lead a healthy life. However, it is not so easy to discern what "health diet" can make us maintain our body in its best state.

Fortunately, the "healthy eating pyramid (Willett 2009)" was established by 40 years of various scientific studies by Harvard University and around the world. It doesn't lean toward specific culture and provides a general guideline as a social medicine of food, so I would like to introduce it as one of the major ways to promote healthy diet (Fig. 2.2):

1. Beware of weight: maintaining an adequate weight or reducing weight can lower the incidence rate of heart attack, stroke, or other types of cardiovascular diseases, high blood pressure, hyperlipidemia, and diabetes. Reducing weight after menopause can also make you less likely to contract breast cancer, endometritis, colorectal cancer, renal cancer, and other chronic conditions. The following are guidelines for "defensive diet," which is to maintain or lose weight:

   - Stop eating before you feel full. It needs practice.
   - Choose: don't eat just because food is in front of you.
   - Eat in small portions, one at a time.
   - Be careful of desserts: a piece of cheese cake is up to 800 cal, and it contains 49 g of fat. Saturated fat takes up 28 g of it, and it amounts to more than 50 % of daily recommended allowance.

- Eat slowly and pay attention to food when eating: when you eat quickly, the digestive system tends to forget to send the signal that "I'm full." Eating in an adequate speed can give our stomach and small intestine to give such message or signal to our brain.
- Make low-fat food in your own creative way.
- Track the calories of food you consume: it doesn't mean you have to calculate all the calories whenever you eat, but you should know what you eat and drink. A glass of orange juice has the same calories as two oranges. Soft drinks are worse because they only give you calories, without any nutrients.
- Try to lose appetite.
- Minimize attractions: in case you really want some snack, always prepare apple, carrot, or cookies made of whole grain, which are all low fat.
- Don't let your guard down: always remember that food companies try their best to win you over, wanting to sell more products.
- Simply maintain "keeping an eye on your weight" through healthy diet and exercise will be beneficial to your vital energy.

2. Eat less bad fat and more good fat: healthy fat is located in the bottom of the "health diet pyramid." It shows that there are changes made to the belief that "every fat is bad." Fats from nuts, various seeds, grain, fish, and liquid oil (olive oil, canola oil, bean oil, corn oil, sunflower oil, peanut oil, and other plant oil) are good fat that can replace saturated fat or trans fat.

   Even if more than 30 % of the calorie intake a day is composed of fat, it is okay if most of it is unsaturated fat (it is liquid in room temperature and is a useful well-being fat that protects our blood vessels). However, saturated fat (fat oil that hardens and induces obesity) should be taken at minimum levels, which are contained much in red meat, dairy products made with whole milk, and butter. Trans fat should be avoided at all times. The following is the recommended fat intake suggested by WHO (World Health Organization).

   WHO Recommendations

   - Fat: less than 30 % of total daily calorie (2000 kcal/66.7 g)
   - Saturated fat: less than 10 % of total daily calorie (2000 kcal/22.2 g)
   - Trans fat: less than 1 % of total daily calorie (2000 kcal/2.2 g)

3. Take less carbohydrate from refined grain but more from whole grain: there are two areas of carbohydrates in the "health diet pyramid." One is located in the bottom of the pyramid and is carbohydrate from whole grain, which is digested slowly. The other is located on the top, which is highly refined and digested quickly (soft drinks and sweets included).

   The more "quickly digested and absorbed" carbohydrate you take in, the higher the blood sugar, insulin, and neutral fat levels. The level of HDL cholesterol (high-density fat protein, the "good cholesterol)" which has protective traits will be lowered. In the long term, it can induce cardiovascular disease and diabetes. However, whole grain food can fight off diabetes, cardiac disease, diverticulitis, constipation, and other gastrointestinal tract conditions the more you consume them and is beneficial to your long-term health.

4. Choose healthier protein products: red meat tops the pyramid, and it is to stress that some parts of red meat, such as the potential carcinogenic substances produced when baked or fried, or the saturated fat, are related to various chronic conditions. The best protein products in the pyramid are beans, nuts, and fish. Poultry and eggs are very good, as well.

5. Take enough vegetables and fruits, but leave potato out of it: vegetables and fruits are essential nutrients that shouldn't be left out in diet. They lower blood pressure and protect our body from heart attack, stroke, and cancer. They also lower the risks of geriatric illness, such as cataract and macular degeneration. Potato is excluded from the vegetable group and should be taken as little as possible, because it can significantly raise the level of blood sugar and insulin.

6. Drink not too much alcohol: adequate drinking decreases the incidence rate of cardiac disease. The best recommended intake of wine is one glass for women and 1–2 glasses for men a day. It can reduce death rate regarding heart attack and cardiac disease and even lower the risk of ischemic stroke resulting from blood clots. However, too much alcohol consumption can induce liver damage and various cancers and increase blood pressure. It also induces hemorrhagic stroke, gradually weakens heart muscles, paralyzes brain function, is harmful to the fetus, and can ultimately take our lives away.

   Adults without history of depression or alcohol addiction, and with a high possibility of contracting cardiac disease, are advised to take a bit of alcohol every day. It is especially effective to people who are suffering from type 2 diabetes mellitus or people who can't lower HDL levels through diet or exercise. If you already drink every day for health purposes, it is important to maintain a proper level.

7. Take multivitamins, thinking it an "insurance": various components of multivitamins, especially B6, B12, folic acid, and vitamin D, play an important role in preventing cardiac disease, cancer, osteoporosis, and other chronic diseases. Therefore, taking multivitamins is similar to subscribing a "life insurance" at a low cost. It can supplement nutrition imbalance even in people who are on healthy diet. People who can't absorb vitamin from food, who can't be exposed to sunlight every day, and who drink can benefit much from taking multivitamins.

   In fact, food we eat has thousands of natural chemical substances in them, and some of them are very well proven through research, while others aren't. We only know what a handful of substances do in our body, compared to the numerous substances contained in food. So the next challenge for us is to collect data on unknown substances and find out what interactions they have with each other.

Health Exercise

As a social medicine to promote healthy life and prevent aging, "health exercise" is as much important as "health diet." Exercise allows people to work out regularly in a systematic way to prevent disease and promote health. Drugs in the infrastructure is based on therapy to save lives, but social medicine in the superstructure focuses on disease prevention and health management, antiaging, and longevity. Therefore, in order to invent social medicine for people expecting to live healthily beyond 100 years, social navigation of physical condition improvement is necessary. In the end, it is linked to public issue based on SHS, which goes beyond individual aspects focused on NHS.

For instance, we can look to National Institutes of Health's (NIH) "Healthy People 2010" for more information. It aims US citizens to live a longer, healthier life. Among the ten principles of the report, the first principle recommended to increase physical activity. It is also stressed in many guidelines for successful antiaging efforts. Some of the symptoms of adult diseases or those caused by lifestyle habits are called "insulin resistance syndrome." Obesity is a big problem to our health as it is linked to a high possibility of developing "resistance against insulin," where blood sugar is not controlled even when insulin is secreted.

"New England Journal of Medicine," a world-renowned medical journal, reports that exercise is the best medicine (this shows that scholars also understand the existence of social medicine, as they formally addressed "exercise" as "drug," even though exercise is not in the category of drugs.) In the course of 4 years, 3200 ordinary people were tested in the following conditions: (1) a group without any special treatment; (2) a group where people took drugs to cure resistance against insulin as a precautionary measure, which is used often; and (3) a group where people changed their lifestyle by exercise. Diabetes was found the most in the first group, followed by the second and the third.

In the website www.exerciseismedicine.org run by American College of Sports Medicine, you can find many contents that stress exercise is the best medicine. What are the good sides of exercise? First, exercise significantly reduces death by heart disease. Second, it decreases the dangers of contracting high blood pressure and is highly beneficial to managing high blood pressure. Third, it develops physique and muscles and increases the flexibility of joints. Fourth, it reduces stress and dispels anxiety. Fifth, it can promote psychological stability and self-confidence. Sixth, it is highly effective in weight control. Seventh, it reduces abnormal blood sugar increase and the dangers of diabetes occurrence. Eighth, it can lower possible early deaths from various reasons. Ninth, it lowers dangers of colorectal cancer and other cancer occurrences. Lastly, it can make people have a healthier silver life (Gong In-Duk and Ye Byung-Il 2012a).

The following is a figure of "health exercise," which is firmly established as health diet (Fig. 2.3).

Keep in mind that the aim of "health exercise" is not a good-looking body but a healthy body that enables people to carry out their duties in everyday life. It is to use your body flexibly so that injuries and diseases can be prevented and that you can enjoy a healthy life, not requiring help or aid from others.

Based on the "health exercise pyramid," let me introduce ten ways to practice exercise regularly in your daily life (Gong In-Duk and Ye Byung-Il 2012b):

1. Set aside time for exercise.
2. Tell your friends that you exercise. Get attention.

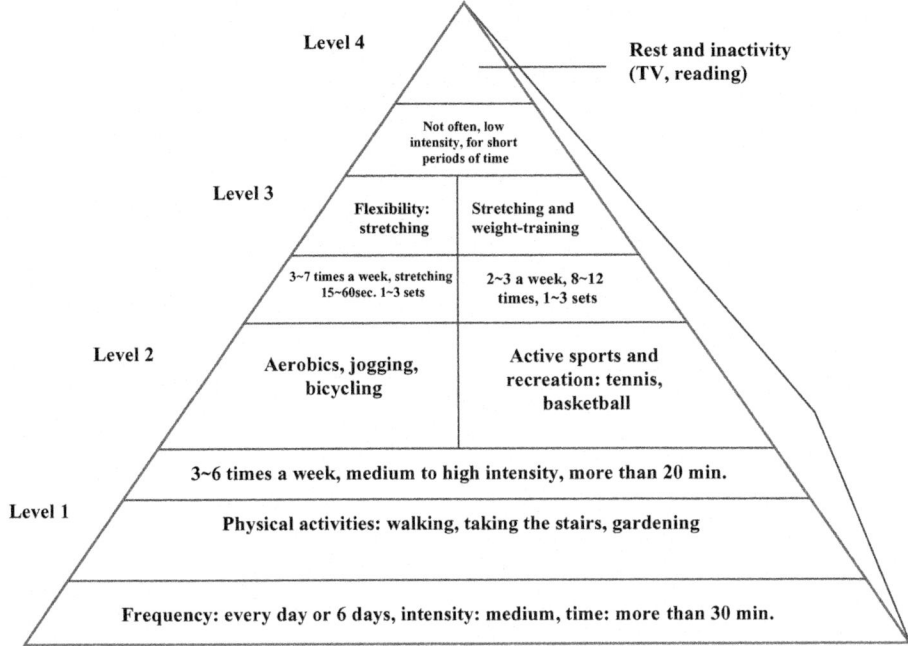

Level 4

Rest and inactivity
(TV, reading)

Not often, low
intensity, for short
periods of time

Level 3

Flexibility:
stretching

Stretching and
weight-training

3~7 times a week, stretching
15~60sec. 1~3 sets

2~3 a week, 8~12
times, 1~3 sets

Level 2

Aerobics, jogging,
bicycling

Active sports and
recreation: tennis,
basketball

3~6 times a week, medium to high intensity, more than 20 min.

Level 1

Physical activities: walking, taking the stairs, gardening

Frequency: every day or 6 days, intensity: medium, time: more than 30 min.

Fig. 2.3 Health exercise pyramid (Source: "Power Physiology of Exercise," 2008, p. 290)

3. Believe exercise will increase vital energy.
4. Self-motivation. Motivating yourself to exercise will give you power to continue.
5. Prevent any injuries by relaxing your muscles before and after the exercise.
6. Concentrate on acquiring skills but don't rush.
7. Find a place that is near and costs a little.
8. Don't be tied down to time or spatial limitations.
9. Use free time to exercise when traveling.
10. Play with your kid.

2.2.1.2 Health Stressor

What is the social medicine that can help you recover from physical, chemical, and psychological stress in daily life? There are many ways of managing stress and it is very important what you choose. Of course, putting them into practice will be the most important.

Humans are made up of body and mind, and that is why there is a saying that "everything depends on how you think." Taking this into consideration, it seems laughter, which gives us health and comfort, is the best medicine throughout all times and all places. Laughter has more than 2000 years of history and recently, it is highlighted along with laughter therapy. Kant was cynical about laughter's positive role of being rational and enlightening, but he highly evaluated laughter in the end because it had a positive impact on health (Kant 1900).

Smiling or laughter as social medicine improves our facial image. It seems like a medicine even more valuable than wild ginseng that heals both body and mind, so I will talk about laughter in a separate chapter. By considering health through the social navigation of "facial image control," we can develop smile and laughter into social medicine, whether it be a natural, beautiful smile or a fake laughter. As I mentioned, laughter has a long history and many important elements, so I will raise the issue once again in "beautiful laughter (BL)." Here, I will stress "health stressor" as social medicine that gives us health and power to overcome stress. The word stress had a negative connotation, so in order to change the perception and to emphasize it as a social medicine, I will call it "health stressor."

The following is from the 38 guidelines of stress management from Benson-Henry Research Institute of MGH or Massachusetts General Hospital (Gong In-Duk and Ye Byung-Il 2012c):

1. Start the day with breakfast.
2. Have some quality time with yourself from time to time.
3. Meditate or listen to music for short periods during work.
4. Choose fruit juice over coffee.
5. Write a checklist and prioritize your work.
6. Get rid of the idea that you have to do all work perfectly by yourself.
7. Do not engage in multitasking.
8. Build a network of people to support you.
9. Reduce noise near you as much as possible.
10. Enjoy lunch, and don't eat at your desk.
11. Have adequate nutrition, relaxation, and sleep for your health.
12. Work out regularly.
13. Enjoy your birthday and holidays, and make many events.
14. If stress is unavoidable, regard it as an opportunity for your growth and transformation.
15. Avoid people who give you stress.
16. Also avoid people who are negative.
17. Don't watch late-night news.
18. Praise yourself and think positively.
19. Try to give thanks in your life with what you have.
20. Give yourself presents.
21. Give your straight answer and say "NO" at times.
22. Be true to your feelings toward your spouse, family, colleagues, and friends.
23. Don't be afraid of asking questions and asking for help.
24. Include enough time in between appointments.
25. Take a deep breath when you think you are under stress.
26. In times of difficulty, think about funny things.
27. Designate a day for your mental health and protect yourself actively from any mental attack.

28. Consider having a pet.
29. Take time to walk and think.
30. Understand that you can't see or do everything at one time.
31. Remember that your life is only a passing moment compared to eternity.
32. Try to be less aggressive.
33. Be considerate and show your kindness to people.
34. When under stress, ask yourself whether it is worth it.
35. Abstain from judging easily or criticizing.
36. Listen carefully to what people say.
37. Be flexible to changes.
38. If you have faith, pray earnestly to God.

2.2.2 Social Medicine from Complementary Alternative Medicine (CAM)

All things from CAM, or complementary alternative medicine, can be selected by ordinary people to be used as social medicine. CAM is not a new therapy and certainly not cutting-edge science. It is an unorthodox medicine emerged to complement problems and limitations of modern medicine, based on naturopathic medicine that manages disease and health in a holistic manner by looking into classic principles of human, environment, and life.

CAM was first established by Western medical experts and by the standards of National Institute of Health, to be more precise. Western medicine is the mainstream of medicine nowadays, and that is why it is referred to as traditional medicine, leaving others to be categorized together as CAM. In the past, CAM was regarded as folk medicine at best, as part of premodern culture due to its lack of scientific data. In the 1990s, CAM received worldwide spotlight when the excellence of traditional medicine, based on biomedical model, was criticized. CAM was referred to as "the third medicine" or "hidden treasure" with rising expectations. There are also movements to integrate CAM into the traditional medical system, calling it as "integrative medicine" or "holistic medicine." However, CAM can't be a silver bullet and it still has to go through strict scientific verification. In terms of understanding and evaluating how diseases work and of comparing ways and effects of treatment, we still have to rely on scientific tools and methods. Some parts of CAM under criticism for reasons of scientific verification shouldn't be ignored for its limitations and problems. Rather, self-imposed efforts to overcome those hurdles will be more necessary.

Oriental medicine is regarded as traditional medicine that is distinguished from Western medicine in Korea. It is not included in CAM, as it holds greater role in Korea, similar to the standing of Western medicine. Still, many other countries see Oriental medicine as CAM.

In short, CAM is a medicine that seeks to cure all diseases and pains of humans according to natural healing power. CAM mobilizes various natural approaches to improve immunity and recovering ability of humans. It looks at patients as holistic beings and doesn't only focus on the injured part but looks after other psychological, social, and environmental aspects in harmony (Oh Hong-Keun 2004). Nowadays, in traditional medicine, CAM is gaining ground as an object of study, and more patients who can't find answers in body-focused traditional medicine are looking toward CAM as an alternative. It goes without saying that such interest will lead to the development of social medicine, which will be a boost to medical experts and ordinary people alike.

There are more than 200 categories that can be included in CAM, but the following 60 are relatively well-known medicines (Jeon Se-Il 2004c). Here, I will list major elements that are the source of social medicine. Other details will be described in the following chapter of social medicine therapy.

1. CAM closely related to the Western medicine

    1. Chiropractic medicine
    2. Podiatric medicine
    3. Chelation therapy
    4. Hypnotherapy
    5. Enzyme therapy
    6. Applied kinesiology
    7. Craniosacral therapy
    8. Iridology
    9. Neurolinguistic programming
    10. Reconstructive therapy
    11. Biofeedback therapy
    12. Mind-body medicine
    13. Magnetic field therapy
    14. Oxygen therapy
    15. Nutritional therapy
    16. Osteopathic therapy
    17. Detoxification therapy
    18. Energy medicine
    19. Orthomolecular medicine
    20. Cell therapy
    21. Environmental medicine
    22. Bodywork therapy
    23. Rolfing
    24. Dream therapy
    25. Recreation therapy
    26. Magic therapy
    27. Neural therapy
    28. Autogenic therapy
    29. Reichian therapy
    30. Guided imagery
    31. Dance therapy

32. Biological dentistry

2. CAM closely related to the Oriental medicine

   1. Ayurvedic medicine
   2. Qigong therapy
   3. Naturopathic medicine
   4. Aromatherapy
   5. Transcendental meditation
   6. Reflexology
   7. Touching therapy
   8. Zen dance therapy
   9. Yoga
   10. Flower remedies
   11. Sound therapy
   12. Horticulture therapy
   13. Bee venom therapy
   14. Psychic healing

3. CAM that combines both Oriental and Western medicine

   1. Herbal therapy
   2. Diet therapy
   3. Fasting
   4. Homeopathic medicine
   5. Light therapy
   6. Hydrotherapy
   7. Sense therapy
   8. Colon therapy
   9. Intramuscular stimulation
   10. Hyperthermia
   11. Quantum medicine
   12. Juice therapy
   13. Urine therapy
   14. Taping therapy

2.2.3   Differentiation of Social Medicine

One of the emphases of the book is that humans are composed of mind and body. Basic premise calls for harmony of the mind and body. That is why health diet and health exercise were introduced as social medicine to help take care of the body. In the same context, health stressor was mentioned as social medicine to look after the mind, where detailed instructions followed. Beautiful laughter (BL), which has a positive effect both on the mind and body, will be dealt separately in the coming chapter to improve facial image. Therefore, the four categories of social medicine are: (1) diet, (2) physical condition, (3) stress management, and (4) facial image control.

When we only consider the taste of the dish or take it as just another ordinary meal, it will be plain food to us. However, when health is considered, which includes the understanding of the correlation between disease and food, along with balanced diet and nutrition, it will be "health diet," a unique kind of social medicine. In the same sense, when you do exercise with no exact plans for the body, it will just be a hobby. However, taking health into consideration and the understanding of the correlation between disease and exercise, it will become "health exercise," also a type of social medicine. "health stressor" and "beautiful laughter" can be developed as essential social medicine in this way.

When you use social navigation, look around your surroundings prioritizing health, and understand the correlation between a possible social medicine material and disease, many ordinary things will become clear to you as social medicine. Until now, hobbies such as meditation, yoga, tanning, bicycling, walking, mountain climbing, swimming, bathing, traveling, talking, watching TV, shopping, reading, citing poems, singing, playing musical instruments, watching art performances, dancing, martial arts, painting, or keeping a pet may have been regarded as simple hobbies. However, when mind and body are considered in these activities, the hobbies will become possible candidates for social medicine. Therefore, you should think about your current health conditions and choose the best for your state. Anything can be developed as your personalized social medicine when they can be planned first and performed regularly.

Another good example of social medicine is pets, as proven recently at a radio show. With the aging of the society, a single household is increasing and so do pets. It has been reported that elderly citizen who live with pets are physically and mentally healthier than those who don't. By living with pets, the seniors tend to feel less lonely and get exercise more, which results in less incidents of depression and heart failure paralysis.

As you can see, various substances and materials near us are used as social medicine. In nature, sunlight, water, forest, and stones are rising as social medicine under the name of therapy. Social medicine is like stem cells that can be specialized in various ways, thereby promoting our health and quality of life. Therefore, candidates for social medicine include everything that can be found around us according to our health condition through social navigation. They include material things such as stones to abstract ones, such as laughter.

Health is something that has to be earned with effort for the rest of our lives. It is the product of self-discipline and control. With this thought in mind, you will be able to choose the suitable social medicine for you. The most important thing before discovering social medicine is to have an accurate perception of your health condition. To help you along the way, the following is suggested as ways to maintain health in certain age groups (Morley and Colberg 2008):

1. From ages 0 to 40

   1. Exercise regularly.
   2. Avoid obesity.
   3. Consume a certain amount of calcium.

    4. Eat nutritious food including fish.

    5. Put on a seatbelt in the car.

    6. Quit drinking and smoking after the age of 21.

    7. Get vaccination.

    8. Do not go over the speed limit.

    9. Avoid violence and unapproved drugs.

  10. Get a breast checkup every month (for women who started their period).

2. From ages 40 to 60

    1. Exercise regularly.

    2. Avoid obesity.

    3. Consume a certain amount of calcium and vitamin D.

    4. Eat fish.

    5. Put on a seatbelt in the car.

    6. Quit drinking and smoking.

    7. Measure blood pressure.

    8. Measure cholesterol and blood sugar levels.

    9. Get medical checkups to prevent breast cancer, colorectal cancer, high blood pressure, and diabetes.

  10. Periodically get medical checkups to prevent ovarian cancer (women).

  11. Do mental exercise steadily and socialize with people.

  12. Avoid too much medication.

  13. Have interest in hormone alternative therapy.

3. From ages 60 to 80

    1. Exercise regularly and do balancing and muscle exercise.

    2. Avoid weight loss.

    3. Consume an adequate amount of calcium and vitamin D.

    4. Eat fish.

    5. Put on a seatbelt in the car.

    6. Quit smoking and drinking.

    7. Get medical checkups to prevent breast cancer, high blood pressure, osteoporosis, and diabetes.

    8. Measure cholesterol levels.

    9. Get vaccination to prevent influenza, pneumococcus, and shingles if possible.

  10. Periodically get medical checkups to prevent ovarian cancer (women).

  11. Do mental exercise steadily and socialize with people.

  12. Avoid too much medication.

4. From ages 80 and over

    1. Exercise regularly and do balancing and muscle exercise.

    2. Avoid weight loss.

    3. Consume an adequate amount of calcium and vitamin D.

    4. Eat fish.

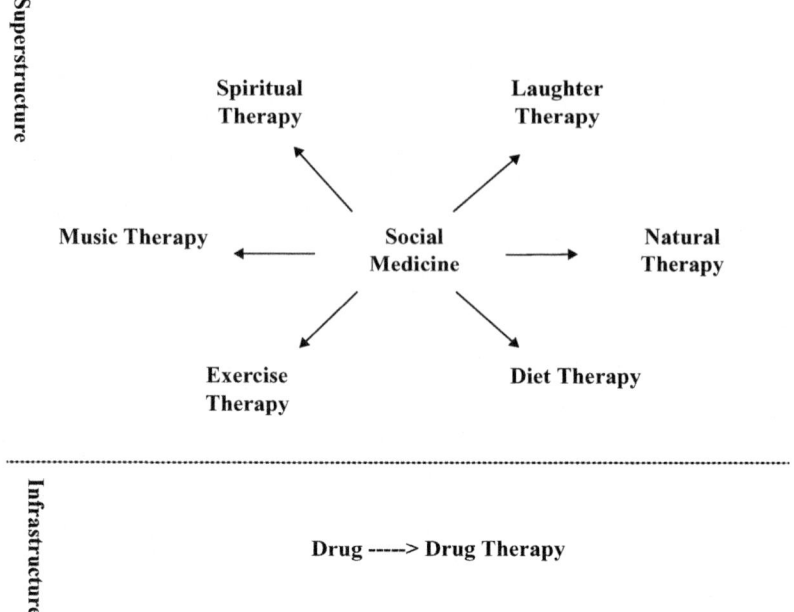

Fig. 2.4 The differentiation mechanism of social medicine

5. Put on a seatbelt in the car.
6. Quit smoking and drinking.
7. Get medical checkups to prevent breast cancer (women).
8. Get vaccination for influenza and pneumococcus.
9. Make your home environment safe to prevent any falls. Use a stick to be on the safe side and wear protection gears.
10. Do mental exercise steadily and socialize with people, and don't get gloomy.
11. Avoid too much medication.
12. Continue to do what you're doing (whether work, hobbies, etc.)

The summary of what I mentioned can be found in Fig. 2.4, which includes how social medicine is discovered to be turned into various treatment methods and therapies. I'd like to stress that when social medicine, which is in the superstructure, is differentiated into "therapy," our experiences, intuition, and imaginations come together to obtain social medicine in a quicker, easier, and cost-efficient way. The process is shown in the "line of arrow" in the picture.

However, drugs in the infrastructure have to go through painstaking, difficult process along with astronomical money in order to obtain its status as new drug. The high-tech scientific phase of the development of a new drug, up to the approval so it can be used in traditional drug treatment, is as follows: looking for source material, extracting olfactory hair substances, preclinical test (animal test) and clinical test, etc. The success rate is only 1/10,000, and I put it as a "dotted line of arrow." In the break of the twenty-first-century, the genetic map of our body was completed, and the three billion pairs of base sequences of the genes, along with the inside structure of the nucleus in human cell, were revealed (it's called "bio-revolution"). Through genomics and proteomics, a "bio-navigation" system is being established to unearth the origin of human life.

In the old days, people used to search for drugs depending on "serendipity." Now the success rate of new drug development has increased, as target discovery based on biochemical mechanism at the nano-/molecular level, and the selective research through drug design, began. Nevertheless, the "dotted line of arrow" tells us that scholars and researchers who put in everything for new drug development experience various failure, and the process is a long history itself, coupled with the sweat and tears of their efforts. Magic Cancer Bullet (2005) shows that the success story of Gleevec (the first-ever targeted anticancer agent in the world) is the "dotted line of arrow."

The development process of drugs in the infrastructure is faced with various regulations. However, the differentiation of social medicine is quite different. After checking your health condition, you can easily discover social medicine in your daily life and surrounding environments. By utilizing the social medicine to find out the appropriate treatment and therapy for you, social medicine can be successfully developed and steadily advance as a specialized social medicine therapy.

References

Association for Applied and Therapeutic Humor (2004) Essence. Retrieved 31 Jan 2005, from http://www.aath.org/home_1.html, p 11

Byun Kwang-Ho, Chang Hyun-Gap (2012) Stress and mind-body medicine. Hakjisa, Seoul, p 24

Cho Byung-Hee (2010) Sociology of disease and medical care. Gypmoondang, p 134

Drucker P et al (trans: Lee Jae-Kyu) (2001) The future community. 21 Centurybooks, Seoul, pp 30–34

Friedman M (trans: Shim Joon-Bo, Byun Dong-Yul) (2007a) Capitalism and freedom. Chongoram Media, Seoul, pp 44–45

Friedman M (trans: Shim Joon-Bo, Byun Dong-Yul) (2007b) ibid, p 82

Friedman M (trans: Min Byung-Kyun, Seo Jae-Myung, Han Hong-Soon) (2009) Freedom to choose. Jayukiupwon, Seoul, p 36

Giddens A (trans: Kim Mi-Suk, Kim Yong-Hak, Song Ho-Keun, Shin Kwang-Yung, Ryu Hong-Joon, Jung Seong-Ho) (2013) Sociology, 6th edn. Eulyoo Publishing Co, Ltd., pp 464–464

Gong In-Duk, Ye Byung-Il (2012a) Body saving prescription for exercise. Thinksmart Press, Seoul, pp 76–77

Gong In-Duk, Ye Byung-Il (2012b) ibid, pp 32–36

Gong In-Duk, Ye Byung-Il (2012c) ibid, pp 44–46

Jeon Se-Il (2004a) Complementary alternative medicine. Gyechukmoonwhasa, Seoul, pp 41–42

Jeon Se-Il (2004b) ibid, pp 37–39

Jeon Se-Il (2004c) ibid, pp 157–159

Kant I. Anthropologie in pragmatischer Hinsicht. Bd. VII. Kap. 76, In: Kant I. Gesammelte Schriften. Hrsg. von der Königlich Preussischen Akadmie der Wissenschaften, Berlin und Leipzig, 1900ff., S. 261f

Kaptchuk TJ, Friedlander E, Kelley JM, Sanchez MN, Kokkotou E, Singer JP, Kowalczykowski M, Miller FG, Kirsch I, Lembo AJ (2010) Placebos without deception: a randomized controlled trial in irritable bowel syndrome. PLoS One 5(12):e15591

Kim Chae-Yoon, Kwon Tae-Hwan, Hong Doo-Seung (2007) Introduction to sociology. SNU Press, Seoul, p 264

Kim Ki-Ran, Choi Ki-Ho (2009) Dictionary of popular culture. Hyunsilmunhwa Research

Kim Yong-Un (1997) Healthcare theory of laughter. Yeyoung Communication, Seoul, pp 60–63

Lee Dong-Seok, Kim Shin-Keun (1997) The history of drug. SNU Press

Lee Min-Joo (2001) A study on the viewers influenced by Canned Laughter in Sitcom. Master thesis, Kwangwoon University, pp 13–14

Lee Yung-Keun, Choi Joon-Yung (2011a) Doctor Detox. Sogeumnamoo (Seoul), pp 229–231

Lee Yung-Keun, Choi Joon-Yung (2011b) ibid., pp 59–68

Morley J, Colberg S (trans: Jung Joo-Yon) (2008) Science of youth. Migibooks Press, Seoul, pp 22–24

Oh Hong-Keun (2004) Medicine of natural therapy. Jeonghan Health Books, Seoul, p 19

Powers S, Howley E (trans: Choi Dae-Hyuk, Choi Hee-Nam, Jeon Tae-Won) (2008) Power physiology of exercise, 6th edn. Lifescience, Seoul, p 290

Schelling TC (1978) Egonomics, or the art of self-management. Am Econ Rev 68(2):290–294

Sen A (2002) Why health equity? Health Econ 11(8):659–666

Smith A, The Wealth of Nations (1776) Edited by Edwin Cannan, 5th edn. Methuen & Co., Ltd., London, 1930. In: Friedman M (trans: Min Byung-Kyun, Seo Jae-Myung, Han Hong-Soon) Freedom to choose. Jayukiupwon, 2009, p 21

Vajella D, Slater R (trans: Lee Choong-Ho) (2005) Magic cancer bullet. Haenamoo, Seoul

Wechsler ME, Kelley JM, Boyd IO, Dutile S, Marigowda G, Kirsch I, Israel E, Kaptchuk TJ (2011) Active albuterol or placebo, sham acupuncture, or no intervention in asthma. N Engl J Med 365(2):119–126

Willett WC (trans: Son Soo-Mi) (2009) Eat, drink, and be healthy. DongA Ilbo Sa, Seoul, pp 28–37

Chapter 3
Therapy of Social Medicine

3.1 Concept and Scope for Therapy of Social Medicine

Man, society, and environment are rich resources of social medicine. When humans discover and utilize social medicine, which uses NHS and SHS as their vital energy, social medicine can be highly valued as therapy of social medicine. As I mentioned differentiation of social medicine in the previous chapter, if social medicine acts both as general remarks and theory, therapy of social medicine is methodology. Usually, theories or principles tend to be one, but the methodologies can be applied in differentiation across many different sectors.

The ground basis of social medicine therapy is utilizing NHS and SHS of each human being. However, it can take various forms in each sector, which is called as "horizontal differentiation." In the case of literature, poem or reading therapy is being developed. In the artistic field, there is music and art therapy. In religion, spiritual therapy or temple stay is gaining popularity, and the same goes for play and laughter therapy in the cultural sector. In environmental field, natural therapies such as sunlight, stone, flower, forest, and fragrance have emerged, while talking, shopping, watching TV, sauna, traveling, and caring pets are practiced as new therapies in lifestyle and hobby sector. As you can see, social medicine therapy is spreading and being distributed faster in a diversified way. Therefore, it is nearly impossible to explain every methodology in the book.

The niche market of social medicine would be the drug therapy market ruled by drug in the infrastructure. When social medicine therapy system is established to the point of physician's prescribing according to each disease (e.g., diet and exercise for diabetes, enforced laughing for cancer, gum chewing for dementia, etc.), patients will be able to do a self-check of activities which they can perform along with medication, which is called as "vertical differentiation." It will become a niche buster. When the methodologies of social medicine therapy in various sectors are studied and completed horizontally and vertically, "the world of social medicine" will be revealed successfully.

© Springer Science+Business Media Singapore 2016
B.-H. Han, *Therapy of Social Medicine*, DOI 10.1007/978-981-287-748-2_3

Social medicine therapy is based on the theory of social medicine, and it refers to intervention activity and an action plan of health management that can bring about disease prevention, easing of symptoms, improved health, and impacts of treatment. In other words, social medicine therapy encompasses all treatment and vitalizing activity that can be helpful to promoting health. In this chapter, I will discuss detailed steps we can take in health diet, health exercise, and health stressor, which can promote disease prevention, antiaging, and longevity in this age of "Healthy 100 Years Old." Later, I will discuss various treatments in social medicine therapy that came from CAM, which is centered on lifesaving activities. In doing so, there may be some overlapping points between treatments in vitalizing and life-saving activities. However, in the aspect of social medicine therapy, it doesn't matter if it is health behavior centered on vitalizing activity or illness behavior focused on lifesaving activity, as both behaviors promote health and healing in healthy and sick people alike.

3.1.1 Social Medicine Therapy: A Formula of Hope

Everyone wants to be happy. There is only once a chance at life for everyone, so all people want to eat well and live well. This has been dubbed as a "well-being life," but it was also hard to understand due to its obscure nature. Recently, studies on well-being reported more concrete concept of the word.

From the mid-twentieth century, researchers in Gallup extensively looked into the elements necessary for a well-being life. As a result, they reported five general points that make up a well-being life. First is "career well-being." It is about jobs that we hold to carry on our lives or to fulfill our calling and how much we enjoy and love our work. Second is "social well-being," which is about strong human relationship and whether our loved ones are with us or not. Third is "financial well-being," related to the effective management of one's money, which gives feeling of stability. Fourth is "physical well-being," and it is about people having enough energy and being in a healthy state to perform everyday routines. Lastly, there is "community well-being," which is about how actively you participate in issues in your local community. It is about what we can do to pay back to our regional society. According to the study, the state of well-being is about living a life that fulfills certain levels in all these five sectors. The results tell us that the biggest threat to well-being is "yourself," as we sometimes damage our long-term well-being by giving over to our short-term desire by impulse, such as buying (Rath and Harter 2010a).

The result of the study gives us important messages about social medicine and social medicine therapy.

1. "Physical well-being" and "community well-being" are included as major elements in the concept of general well-being most people want.
2. Western people also regard "physical well-being" as "vital energy."

3. And a well-being life goes beyond personal health, which means it entails participatory works and contribution (sharing and volunteering) in the regional community.

This shows that social medicine and its methodology, social medicine therapy, which represent the superstructure, are based on vital energy that sends off NHP, which is made up of NHS and SHS. This reaffirms us that the universal stream, which has the traits of fusion energy, appearing in the unity stage of sublimation of SHS, is essential to our well-being. The universal stream is made up of small efforts and love that can arise when we pay attention to others, and it is composed of sharing and volunteering works.

There is another study to be cited called, "Is there a formula for a happy life?" From the late 1930s, a team of researchers in Harvard University had tracked the lives of 268 sophomores for 72 years until Jun. 2009 (the "Study of Adult Development," is still ongoing, which was the foundation of the study). The result and implications of the study is included in the book, *Aging Well*. In the book, the author George E. Vaillant, a professor of psychiatry at Harvard University, declares that the most important thing in life is human relationship. This shows that "loving our neighbors," based on SHS, is very important in your well-being and health (Vaillant 2012).

Aging can be defined as functional, structural, and biochemical degrading process in the cells and tissues of humans as they age. Human beings age from 20, and the ultimate reason why we age is still a mystery even to the scholars. The secretion of hormones decreases sharply around 50, and people just guess that disharmony of homeostasis, a symbol of healthy body, is the problem. It is believed that the evolution of our body is yet to catch up with the increased life span. Aging not only has an impact on our physical health but also on our mind and spirit. That is why Henri Amiel (1821–1881), a scholar and poet to Switzerland, said that "To know how to grow old is the master-work of wisdom, and one of the most difficult chapters in the great art of living (Amiel 1985)."

We still don't know the exact cause and mechanism of the cells, but now I will introduce five useful theories on aging. By doing so, we will be able to find ways to deal with diet, physical condition, stress management, antiaging, and longevity (Kwon Yong-Wook 2004).

First is "Wear and tear theory." Cars will become rusty when used for a long time. In the same sense, when our body is used for a long time, it will suffer damages which will lead to aging. In other words, our cells and tissues have no choice but to become old and rusty due to the toxic elements coming from food and the environment. In the younger days, NHP operates actively, which offsets the damages of wearing and tearing. However, aging deters the recovering ability of NHP, which exposes us to diseases, finally leading to death. Therefore, eating healthy food, living a regular life, and diminishing exposure to harmful environments will delay aging. The theory is in line with social medicine therapy in that it promotes self-control in the long term.

Second is "neurohormone theory." It means that neurons and hormones that are the network of biochemicals inside our body play an important role. Hormones are synthesized in a certain part of our body and move to other parts through blood flow. It then controls the functions of cells and tissues there, acting as a "body signal transmitter." Neurons and hormones cooperate to control metabolism and the function of the body, and they are critical to recovering damaged parts. When people age the secretion of hormones decreases, which deters recovering abilities, bodily functions, and control abilities. Therefore, a natural hormone therapy to stimulate the body is the major solution to actively pumping out hormones. If natural hormone therapy is not sufficient, hormones can be injected as a supplementary measure or as a stimulus of secretion, to delay the aging process. However, side effects may occur so it is important to consult an expert beforehand.

Third is "free radical theory." Almost all living beings need oxygen to sustain health. As I mentioned, mitochondria are where energy is made in cells, which is why it is often compared to the engine of a car. The theory presumes that the "engine" is incomplete. In other words, when mitochondria are making energy, it combines oxygen with chemical substances and emits water and carbon dioxide. In the process, about 1–5 % of oxygen turns into free radical which destroys cells. Just as the free radical rusts iron, cells are oxidized, diminishing cells' protein functions. By damaging DNA, it also raises genetic mutation, ultimately resulting in cancer. Free radical's mechanism to recover from injuries also works well when we are young. Therefore, the damages may be a little blow to us. However, as we age, the damages accumulate, and antioxidant activities to counter free radical diminish, which causes cells to age. Free radical attacks collagen and fiber that maintain our skin, joint, sinew, tendon and muscle and turn them into a soft and flexible state. It is the main culprit of aging skin, making it loose and increasing its wrinkles. Joints also become stiff, making our body less flexible.

Therefore, it is important to cut down free radical as much as possible. Smoking and stress should be avoided. It is desirable to relieve stress immediately if possible, and a healthy dose of exercise is recommended. Exposure to hazardous environments such as air pollution, ultraviolet rays, and food additives should be prohibited, and it is advised to eat less, as food produces much free radical. Taking antioxidants is another way to decrease free radical. Fresh vegetables and fruits are recommended and green tea over coffee. As we age, it is hard to cut down free radical with only vegetables or fruits, so one way to fight aging and oxidation is by taking vitamin C and E, beta-carotene, selenium, melatonin, polyphenol, and propolis in pills.

Fourth is "program theory." The theory presumes that all humans are programmed in their DNAs to age, and it is similar to the Eastern concept of the phrase "Life and death are providential" and the way of vitology. In the past, people used to think that DNA had a dominant effect on aging and longevity, but according to mechanical studies nowadays, it is believed that acquired factors such as diet, exercise, and stress have a bigger impact. That is why controlled and regular lifestyle and habit are important. The theory reports that there are DNAs which control aging, and if the DNA can be named and controlled, humans can be freed from aging. However, it is not quite certain whether people will be able to live forever by manipulating DNAs.

Fifth is "telomerase theory." Telomere is the tip of a chromosome, and its shape is different from other parts of the chromosome, as it is composed of different substances. Furthermore, the telomerase enzyme forms telomere structure, thereby oppressing the aging of cells by protecting the tip of the chromosome, acting like plastic caps that are found in both ends of shoelaces. Telomeres are not duplicated even when chromosomes are reproduced by cell division, and their length shortens as cell division takes place. This means when telomeres wear out, the cell can no longer be divided but die out. Therefore, the length of the telomere is the barometer of how much longer the person can live.

Telomerase is the enzyme that reproduces the telomere. When cells are injected with telomerase, telomeres don't get shorter even when cell division takes place. This means that cells don't wear out and die after going through cell division. This is possible in laboratories, but not yet sure in real life, so the efforts to integrate it into the human body are actively ongoing. One tricky part of the enzyme, however, is that it increases the risk of cancer. Cancer cells are the ones that grow with infinite cell division. Telomerase is active in cancer cells, which helps maintain the length of the telomere even if cell division occurs. As telomere doesn't die out as well, the unlimited proliferation of the cells threatens our lives. The aged cells, however, don't have any telomerase left, which shortens telomere repeatedly after cell division, causing deaths in people. Therefore, telomerase is actively being researched in both cancer treatment and antiaging fields. Telomerase can stop or at least delay the time of telomeres' shortening length in healthy cells. Oppressing telomerase can also stop the growth of cancer cells.

As you can see from the five theories, the key to maintaining health and vigor is not by maintaining youth. Aging in a healthy manner (antiaging) is more important. It is believed that good antiaging efforts will lead us to longevity. Each theory has its own points, so by looking at each crucial point, we will get an opportunity to take a step closer into disease prevention, antiaging, and longevity in a holisticsense.

If social medicine is the origin of humans, social medicine therapy is said to be connecting the three dots of man, nature, and society, a humanistic and naturopathic methodology that is based on humanism. Social medicine helps us to manage our health in daily life and also make us depend on each other as members of nature. Social medicine therapy deals with diet, physical condition, stress management, and facial image control, for a more profound and fundamental change. Social medicine therapy is a formula that uses both detoxification and nutrition supplement to grant us health, well-being, and happiness.

3.1.1.1 Diet Improvement

Today, we are living in a world where news about well-being and health flood us. However, sometimes the contracting news and information confuse us:

> People are curious about the recent results (although they don't always mean the best) to get to the keys of a healthy life and longevity, whether they are food, vitamins or supplements, or ways to control their diet. Mass media provides new information about health to fulfill

peoples' desires. The problem is that newspapers, TV, Internet and other means of media report studies that are yet to be confirmed, in big headlines, such as "great achievement," "remarkable discovery," or "possible treatments." Their titles confuse the public, and it is similar to reading some parts of the book randomly, rather than seeing the whole picture. (Willett 2009)

Therefore, it is not wise to get rid of dietary habits that you have kept because of a single research result or a newspaper article. The words of Mark Twain, "Be careful about health books – you may die of a misprint," are still effective today.

Carbohydrates were believed to be healthy, but it is found out that the carbohydrates in white bread, potato, or rice cause blood sugar to rise and fall rapidly. As a result, it has an impact on the rapid rise and fall of insulin, making people to feel an empty stomach soon. Carbohydrates that can be easily digested have a severe bearing on overweight people. However, carbohydrate in beans and whole grain is hard to digest and has a slower impact on the rise and fall of insulin and blood sugar, and it prevents you from feeling hungry soon. Carbohydrates in beans and whole grain are full of cellulose and minerals, which prevent heart disease and diabetes. By turning on social navigation, false information can be corrected, which is the first step to diet improvement.

3.1.1.2   Physical Condition Improvement

Physical condition improvement is essential for disease prevention, healthy aging, and longevity on the members of the society. Just like diet improvement, strengthening your physical condition should be conducted with a long-term perspective. If desires to sleep more and lie-down take over, it is hard to expect that one would continue long-term behavioral changes needed for physical condition improvement. If you know from experience how 20 min of exercise a day can brighten up your mood for the next 12 h, or how your friends with abdominal obesity contracted chronic disease, you can easily opt for exercise by waking up a bit earlier to exercise in the morning.

Until some time ago, experts believed that strong exercise is necessary to maintain a healthy heart and circulation system. However, study results show that walking or jogging has the same effect of working out at the gym. Small changes in behavior and habit have a long-term "butterfly effect," which increase not only health but also our quality of life.

The aging speed of tissues and organs differ as we age. If we know the general biomarker of aging as the following shows, continuous efforts to improve physical condition will be made, which will be helpful to decelerate to antiaging (Table 3.1).

Interestingly, a study result was released that said exercise prevents shortening of telomeres, which is caused by stress. This means exercise can oppress aging of cells, as it prevents mental stress's negative effect on telomere. For modern people under a lot of stress, physical condition improvement by health exercise has a direct and positive impact on longevity.

Table 3.1 Biomarkers that show biological age	Functions of the heart and blood vessels (strength of blood pressure and heart)
	Metabolism (blood sugar and cholesterol)
	Maximum aerobic capacity (exercise tolerance test)
	Muscle strength (pharmacodynamic strength)
	Lung capacity (FVC and FEV)
	Bone density
	Skin elasticity
	Psychological functions (cognitive abilities including memory)
	General inflammatory reaction (measured by blood test)
	Reaction time (speed of neurotransmission)

Source: *The Science of Staying Young*, 2008, p. 29

The CDC, or Centers for Disease Control and Prevention in the USA, recommends that adults engage in strong exercise for 75 min a week or a medium-level exercise for 150 min. Adolescents are advised to exercise for 90 min a day. With the advice, the CDC is seeking to raise the physical condition of US citizens across the country (Gong In-Duk and Ye Byung-Il 2012a).

3.1.1.3 Stress Management

In general, stress is divided into physical stress and mental stress. The former is raised by objective elements such as environment or outside stimulus from house life and workplace. The latter is often related to subjective elements such as how we view and interpret the world. Mental stress occurs when our expectations, beliefs, and faith from the past differ from the reality.

In order to manage stress that can't be seen with our eyes, we need to understand the mechanism on how stress occurs in our body. Therefore, the following explains how mind, brain, and body are related to stress:

The stress arousing stimulus is accepted by the corticolimbic of cerebral cortex, which is part of the brain, and is interpreted by past experiences and memory. Corticolimbic of cerebral cortex is made up of frontal lobe, which controls cognition and forecast, hippocampus, related to memory, amygdala that controls emotions and septum, which oversees behavioral reactions.

When the stimulus is recognized as stress in this part of the brain, CRH cells, or corticotropin releasing hormone cells of hypothalamus, which is neuroendocrine adaptive system, and the secretion cells of norepinephrine (called noradrenalin in England) of LC (locus ceruleus) of the brain stem, are activated. (Brain stem refers to all parts in the brain excluding the left and right of cerebral hemisphere, and cerebellum. It is the bottom part of the brain which is composed of midbrain, the pons and myelencephalon.) In short, neurotransmitters or neurohormones such as sympathetic nervous system, serotonin, dopamine and beta-endorphin and cytokine (refers to all protein and sugar protein secreted by immune cells, and controls immune ability. It is also called as lymphokine orinterleukin) secretion cells are activated. CRH secreted from hypothalamus stimulates adenohypophysis (it has five types of cells and each synthesizes and secretes different hormones), giving off ACTH or adreno-corticotrophic hormone. ACTH in turn stimulates adrenal cortex, which is situated right above the kidneys, secreting cortisol which is a type of glucocorticoid. The process is called, "the axis of HPA or hypothalamic-pituitary-adrenal."

The stress hormones that are made in such stressful situations make various physiological responses in many organs, including cardiovascular system (end-organ), immune system and endocrine system. The essential elements in reactions to stress are hypothalamus' CRH/cortisol system and the sympathetic nerve system of LC. The two systems stimulate each other and are activated, which is called the positive feedback. Serotonin (which is produced from tryptophane) and acetylcholine (works as neurotransmitter between exercise nerve and parasympathetic nerve) also stimulate the two system. Peptide of GABA (gamma-aminobutyric acid) system, beta-endorphin and cortisol, the products of POMC (pro-opiomelanocortin, a type of prohormone, which is a precursor of peptide hormone, and it is a nerve cell that oppresses feeding), oppress the stress reaction.

To summarize, the main role of sympathetic nerve system is to activate and awaken the body in times of acute stress, so that we can better prepare for danger. Some researchers report that sympathetic nerve system usually acts on positive stress reactions. HPA axis secretes cortisol to preserve energy, and oppresses CRH, and also represses the activation of sympathetic nerves in LC to soothe acute stress reactions. However, cortisol is the main culprit in chronic stress and negative stress reactions, and cortisol is believed to cause various damages in our physiology as its blood level is maintained at a high level. (Byun Gwang-Ho and Chang Hyun-Gap 2012)

Stress stimulus induces unique and various physiological phenomena in each human through their brain. There are about 100 billion neurons related to the process, and each neuron is linked to numerous other neurons, which make up more than 100 cases of nerve connections.

Therefore, to understand stress reaction in a more fundamental way, we need to know how our brain works. The level of manifestation can be different on each person, so we need to see ourselves as health prosumer and develop social medicine (the health stressor) suitable to us. Facial image control will be dealt in the next chapter of laughter therapy.

3.1.2   Complementary Alternative Medicine (CAM) and Social Medicine Therapy

As I mentioned, NHP of humans refers to vital force, which combines NHS that aims to maintain homeostasis with SHS, which is based on reciprocity. So what social medicine therapy is working toward is to look for solutions to health and disease-related problems in the modern society by recovering NHP.

Many people nowadays suffer from adult diseases, and it doesn't occur from infection but from bad lifestyle and habits. Adult diseases come from deteriorating environments from the outside and lowered level of immunity in the inside. When we look closely into patients' cells who suffer from adult disease (with social navigation), there are two fundamental reasons why NHP is lost on us. First, there are toxins which hinder the function and chemical reaction of cells. Second is the shortage of nutrients that are needed for the process to happen (Junger 2013a). Through CAM, we now know that medical experts and ordinary people alike have not given much thought to the importance and impacts of toxins and nutrients:

> Among many toxins, endotoxin is waste resulting from normal activities of cells. Uric acid, ammonia, lactic acid and homocysteine are well-known toxins. When these accumulate in the body, it can cause diseases. For instance, when concentration of uric acid increases in the blood, one may have gout.
>
> Exotoxin and xenobiotic are artificial toxins that are emitted either intentionally or accidentally. Every year, various chemical substances are made, and when the substances meet together (or alone), they hinder the functions of healthy cells. (Junger 2013b)

All our outside environments such as the air we breathe, the food and water we eat and drink, cosmetics, houses, office buildings, and electromagnetic waves all contain chemical substances and toxins that harm us. In our daily lives, we are exposed to an excessive amount of toxins. Sometimes the drugs that are prescribed to cure disease act as toxins in our body. Toxins mingle with chemical substances that are useful and necessary in our body to hinder their functions. Furthermore, they stimulate cells continuously to induce inflammation and allergies. Studies show that standing in a severely air-polluted area for several hours can raise the risk of contracting heart attack (Junger 2013c). The chemical substances that humans have invented for a more convenient life are now threatening us.

Precautionary measures and treatment are needed for us to respond to such risky circumstances that stem from the loss of NHP. The reality is harsh, and our body is becoming weaker. What we lack much are nutrients found in food, such as minerals and vitamins. The plants and vegetables grown in barren ground don't have much high-quality nutrients in them to grant us vital energy.

The most recent cure to recovering NHP is very simple. Just like Rousseau, Jean Jacques (1712–1778) said in the eighteenth century that we should "go back to nature." How can we do this? We should cleanse our body from toxins and fill it with good nutrients.

Therefore, social medicine therapy that stems from the popular CAM nowadays is similar to traditional nature therapies. In order for the social medicine therapy to go along with natural healing cycle, it focuses on detox programs and development of systems. Diet improvement and various methodologies to harmonize necessary elements to supplement nutrition are its meaningful focus.

Furthermore, approaches taken by Western medicine are thought of as being too uniform, and academics criticize that most of the drugs only have half the effect than it should have on patients. People are also concerned about the misuse and abuse of drugs, which is why the era of personalized medicine is dawning, breaking from an allopathic health management system that emphasized drug treatment. Prior to prescribing costly medicine, tests to check patients' genetic dispositions or the level of vitamin D are being conducted. As the tests and the technologies to make them possible are becoming popular, it seems personalized medicine will spread more widely.

Oriental medicine stresses that not all people can be cured by the same formula. It has stuck to the principle of "individualized medicine" that adapts to each person's physical condition. For instance, an Oriental doctor can give as many as seven different types of diagnosis on the same patient suffering from similar conditions. This means that the doctor is able to prescribe the best possible cure for the specific needs of each patient (Junger 2013d).

What we should keep in mind is that all people have different aims, hopes, specific health problems, ages, and body shapes. If one can experience NHP through detox program, he/she will have the wisdom to choose from various theories and methodologies in the world. They can become wise patients who can decide the cure for themselves. This gives us an opportunity to look back upon ourselves as health prosumers.

3.1.2.1   Detox

As I mentioned, if toxins in our body go ignored just because they aren't visible, and if we keep sticking to the unhealthy lifestyles and environments, our body will be damaged. Therefore, now I will talk about the mechanism of detox and identify the substances that cause toxins to occur. Then I will discuss ways to eliminate the toxins thoroughly and give you seven daily detox guidelines.

The Mechanism of Detox

Our body finishes digesting process in 8 h after eating. Then a signal is turned on, urging the emitted toxins to be moved from tissues to the circulatory system (blood flow and lymphatic system). Signals to start the detox process differ on the quality and quantity of food, varying from 6 to 10 h after eating. Generally, the more you eat, the more it takes for the detox signal to be turned on. If food is taken in as solid food, it has to be dissolved for easier digestion, so it requires more time and energy. Liquid food, however, can be absorbed without decomposition and requires not much energy. If our body has to make enzymes for digestion, the energy needed for digestion increases, which naturally hinders detox process. Therefore, taking natural food as itself such as vegetable, fruit, and nuts that have enzymes in them is the fastest way to detox.

If foods that cause allergic reaction are taken, more time and energy is needed. When GALT (lymphatic tissue related to bowel), the immune cell on the wall of the stomach, is stimulated, it starts to produce histamine and immunoglobulin in large amounts, which are substances that regulate allergies. The substances activate the reactions that spur inflammation. Therefore, foods that induce allergic reactions activate three systems in our body, which are alimentary, immune, and allergic systems. All three consume energy a lot, and as their effect grows, their action induces chain reactions that engage other cells. It triggers cough, itching, vomiting, and blood vessel expansion. The process requires a lot of energy, which naturally delays the detox process. In the worst case, it results in energy depletion, making the body to malfunction.

If we can avoid food that is hard to digest and is known to invoke allergic reactions and hypersensitivity reactions, our body can start the detox process. As soon as the process kicks in, toxins and mucus have to be neutralized and ultimately eliminated. The toxins include free radical, and the molecules that were electrically charged go into tissues to damage cells that were contacted. Other toxins hinder processes such as cell division, reproduction, hormone secretion, and increased sensitivity of receptors. This means that the fundamental cause of toxins in the body is free radical. Now let's look at how the detox process goes on in our liver in the molecule-biochemical level:

> Toxins affect the manifestation of genes, change the way how central functions of the body are ruled, and it literally changes the process of the manifestation of life when the order is executed. Furthermore, toxins, and especially artificial toxins like fat (has lipophilic property), move around the body for a long time without being neutralized, looking for fatty tissues to settle into.
>
> As you know, toxins accumulated in the fat is hard to come out, and that is why toxins that entered circulatory system, or the toxins that are freed, have to be transformed from a fat-soluble molecule to a water-soluble molecule. In that way the toxins can be emitted more easily and liver plays the central role in the process. Liver cells have enzymes called cytochrome P450 system. It provokes a chemical system that is necessary in the neutralization process that changes fat-soluble molecules to water-soluble molecules. The chemical process takes place in the first and second stage of the detox of the liver.
>
> In the first stage, the structures of toxins that are being neutralized are changed de facto, turning them into "intermediary metabolite." Sometimes the metabolite can become more toxic than the original toxins. In this case, the second stage of liver detox kicks in rapidly. In the second stage, the characteristics of the toxins are neutralized, turning them into water-soluble ones. This is needed so that they can enter kidneys through blood vessels. Kidney cells capture the water-soluble-turned toxins from the blood, and ultimately let them out in the form of urine. When the urine is released, the journey of the detox process ends. (Junger 2013e)

The prerequisites of the detox process of the liver are as follows: First, energy is needed. Second, antioxidants such as vitamin A, C, and E, selenium, copper, manganese, coenzyme Q10, flavonoid, silymarin, anthocyanin, and thiol to neutralize free radical should be supplied constantly. Third, other minerals, vitamins, and nutrients are needed to prepare the necessary ingredients for the first and second chemical procedure. With all the conditions ready, the detox process can take place safely.

In addition, it takes little time to move on from the first (the detox process by the overall cytochrome P450 enzyme system) to the second stage (the detox process by combination reaction). Therefore, it is hard for the compounds made in between the processes to be escaped. If essential amino acids and other necessary outside supports are absent, the second stage can be hindered. When substances are not neutralized enough in the second stage and if partly transformed toxins come from the liver to move onto blood and lymphatic circulation system, they can move about freely in the tissues and cells and ultimately cause damage.

The problem is that there is no other organ that can substitute the role of the liver. Even if toxins are emitted rapidly from the tissues, when liver can't detox adequately, diet program to facilitate the detox process can be harmful to health. This is because no nutrient can conduct toxin eradication and neutralization process after the emission of toxins. If a person feels tired due to overwork and doesn't eat enough, nutrients can't be supplied, which in turn would cause liver damage, affecting the detox process. As a result, his health condition can be deteriorated.

Detox Guidelines

People nowadays live in an era where everything is ample. We are exposed to various foods, which maybe a burden to our stomach, as much energy is needed to digest food. Our body would have to concentrate only on digestion, absorption, and transportation of food and nutrients, and there will be no energy left to use for the detox process. If fasting is done inadequately to emit toxins, our body can suffer even more. When toxins are not emitted properly, it works like a magnet, being absorbed again into our body. Toxins that come into our body in this way can be more fatal, and we should be careful.

The purpose of fasting is to cleanse our mind and body, so in general sense, fasting means detox. According to the natural order, all members of nature have their periods of growth, activity, and rest and maintain balance. In short, there is a time for working and resting and also time for eating and fasting. It all amounts to strengthening of our body.

However, if fasting is carried out by starving oneself, it may hinder daily activities and it will take a long time for the function of the body to recover its normal level. Therefore, it is important to find out a way to fast that can aid the emission of toxins and also maintain the functions of the body. When blood becomes cleaner due to fasting, blood circulation is facilitated in each cell. It results in the increased immune power of the body and strengthenedNHP.

How you fast is important. Reckless fasting where one only drinks water or takes salt, ignoring the essential nutrients that are necessary for the detox process, can cause great side effects. Fasting to lose one's weight can bring about yo-yo syndrome as well. It will be helpful to understand the guidelines for fasting with an aim to detox, which are as follows:

1. Find diet that is suitable for your body. There are various types of diet, such as water diet, grape juice diet, yogurt diet, agar diet, clear soybean soup diet, and meat diet called, "Atkins diet." Water diet is fasting by drinking more than 2500 cc of water a day. Sometimes it is conducted by drinking water alone or by drinking it with a small amount of bamboo salt to supplement salt. In order to supplement vitamin C, fermented liquid of native grass and apricot can be used. *Salicornia herbacea* can be taken to supplement salt and minerals. The water diet varies from a 1-day program to a 9-day program. When the duration is long, it can become dangerous. Therefore, preliminary fasting, fasting, and the end fasting should be conducted thoroughly.

   Juice diet using grape or yogurt diet literally refers to diet that is conducted by one type of fruit juice or yogurt. Agar diet utilizes agar, which is a water-soluble fiber. It prevents intestinal obstruction where stomach cling together or volvulus, where stomach is twisted or is made into a knot. Agar diet is good as it makes you feel full. Eating boiled cabbage is also a similar type of diet. Clear soybean soup diet is going on a diet by drinking watery soybean paste soup, and it is frequently used as it tastes good and makes you feel less hungry. There is also raw food diet. It is a diet on raw food powder, vegetables, and fruits. There are many enzymes in the ingredients, so it is helpful to the decomposition and emission of toxic agents. It is recommended if you want to change your diet.

There was a time when meat diet, the diet where you only eat meat to control your weight, was popular. The diet started from the west, and it is a very dangerous diet that ignores the basic principles of diet. Why? First, meat diet intensifies leaky gut syndrome, or LGS. Second, it rapidly acidizes the body. Besides the aforementioned diets, there is a nutrient diet where you drink powders that are ground with natural minerals, vitamins, nutrients such as antioxidants, and small amounts of carbohydrate, fat, and protein. The powder is mixed with water in the form of shake to be drunk, and it is referred to as the so-called medical food or nutrient cleans. Nutrient diet is the most recommendable as it balances the nutrients in our body. A similar "enzyme diet" became popular in Korea recently.

When people lose weight by skipping meals, our body has a tendency to store nutrients as fat for a future rainy day. So even if you lost 6–7 kg, our body tends to store up 7–8 kg of fat right away, which is called the "yo-yo phenomenon." Moreover, diet makes us short of carbohydrate. Ketone, which is made when fat is burned, is secreted and acidifies our body. To neutralize our body, strong alkaline calcium that is in our bone is extracted to be used, and that is why people who were frequently on diets suffer from osteoporosis. Diet makes us lose weight and the fat on the jaw can be lost due to fat decomposition. However, wrinkles on the face can't be avoidable in return. Therefore, when diet is administered in a wrong way, our body can be aged and can make us look older.

When you have found the suitable diet for you, then for a limited amount of time (usually 3 weeks), you should write a diet diary every day. It is preferred to take a photo of yourself before and after the diet, in the same angle and position, so that the changed status of yourself can stop you from going back to the bad eating habits of the old days. In particular, it is useful to remember the 12-h diet rule. Detox signal comes on about 8 h after your last meal, and you need at least 4 h to conduct the detox process. If you fill up your stomach with late-night snacks and then have breakfast early in the next morning, your body will concentrate on the digesting process, and there will be no room for detox process. So for the 3 weeks you are on a diet, you are advised to sleep a little bit earlier than usual.

2. Emission of the toxic ingredients can be helped by detox. Most body wastes and toxic agents from food are emitted from our body through excrement and urine from the colon and kidney, respectively. They are also emitted from the skin (sweating) and lung (breathing) and from the circulatory system (lymphatic system). Toxic agents, in particular, are emitted when the body temperature rises above 36.5 °C, and people with cold hands and feet have a hard time emitting

toxic agents. In this case, gas emitted from the toxic agents can fill up the body, and it becomes painful, sometimes ending up as disease. These are the methods to get rid of toxic agents from our body:

1. Help the normal function of the stomach by getting rid of the old feces. The number of times you go to the restroom and the color of the feces have a close correlation with your health. Usually, healthy feces take on a similar color as yellowish brown peanut butter in its color and concentration. The color becomes darker when red and green vegetables are taken, which are good for the body. Defecating once a day is normal, but a healthy person who isn't exposed frequently to toxic agents will go to the restroom after each meal. The best way to defecate is to go the restroom as much as you can to get rid of the negative substances that can affect your body.

   Asians who usually eat more vegetables than meat-consuming Westerners have a longer intestine. The reason is to get more nutrients from vegetables as possible. In the case of Westerners, meat produces much toxic agents, so the intestines are made shorter to prevent the absorption of toxic agents. We can see that the principle of "natural selection" took effect.

   Fast food, junk food, and those that lack fiber because they are taken without the covers (such as white rice, white sugar, and white bread), the food that induce leaky gut syndrome (alcohol, coffee, artificial sweetener, trans fat, etc.), and when the feces mingled with the toxic agents aren't emitted right away and remain in the stomach due to stress, and they cling to the stomach walls to be thickened after a long time. This is called coprostasis. When it is not emitted, the toxic agents in the coprostasis penetrate the tight junction to go deeper into the body and contaminate the blood. Pathogenic bacteria that are in the stomach also feed on the coprostasis on the stomach walls, and they make the stomach worse by emitting stronger toxic agents. As a result, skin problems will arise, and you may feel chronic fatigue due to the gas filling up in the stomach. One of the main causes of leaky gut syndrome is coprostasis.

   When olive oil, which is highlighted in the health diet, is taken at night, it makes your stomach smooth, and it will be easier to go to the restroom. It kills germs and increases burning fat. With the help of the olive oil, the gall bladder and liver are stimulated to move the bile that cleanses the liver system. It promotes the formation of bones, prevents blood clots, and strikes a balance between the hormones. Each night before you go to bed, you are advised to take two spoonfuls of olive oil along with a glass of lemon water. By eliminating toxic agent-filled coprostasis with detox programs such as diet, you can recover from certain disease along with promoting body condition. In short, social medicine to get rid of coprostasis is related to olive oil.

2. Drink much water to get rid of the toxic agents in the urine. Seventy percent of our body is made up of water. Feces can move easily in the stomach to be emitted when there is ample moisture in the body. Carbonated drinks, coffee, and alcohol all have dehydration effect and make it harder for you to go to the restroom.

Moreover, toxic agents like fat, and it changes the toxic molecules that cling to the fat into temporary water-soluble molecules. The new temporary water-soluble molecules should be filtered through the kidneys and emitted in the form of urine. Therefore, it is recommended to drink plenty of water to facilitate urine activities. When you go on a diet, you are advised to drink up to 2~3 liter of water a day, which bears oxygen and living enzyme. In this case, living water is the social medicine.

3. Help the emission of toxic agents with abdominal breathing. Taking two deep breaths and letting out two deep breaths is called abdominal breathing. The aim is to make you take a deep breath. It is hard to get rid of the toxic agents in the body with the shallow breaths we usually take.

The deeper breath you take, the more oxygen flows into the lung. Then much endorphin is emitted, and it is good to relieve stress. The following is one way of abdominal breathing:

Step 1: put both of your hands on the stomach. Breathe slowly with your nose for 7–10 s. Make sure to move the air to the stomach so that the stomach swells up. You should close your mouth and only use your nose to take deep breaths.
Step 2: stop breathing for 1–2 s and maintain the status.
Step 3: imagine you are letting out all the toxic agents filling up in your body. Press your stomach so that it goes in as much as it can. Breathe out for 7–10 s. This time, use both your mouth and nose to breathe out.

In this case, deep breathing is the social medicine.

4. Sweat a lot to help emission of toxic agents in the body. Sweating helps us emit extra moisture, minerals, and salt in our body. After you exercise, you sweat a lot and feel refreshed. It is because you let out the toxic agents and wastes that were in your body through sweating.

Therefore, sweating much is good for the body. Opening up the closed hair holes and sweat holes through exercise or cold or hot bath and facilitating sweating through far-infrared radiation sauna are all good ways to sweating. In far-infrared radiation sauna, the invisible infrared radiation makes radiant heat and is different from the usual sauna which heats up moisture into air. The radiant heat can penetrate deeper into the skin layers rather than ordinary sauna heat. It stimulates fat molecules and emits the toxic agents.

Through sweat, toxic agents and wastes are emitted. When heat and bad energy are emitted through the skin, body temperature goes down and cleanses the blood. In this way, immunity and natural healing power (NHP) also strengthen. In this case, sweat is the social medicine.

5. Help emission of toxic agents by stimulating the skin. Massage is important for skin management. Massage stimulates the lymph to emit toxic agents. Through the lymphatic gland, wastes, toxic agents, and sick cells are moved. Lymph is the liquid that eliminates sick cells, fights virus and bacteria, and acts as a filter to get rid of the toxic agents. Therefore, for health purposes, it is more helpful to get a body massage than a facial massage, as it can stimulate

the entire body. In reality, when the back, armpits, and chest are massaged, facial color can be brightened. For sure, a steady massage is good for detox.

Before taking a bath or a shower, it is good to use a brush made of smooth, natural animal fur to brush the dry skin from the tip of the feet to the top of the head. When the skin is smoothly stimulated by brushing in circles, the closed pores on the skin opens up, and the dead cells come off easily. It stimulates the lymphatic and the hormone system and helps emit toxic agents. When massaging the front and back of the body, arms and neck should be included. When brushing, it should start from the bottom to the heart and from the outside to the inside. Five to ten minutes of massaging every day is very good for the body.

Cold and hot shower stimulates the skin by chilling and letting out heat and through contraction and expansion. It promotes blood circulation and emits toxic agents by opening up the closed pores. It quickly gets rid of the dead cells and neutralizes the body fluids. The skin is the largest organ of our body. Under the skin, there are blood vessels that are more than several kilometers long. Arteriole and veinlet full of blood are vessels. Veinlet is loosened and expanded when it is hot, and it contracts when it is cold. When expansion and contraction occur, the skin lets off as much blood as the heart.

Sprinkling cold and hot water alternatively for 1 min on the skin when taking a shower everyday will make you feel the difference. Five to seven times of alternatively sprinkling cold and hot water on the body is recommended. After taking a bath, coconut oil and natural oil should be applied to the skin rather than body lotion, to keep the skin from dehydrating. In this case, massage is the social medicine.

3. Maximize the emission of toxic agents by exercise. As I emphasized in health exercise, it is never too much to stress the importance of exercise. Exercise promotes the circulation of blood and lymph and facilitates emission of bad substances through sweat and the skin. It also stimulates the stomach to help defecation. When you exercise, much calorie is used, so obesity is prevented and repressed. Taking long breaths becomes easier, and you can supply your body with enough oxygen, advancing the cardiac functions. Exercise is a natural antidote that eases your mind and relieves stress.

Let's look at the exercises that are helpful to detox. First, there is yoga. Hatha yoga, where you consecutively twist and bend your body, is a good way to massage every organ in your body. It promotes the organs to do their functions. Skipping ropes also stimulates the circulation of blood and lymph, as you jump up and down. It is good for detox as well. The best way to relieve toxic agents is massage where you can stimulate every corner of the organ.

4. Take enough rest and sleep. The best medicine for modern people who lead a hectic life is sleeping. Diet is a way to give rest to our organs in the body which has no rest in our everyday lives. When we eat and go to sleep, our brain and body are at rest, but organs decompose food and move them, and they have no time to rest. Organs can enjoy comfortable rest when we go on a diet and have an empty stomach. Therefore, it is good to go on a diet for a limited period of time.

Enough rest and sleep help refreshing your body, along with emission of toxic agents. Therefore, rest and sleep are social medicine.

5. Get rid of stress. As I emphasized in health stressor, the root of every disease is stress, and it is something to be overcome along with toxic agents. In terms of detox, the bodily detox process promotes the detox process of our mind, which is invisible. It works the other way, too. Some time ago, "thinking positively" and "the force of positivity" used to gain worldwide popularity. They are better than negative thinking, but concentrating too hard on positive thinking on purpose can cause stress and take away concentration and energy.

   Therefore, it is advised to "focus on the present" rather than thinking what is positive or negative. Chronic stress is the main culprit that produces all kinds of disease, so it is good to engage in efforts to get rid of stress. I will talk about this more in the following chapter on "social medicine derived from health stressor."

6. Learn to cohabitate with feelings of hunger. With increased living standards, people nowadays are surrounded by food, unlike the past. There are so many things to eat when you turn your head around, and it is difficult to choose what to eat. We may be preoccupied with "fake appetite" in the midst of our hectic lives. Therefore, we tend to eat out of habit, not on how hungry we are and not based on the pleasure of eating.

   When we consume less food, the biggest problem is the feeling of hunger. People have a fear of being hungry, and it prevents them from going on a diet or detox program. However, our body can go without food for a couple of days. Our body can easily adapt to the changes of the amount of food we eat. When food stops coming into the body, our digestion system can take a rest and can save much vital energy that used to go into the digestion process. When the body can take such changes, there won't be much problem.

   However, the problem is the resistance from the mind. When you feel hungry, drink a glass of water slowly. Learn to endure the feeling of being hungry, rather than getting rid of the feeling. When we can handle this problem, we can take a control over ourselves on what to eat, when to eat, and how much we have to eat to satisfy ourselves. Anyone would feel comfortable with an empty stomach and uncomfortable with a full one. By conducting diet program for detox, we can learn to cohabitate with the feeling of being hungry.

7. Regard food as medicine. The modern culture of eating good food and enjoying life has become a trend. Television programs, newspapers, and the mass media are in a hot competition over introducing food and good restaurants. They all heatedly scale up people's appetite and their obsession of food. In particular, restaurants use much seasoning, sugar, and salt to stimulate people's tongue. Therefore, we know that food from eating out is not good for the body compared to the food homemade. However, in reality, we have no choice but to eat out as a part of working life and business. In terms of detox, it is not good to keep eating bad food and sticking to bad eating habits. It is wise to distinguish which food is good for the body, thinking food as a kind of medicine, rather than viewing it as a mere tool to fulfill the demands of our appetite (Lee Yung-Keun and Choi Joon-Yung 2011a).

We looked into the detox mechanism, the kinds of diet program, and the guidelines for detox. In the process, we once again found out the importance of health food, health exercise, and health stressor as social medicine. I think it is a good starting point to detox as we talk out "social medicine to catch three birds with a stone," which I will address in the next chapter.

3.1.2.2 Supplement of Nutrients

The aim of detox is to get rid of toxic agents from our body. On the other hand, supplementing nutrients is a way to fill up the necessary nutrients in our body. It is hard to get rid of bad eating habits only with mental power or positive thinking. Improving the absorption of nutrients in the body, metabolism, defecation, and the environment can be much more efficient. Any healthy person will want good-quality food that can help maintain health.

It is estimated that about 100 trillion cells comprise our body. In each cell, there is nucleus in its center and the important substances in the cell nucleus are DNA (deoxyribonucleic acid) and RNA (ribonucleic acid), which hold genetic information. Nucleic acid including DNA and RNA are in all living creatures that conduct cell division, and they are essential to body metabolism and genetic treatment. Human cells repeat the cycle of birth and death till we die, and cells that are produced in old age lack nucleic acid, resulting in aged cells. In this case, when ample nucleic acid is provided along with enzymes, vitamins, and minerals, nucleic acids turn into young, healthy cells. This means that nucleic acid changes the incorrect DNA that is in the cell nucleus. Therefore, I would like to talk about enzymes, vitamins, minerals, and probiotics as essentials for nutrition supplement.

Enzymes

Any food that is cooked in over 48 °C will have its enzyme destroyed. Enzymes are the most important factors in digestion. As too much energy is needed when large amounts of enzymes are made, nature makes them and supplies them to us. In vegetables that are not boiled and in fruits, nuts, and seeds, there are already much enzyme contained to aid the digestion process. Therefore, when these products are eaten after boiling, it is just like throwing away useful resources and nutrients in the products. If we follow the law of the nature, nature gives us enzymes to aid the digestion process through products that have ample enzymes.

The three major nutrients are carbohydrates, protein, and fat, and adding vitamin and minerals in the group makes them the five major nutrients. Furthermore, people sometimes refer to it as the seven major nutrients when water and other fibers are added. However, the most important nutrient, enzyme, is nowhere to be found in the group. Vitamins and minerals are coenzyme, which help the enzyme. Therefore, I believe it is not right to group carbohydrates, protein, fat, vitamin, and minerals as the five major nutrients when enzyme is not.

Until now, the importance of vitamins and minerals were stressed but not so much for enzymes. This is because vitamins and minerals are not made in our body but have to be taken from the outside, but enzymes can be made inside of our body. Enzymes have many functions, as they can be used in food, metabolism, and digestion. Depending on where they work, enzymes are categorized into two: ones that are taken in the form of food or drug and the ones that can be produced in our body. Generally, food enzymes are used in the digestion process of our body, and other enzymes that are largely concentrated in specific plants are used in medicine. Enzymes that can be made in our body are used in metabolism that accelerates the process.

As I mentioned earlier, this chapter will focus on detox and harmony in the metabolism process, so I would like to talk about essential metabolism enzymes that are related to this. Metabolism enzymes in our body are produced by microorganisms in the liver, pancreas, and stomach. Microorganisms living in the stomach that amount to as many as 100 trillion in numbers absorb nutrients, vitamins, and minerals to produce enzymes. In short, the productivity of the metabolism enzymes depends on the environment of the microorganism in the stomach, so a good number of enzymes are useful for good metabolism. As vitamins and minerals that help the enzymes are not produced in the body, they have to be taken from food in a balanced manner, and it is desirable that probiotics, which are determinants in the harmony of the environment of the microorganism in the stomach, are stressed nowadays.

Enzymes are substances that catalyze fermentation, which links it directly to yeast. Fermentation is the process of leaving food as it is for a lengthy period of time. Yeast kicks off the fermentation process, and enzymes are special substances that make fermentation come true. Enzymes are proteins that catalyze various biochemical reactions in our body, and they help metabolism and body reactions, different from other catalysts in general chemical reactions. In short, enzymes start the reaction process as the middleman when substance A has to be turned into B in our body. When enzymes are used as catalysts in this way, the biochemical reactions start the changing process very rapidly. There are thousands of enzymes in our body, but only one enzyme works in one situational change, and it is called "enzyme specificity."

As you can see, thousands of biochemical reactions in our body are impossible if we don't have enzymes. Any person without enzymes will not be able to sustain even for a couple of hours. Foods we consume are decomposed by the digestion enzymes and are turned into nutrients, and they provide vital energy that is necessary for our everyday lives such as talking, eating, sleeping, and working. The nutrients also make up the cells that compose our body, for instance, the skin, muscles, brain, various organs, and nails.

Every cell in our body turns into new ones after 10 months. Cells in the heart, brain, bone, and skin turn into new cells, too. Five senses that are received from our sensory organs are delivered to the brain through neurons. In the brain, information is processed, and conscious and unconscious reactions are aroused. The rapid movements and functions of the brain and neurons are also possible due to enzymes. When we lack enzymes, digestion of food is hindered, and we feel full. Food wastes that are not yet fully digested rot in the colon and let off toxic agents. Therefore, enzymes play an important role in the detox process, and "half-enzyme diet," which is getting rid of toxic agents by taking enzyme food, is good for detox.

When wounds or inflammation by infection occur in the body, enzymes to decompose protein are needed to cure the wounds and reproduce new cells. When much enzyme is taken in the period, the process can be shortened. In particular, much enzyme is needed to get rid of free radical. Free radical, the main culprit of cell destruction and aging, also works as toxic agents in the body. Enzymes not only eliminate free radical but also make our skin healthy. It facilitates the circulatory system to delay aging and has a stark antiaging effect.

Rheumatism, lupus, and atopic and allergic conditions (which are all chronic diseases) are called "autoimmune disease," where healthy cells are attacked by the abnormal function of the immune system. The toxic agents that come into the stomach combine with antigen and antibody to form immune complex. It moves around the blood vessels and makes inflammation in various organs. When enzyme combination therapy that uses hydrolysis enzyme is prescribed, immune complex can be dissolved. In the early twentieth century, Doctor John Beard found out that pancreas extracts deter the growth of the cancer cells. He later filtered the pancreas of newborn piglets and sheep and injected concentrated enzyme liquid taken from them to the cancer patients. He confirmed that the cancer growth was repressed and the patient lived longer. Later, enzyme therapy in the medical world is frequently used along with operations and chemical therapies.

For humans, it is natural for food to be decomposed and digested of itself by the enzymes in the food. When the enzymes in the food are insufficient for the digestion process, enzymes that are made in the body participate as well.

The problem is that foods we take nowadays don't have enough enzymes in them to digest food. When we take foods that are cooked with fire, no enzyme exist in the food, so the food should be solely digested with the enzymes that are already in the body. Enzymes are used for food digestion, and there is a lack of enzymes that have to be used for metabolism and immune system. That is how various diseases, such as degenerative condition, chronic diseases, and conditions that stem from everyday habit, are produced. In short, eating food cooked with fire that kills enzymes in foods is the problem.

The reason that humans have the biggest pancreas in proportion to their weight compared to other animals is that we take foods cooked with fire, where digestion enzymes no longer exist. The pancreas is the organ where digestion enzymes are secreted. For the digestion of food that lack enzymes, the pancreas has to supply all the necessary digestion enzymes. The result is the abnormal big size of the pancreas. People who eat ample amounts of fresh vegetable and fruits don't have lagging fat. The main cause is that the digestion activities in the person are good, that their immune systems are strengthened, and that the metabolism is stable. It results in healthy internal organs and skin.

Therefore, we need to consume vegetables and fruits that have sufficient digestion enzymes. Also, protein-based food, essential for making enzymes, should be supplied. However, it is not easy to eat large amounts of vegetables and fruits every day. Furthermore, changes in the soil make it harder for us to take in enough vitamins and minerals, even if we take the same amount of vegetables and fruits as in the old days. Lack of enzymes, vitamins, minerals, and other nutrients are reasons modern people suffer from so many conditions.

After mid-life, people may feel fatigue without special reasons and may feel low. In this case, problems in energy metabolism can be one reason. An easy way to counter the situation is to supplement enough enzymes, vitamins, and minerals. We should recognize that the lack of enzymes and the lack of vitamins and minerals, which work as important second enzymes, induce diseases that are hard to find out the cause. It ultimately undermines our health.

Vitamins

Vitamins control various functions in our body, though they can't produce energy like carbohydrate, fat, or protein. Most vitamins work as aides to enzymes or their roles and take part in the metabolism of carbohydrate, fat, protein, and minerals. Unlike hormones that are synthesized in the endocrine organs of our body, vitamins can't be made in our body. Vitamins are essential nutrients that have to be taken in from the outside. Although only small amounts are needed, they control the metabolism or physiological functions, so they are similar to hormones and as important. There are more than ten types of vitamins now, and there are "provitamins," which are substances that turn into vitamins. For instance, carotene turns into vitamin A in the body, and ergosterol turn into vitamin D when it is exposed to infrared lights.

Water-soluble vitamins such as vitamin B complex and vitamin C melt into water and are emitted through urine, so not much harm is done when overtaken. However, fat-soluble vitamins such as vitamins A, D, E, and K can cause various side effects when they are piled up in the body. Absorption rates for each supplement are different, so this should be taken into consideration as well.

Taking too much nutritional supplements can cause side effects. For instance, absorption abilities are hindered when calcium and iron are taken together, so it is advised to take them separately 1 month after another. If not, taking some time space between the two is recommended. For instance, taking calcium before meals and iron after meals is good. *Chlorella*, *Spirulina*, and amino acid, which are all protein supplements, shouldn't be taken with calcium, for protein hinders the absorption of calcium.

However, there are supplements that have synergy effects when taken together. Vitamin C increases absorption rate of iron or vitamin E when taken together. The same goes for vitamin D and iron and calcium and also for omega-3 fatty acids and fat-soluble vitamins. Vitamin E in omega 3 not only increases the absorption rate of omega 3, but it also delays the oxidation of omega 3 by antioxidant activities.

Before or after climacterium, or menopause, a large amount of calcium is taken from the body, and it accelerates both osteoporosis and aging. Therefore, it is important to take vitamin A and calcium in this period. Middle-aged men also need calcium intake. Smoking men have 1.5–4 times of higher risk of suffering from osteoporosis than nonsmokers, and degraded absorptive function can lead to lack of calcium. Vitamin D plays a vital role in calcium metabolism, and that is why lack of vitamin D can lead to osteoporosis and fracture, even if calcium is sufficient in the body.

Recently, vitamin D has been recognized to play an important role in maintaining physiological function of the body and strengthening of immunity. Some regard it as a fundamental solution, better than the flu vaccine. Vitamin D controls more than 60 genes and shows specialization induction, genesistasis, and metastasis blocking effect in cell cycle. It also helps cell growth, preventing normal cells from turning into cancer cells, and produces protein that acts as antibacterial substance and oppresses inflammation. There are also reports that lack of vitamin D can lead to diabetes and even worsen the condition. That is why genetic modification of vitamin D acceptor is presumed to be related to diabetes. It seems that personalized medicine will be the trend in the near future, where checking one's vitamin D level will become a norm.

Seniors are advised to take calcium, magnesium, and vitamin D to prevent osteoporosis and strengthen muscle. Omega-3 fatty acids and vitamin E help prevent stroke, dementia, and hardening of the arteries. It seems "personalized prescription of nutrients" will also be in trend soon.

The most effective way for people to take nutrients is to take them little by little after meals. In case you have to take a lot of supplements at one time, it is effective to take it after you had the biggest meal in the day. Mineral is necessary to digest vitamins well, so it is recommended to take minerals and vitamins together (Kim Hye-Yun and Lee Yung-Keun 2013a). I will talk more about each vitamin in more detail in the next chapter, "social medicine therapy from health diet."

Minerals

Minerals only take up about 4 % of our weight among all other substances that compose our body. Minerals found on the ground don't have carbon in their molecular structures, which means they can't produce energy on their own or synthesize them in the body. Therefore, minerals have to be taken from food.

Minerals can be divided into two types according to the content in the body, the major element and the minor element. Major elements account for about 3.5 % of the weight and include the seven following elements: calcium, iron, sulfur, potassium, sodium, chlorine, and magnesium. Minor elements include iron, iodine, ion, copper, selenium, manganese, chrome, molybdenum, cobalt, fluorine, boron, arsenic, tin, quartzite, vanadium, nickel, etc. They only take up 0.5 % share in our body, but even the absence or lack of one single element causes problems in our metabolism. Disease of unknown cause or chronic disease may occur, so the elements are not to be ignored.

Minerals in the air and soil are mostly inactive minerals that can't be digested or absorbed by humans. Only minerals that are in vegetables, animals, and fisheries are active minerals that can be digested and absorbed by people. Active mineral can only be digested in the human body when they are turned into organic materials by going through photosynthesis of plants. Metal minerals that are directly received from soil can't also be easily absorbed and digested in our body. Only 5–8 % of the intake amount are absorbed, and the rest are all emitted out of the body.

Recently, scholars began to understand that minerals, which only take up 4 % of our body, play a very important role in not only maintaining life but also preventing disease and antiaging. Now, the following is the roles of minerals in our body:

1. Minerals compose each part of our body. Calcium and phosphorus make up hard tissues such as bones and teeth. Maintaining an apt concentration of calcium, phosphorus, and fluorine is very important. Furthermore, manganese, copper, and ion are essential for the formation of the connecting parts of our body. Hormones, enzymes, and vitamins can't entirely do their job if there are no minerals.
2. Minerals also strike a balance between acid and base. They control the level of acidity and basicity to be normal, as they are essential for various metabolisms in our body. Some minerals stabilize pH levels in our body, and other minerals control base. As you can see, minerals make the balance of metabolism by maintaining acidity and basicity of blood, tissues, and cells.
3. Minerals control osmotic pressure. Osmotic pressure is necessary to move the bodily fluid in the blood vessels and cells to another part. Moving the fluid includes passing quasiprojective cell membrane. In the process, the concentration of minerals determines the direction and quantity of water that move in and out of the cell membrane. Therefore, when the balance of minerals is broken, bodily fluid may pile up in one place or cause dehydration.
4. It acts as a catalyst for various metabolism activities. Magnesium is necessary for decomposition and synthesis of carbohydrate, fat, and protein. Various kinds of minerals such as copper, calcium, manganese, and ion are used as catalysts in the catabolic and assimilation processes of the body. Furthermore, minerals are coenzymes and are needed as a part that makes up the enzymes. The absorption rate of nutrients goes up with the help of minerals. In short, minerals are used as "catalysts" in the function of our body when it uses amino acids, fatty acids, and vitamins. Therefore, if there is no interaction or catalyst process of minerals, the efficiency of nutrients will not go up, no matter how much nutrients you take in.

Modern people nowadays lack minerals. This is attributed to the fat that the soil has been weathered and eroded for a long period of time. Furthermore, minerals have become scarce due to the changes of the soil, as chemical fertilizers had been used in the process of industrialization and cultivation of the land. It is impossible to get enough minerals from vegetables and grain that are harvested from land nowadays. In order to live a healthy life without disease, people steadily have to supplement minerals by themselves.

Now we will be looking into essential minerals. Calcium, iron, magnesium, potassium, sodium, selenium, and ion are not dealt here, as they will be introduced in the next chapter of "social medicine originated from health food."

1. P, phosphorus: phosphorus is the mineral element that takes up the second-largest portion of our body, following calcium. Eighty-five percent of phosphorus in the body exists in the form of "calcium phosphate" and is combined with calcium. It is included in the bone structure and teeth tissues. Phosphorus, which is evenly distributed in almost every cell in our body, is used as nutrient that is necessary for the workings of cell energy circuit in the combination of phosphoric acid. In addition, phosphorus is a component of nucleic acid material that exists in the cell nucleus and contains in itself the genetic information that determines the amino acid sequence of protein. Phosphorus also works as accessory factor of numerous enzymes that are in the body. It maintains the level of pH of the body fluid. Other works of phosphorus include hydrogen ion defecation process in the kidney, buffering of cell sap, and the changes of effect of vitamin B complex.

   If you have a healthy meal, there is no need to worry for lack of phosphorus, as it is in animals and vegetables. In order for phosphorus to function well in the body, it is desirable to maintain a ratio of 1:1.5. Overly consuming phosphorus can be a problem sometimes, and in this case, calcium comes out of the body, melted in the blood. Most of the processed foods such as ham, clam, sweetener like canned juice, and meat have too much phosphorus in them. If you tend to overconsume such processed foods, the balance of minerals is broken due to lack of calcium.

2. Cl, chlorine: chlorine is an important anion of extracellular fluid. Along with sodium, it controls the balance of bodily fluid and osmotic pressure in the extracellular fluid. It also maintains the level of pH of the bodily fluid.

3. S, sulfur: sulfur is a component of cell protein, and it exists in every cell of our body. Sulfur is mineral that takes part in the biological oxidation process and flowing process of cell tissues. The sulfhydryl group of sulfur forms the sulfur combination that has high energy. By combining with sulfate, a toxic substance, it turns it into a toxic-free material and lets it out through urine. So it is very important in the detox process. Sulfur is sufficient in cabbage, garlic, fish, kale, and meat.

4. I, iodine: iodine is a mineral that is closely related to thyroid functions. About 70–80 % of iodine is found in the thyroid. It is a component of thyroxin that is secreted from thyroid. Iodine not only produces energy by burning fat but also takes part in the promotion of basic metabolism such as the physical, mental, and sexual growth of children. Lack of iodine hinders thyroxin synthesis, and our body expands thyroid tissues to make up for it. This is why thyroid hyperplasia comes about. Goiter or malfunction of thyroid can result in anemia, low blood pressure, slowing of pulse, obesity, and even miscarriage.

5. Cu, copper: copper is used when iron is synthesized with hemoglobin in our body, making inactive iron turn into active iron so it can be used in our body. Therefore, when copper lacks, it can't be used in the synthesis of hemoglobin, which results in anemia. In this case, the condition doesn't get better even if you take in much iron. Copper has to be supplemented together to ease the condition. As a mineral that produces energy in the cell, copper strengthens the elasticity of blood wall, protects nerve membrane, and maintains immunity. It also cures injuries and plays a pivotal role in controlling central nerves and making of melanin coloring. Copper is also an essential nutrient in composing the combination tissue of collagen and bone cellular matrix. Lack of copper raises the risk of contracting osteoporosis. However, when there is too much copper in the body, it can lead to depression, erythrism, nausea, vomiting, muscle pain, and arthralgia. Copper is rich in almonds, barley, beans, broccoli, garlic, mushrooms, dried grape, salmon, and orange.

6. Mn, manganese: manganese is a mineral that plays an important role in growth, formation, and development of bone structure, growth of testicles, and the functioning of the ovary. It works in physiological strain and the central nerve system, and it is one of the compositions of enzymes that control the synthesis of fatty acids and cholesterol. Working as a catalyst, manganese plays an important role in the formation of elements, emission of fat matter, and functions of a cell's mitochondria. In short, manganese is essential in energy emission.

    Therefore, lack of manganese results in growth problems, abnormality of bone structures, lowered fertility, and infant ataxia. Manganese is concentrated in whole grains that are not cracked, blueberry, the yellow part of an egg, pineapple, spinach, and green leafy vegetables.

7. Cr, chromium: chromium is well known to be a component that controls the function of insulin in cell perspective, which is essential in controlling the level of glucose. Chromium is a mineral that is absolutely essential in maintaining the level of cholesterol and metabolism of fatty acids and carbohydrate. In particular, insulin has to take its unique form in order to function well in our body. Chromium is needed for insulin to take the right form. Therefore, chromium increases usage rate of sugar in the blood by helping the function of insulin. Chromium also takes part in fat metabolism and is used in weight loss and acme treatment.

    Abnormality in glucose metabolism after mid-life can be treated easily, so it is usually used in diabetes and hypoglycemia. Lack of chromium results in diabetes, hypoglycemia, arteriosclerosis, and increased cholesterol levels. Other diseases that can be induced include abnormal increase of insulin due to diabetes, increased impaired glucose tolerance, disorder of amino acids metabolism, decreased adaptability to stress, growth disorder, corneal opacity, headache, fatigue, weariness, concern, and anxiety. Chromium can be found much in the yeast of beer, brown rice, meat, and cheese.

8. B, boron: boron is a mineral that is needed in trace amounts, essential for the growth and stabilization of bones. It is a nutrient related to calcium and magnesium. Boron is needed for the function of cell membrane, and it helps the

absorption of calcium and activates vitamin D. At the same time, it decreases the amount of calcium and magnesium that is lost in urine.

Lack of boron in women results in osteoporosis and osteoarthritis. It increases calcium loss through urine and decreases estrogen hormones. Boron also promotes brain functions and makes people agile and prevents osteoporosis and the damages of muscles after menopause. When boron lacks, it induces deficiency of vitamin D. Boron is included much in vegetables, fruits, and grain.

9. Other essential minerals: Si, silicone, is one of the minerals that is most widely distributed on earth. It prevents atherosclerosis and cardiac diseases. It has anti-inflammation effect and can protect our body from infections. It also prevents aging of cells and cell tissues. Co, cobalt, is a mineral that is essential for the composition of vitamin B12, and lack of it can result in aplastic anemia. Ni, nickel, is an important component in the stabilization of DNA and RNA of a cell nucleus. It is related to the metabolism of carbohydrate and overconsumption of it induces contact dermatitis. Lastly, Mo, molybdenum, is an essential vitamin that works as a facilitator for enzymes in our body, and it is used as a catalyst for enzymes of oxidase, sulfide oxidation, and dehydrogenation (Kim Hye-Yun and Lee Yung-Keun 2013b).

Probiotics

Lactobacillus acidophilus and *Bifidobacteria* are useful germs that are frequently found in the human stomach. They are called "probiotics," and it means that they are "probiotics" that make acid to hinder the growth of bad bacteria and help the growth of good bacteria. Foods that have much probiotics are garlic, asparagus, barley, and oatmeal (Morley and Colberg 2008a).

The origin of probiotics comes from the Greek word meaning "for life." It is the combination of "pro" (for something) and "biotics" (related to life). Considering that the word "antibiotics" is composed of "anti" and "biotics" (related to life), probiotics mean it's favorable to life. In short, probiotics use the good characteristics of germs to promote our health, especially the condition of the stomach.

In the late nineteenth century, Metchnikoff referred to yogurt as the wonder drug, the elixir of life. He argued that large numbers of rotten germs in the stomach let out much toxic gas and result in disease and shortened life span. He said that drinking much yogurt makes *Lactobacillus* to protect good germs in our stomach and repress bad germs. Later, the belief in the effectiveness of fermented food was passed down as folk remedy. Nowadays, scientific research reports that *Lactobacillus* and fermented food play an important role in our health. WHO and FAO define probiotics as living germs that are helpful to health when taken in suitable amounts.

These days, probiotic bacteria are the same ones that are used in making yogurt. They are resident germs that are frequently found in healthy peoples' stomach. *Lactobacillus* and *Bifidobacterium* take up the lion's portion. When the environment of the stomach is undermined due to various reasons, good germs decrease and harmful germs increase exponentially. They damage intestinal mucosa and the increased penetration rate (leaky gut syndrome) induces diseases in the digestion system and causes allergies. Intestinal mucosa is where the most immune system is located in our body (about 70 %). The lymphatic tissue in the inner part of intestinal mucosa (GALT) steadily communicates with the stomach environment. In this process, probiotics maintain the balance of Th1 and Th2 cells that are related to anti-inflammation. Therefore, it boosts immunity and effectively controls hypersensitive immune response.

If you eat too much fruit, glucose is increased, and dysbiosis of intestinal microorganism can be promoted due to the harmful germs in the stomach. When carbohydrate and dairy products are taken too much, which are hard to digest, the mucus of intestinal mucosa that eases stimulation gets thick. It only absorbs some part of food and the half-digested food gets to remain in the stomach. Therefore, it gives time for the yeast and the harmful germs to eat up more food. As a result, the activity of harmful germs is facilitated and lets out more toxic wastes. It nullifies the nerves, weakens large intestine muscles, and increases constipation. The problem in this case is that constipation results in the reabsorption of toxic agents. Other diseases such as headache can be induced. Therefore, probiotics are a living microorganism that is helpful to antiaging and that prevents damages from disease and inflammation, when taken adequately.

However, the concept of probiotics in Korea is not yet generalized. *Lactobacillus* has been regarded as one of the intestinal drugs and didn't receive the rightful attention. One food that represents probiotics in Korea is "kimchi." The probiotic germ ferments the spicy white radish and cabbage. Now, probiotics are getting more attention, and in some hospitals, it is prescribed to the patients as healthy functional food.

Probiotics can be applied to the following diseases: diseases in the digestion system, allergies, and infectious diseases. First, let's talk about diseases in the digestion system. There can be secondary diarrhea when antibiotics are taken or when patients suffer from infectious diarrhea. In this case, there is a report that giving probiotics with five billion living germs a day to a child patient has significantly reduced his diarrhea by antibiotics. In another clinical research, probiotics and mesalazine, a medicine for ulcerative colitis, were provided for 12 months to the two groups of 327 ulcerative colitis patients, respectively. The result showed that the effect of the two was similar on each group. In the case of liver condition, there are reports that the intake of probiotics decreased the level of pH in the feces and the ammonia levels and inner toxic agents in the blood. Yet in another research with 58 hepatocirrhosis patients, it was revealed that the probiotics and fermented fiber reduced the level of inner toxic agents and hepatocirrhosis.

Second, in terms of allergies, probiotics were revealed to have an effect on the prevention of atopic condition, but not on its treatment. Third, it was reported that probiotics can't prevent the infection but can reduce the period for about 2 days and lessen the severity of the condition. Fourth, by decreasing the concentration level in the blood lipid, probiotics had effects on the hyperlipidemia and was also helpful to the disease in the cardiovascular diseases. Fifth, when treating vaginitis, alternating vagina insertion, oral administration of probiotics, and the existing urologic procedures proved to be effective. It is noteworthy that only the oral administration has an effect, too. There are other examples that show the effectiveness of probiotics: first, decreasing the complications before and after operations and second, increasing the treatment effect by using it in the eradication therapy of *Helicobacter pylori*.

Probiotics can be very helpful in aiding elderly's health. In a study in the USA, 360 senior citizens with ages more than 60 were organized to take milk with probiotics and just ordinary milk to see their resistance ability against cold. The group that was on milk with probiotics had 20 % higher rate on average of recovering from cold. In another study, senior citizens with ages more than 70 took *Lactobacillus* (beneficial germ) for 4 months, and the result was encouraging. The activity of immune cells was boosted, and there was more than 89 % improvement in constipation.

Probiotics are more useful when it is prescribed in various types. Adequately combining anaerobe and aerobe can increase efficiency. Representative anaerobic bacteria are *Lactobacillus* and *Bifidobacterium*. *Bacillus subtilis*, which is the main ingredient for fermented bean paste in Korea, represents aerobic probiotics. As the aging process takes place, it is natural for the beneficial germs in the stomach to decrease. There are reports that senior citizen patients aged more than 65 have 26 times less lactose germ than the young people (Lee Yung-Keun and Choi Joon-Yung 2011b).

Helicobacter pylori were found as causative agents that can contact stomach cancer back in 1982. Currently, more than 50 % of the entire population in the world is reported to be infected. Therefore, there are guidelines in each country, and the Japanese government took action so that the patients can benefit from insurance since 2013. *Helicobacter pylori* can be wiped off by taking 3–4 types of medicine along with strong antibiotics for 1–2 weeks. However, tolerance against antibiotics has increased recently, and the ability to control germs fell to below 80 % levels. Other ways to counter the situation is being sought out. Among the *Lactobacillus*, *reuteri* is known to produce reuterin and significantly repress the growth of *Helicobacter pylori*. When *reuteri* is taken with omeprazole, which is included in the three types of medicine, a clinical test confirmed it can increase the treatment rate than when medicine is taken alone. I believe it can increase its standing as one of the probiotics helpful to the stomach.

As you can see, probiotics are a representative nutrient that can strike a balance in our body and that exists peacefully with other materials. That is why probiotics' role is expected to become more important, in terms of vitalizing or lifesaving activities. If modern people use probiotics to keep to the principle of Mother Nature's "Get rid of toxic agents and fill up the body with nutrients," their health will benefit greatly in terms of health management. Globally, there isn't a special medicine that can completely get rid of cold or *Helicobacter pylori*. As aging is one of the buzzwords of our era, I believe probiotics, which as a sure resisting power against *Helicobacter pylori*, will prove to be very useful. The future of probiotics is very bright.

Nowadays, health-related TV shows in Korea heatedly introduce various ways to restore peoples' natural healing power. I think most of them can be included in the social medicine and its therapy, which is a complementary alternative medicine. Interestingly, there is one common factor of the "patients that experienced miraculous results" that went beyond the imaginations of medical experts. Those patients totally got rid of their old life pattern in order to fight the disease. Some became a fervent believer of religion from an atheist. Others went to live in the countryside to meditate, after ending their stressful city life. Still others turned into a vegetarian after clinging to meat and fast foods. In this respect, we can say that almost any disease can be ruled and that there are sick people who can't change themselves.

Let me put it this way. Whether it's current or traditional, if you want to seek ways to maintain health by natural healing power, you have to think outside the box and break free from the boundaries of Western medicine that was defined as the traditional medicine. We should look into social medicine based on the organic combination of the human and Mother Nature. Discovering social medicine therapy is the way to find ways to make our body and mind cure themselves.

There are about three ways of social medicine therapies that have been handed down from generations as complementary alternative medicine. First, you should be the main player of your health, and get results by continuous meditation, training, and performing actions by yourself (e.g., horticulture therapy, Qigong therapy, yoga, etc.). Second, you become an object and get results by exposing yourself to another object or action (e.g., bee venom therapy, intramuscular stimulation, etc.). Third, you don't do anything, but have the expert (a third person) with great powers or specially designed machine to do it for you (psychic healing, homeopathy, quantum medicine, etc.). The detailed explanation will follow in the next chapter.

3.2 Classification for Therapy of Social Medicine

3.2.1 Therapy of Social Medicine to Catch "Three Birds with One Stone"

3.2.1.1 Therapy of Social Medicine Derived from Health Diet

As I mentioned, the "three birds" that people want to catch with "one stone" are disease prevention, antiaging, and longevity. To do so, health diet is the number one factor to be considered. However, it is hard for us to come up with the right decisions in the long term, as there are many options that lure us. As long as short-term desires such as gluttony overtake, it's hard to expect long-term behavioral changes in health diet.

However, we can still find out the short-term incentives that can get us to the long-term "three birds" goals. It will make us easier to make the right decision. For instance, the healthy people shouldn't feel that they are safe from obesity or diabetes, which is a dangerous factor in the long term. When the uncomfortable truth dawns upon them (that they will suffer from a full stomach the next day, if they sleep after having oily night snacks), they will eat less hamburgers and fries.

As you can see, if we can see the results of our everyday life habits, what they will give us in the long term, we can take one step at a time to the goal that we want, which is disease prevention (cancer or other diseases stemming from our everyday habits), antiaging, and longevity. Therefore, I would like to talk about detailed ways centering on health diet. The contents to be followed are mainly quoted from the book by Walter C. Willett, *Eat, Drink, and Be Healthy: The Harvard Medical School Guide to Healthy Eating* (2009).

Fat

For the last 40 years, fat was the number one enemy to be avoided at meal time. Adequate amount of fat intake is important because first, dietary fat is the number one cause of death in most advanced countries, and second, it is the main culprit that causes cardiac diseases. The fat and oils in our average meal nowadays take up about 33 % of the total calories. If the intake of fat is reduced and saturated fat is replaced with carbohydrate, the level of total cholesterol can be lowered. However, the problem is it can lower the level of good cholesterol, HDL. So it isn't a good idea. If the total calorie is maintained and the saturated fat and carbohydrate are reduced and unsaturated fat is taken more, weight won't go up. So let's look at the types of fat (fatty acids) first.

1. Saturated fat: "saturated" means that the carbon atoms in chains have the most number of hydrogen atoms that can be combined together. It can only be possible when each of the carbon atoms is connected to the next carbon atom in a single bond. Therefore, it forms a lineal chain shape. In nature, there are more than 20 types of saturated fat. They are included in the meat, animal fat, and milk products and in some vegetable oils such as palm oil and coconut oil. At room temperature, it is solid, and it's like the oil from bacon or hamburger that is stuck on the pan when dried.

   In terms of cholesterol and atherosclerosis, saturated fat is bad. Saturated fat that increases the bad cholesterol LDL the most is the saturated fat in butter and other milk products. Next comes beef, and the saturated fat in chocolate and cocoa butter has little bad effect.

2. Monounsaturated fat: it is formed as two carbons in a double bond at some part of carbon structure. It has little difference from the former one on the outside but produces many significant differences. It reduces two hydrogen atoms that the carbon chain can have, and the form is in a stick where the lineal one is bent once. Monounsaturated fat makes fat liquid at room temperature. Monounsaturated fat is liquid oil, and it can be found much in most nuts, olive, peanut and canola oil, and avocado.

3. Polyunsaturated fat: when there are more than two double bonds, it is polyunsaturated fat. It has less number of hydrogen atoms than the monounsaturated fat that has the same number of carbon structure. The form of polyunsaturated fat is a stick which is bent twice. It is divided into "omega-6" and "omega-3" types.

The number shows how far the first double bond is located from the tip of the carbon chain. At room temperature, it is liquid. As our body can't make this, necessary fat such as polyunsaturated fat should be taken from vegetable oil, which include corn or pea oil, or from seeds, whole grain, salmon, and tuna.

※ Omega-3 fat: omega-3 fat is a polyunsaturated fat. It is necessary fat that is needed for the normal functioning of the body. It has to be taken from the outside, as our body can't produce it. The three main omega-3 fats in food include ALA, EPA, and DHA. Various vegetable oils, nuts, leaf vegetables, some animal fat, and fat of the cattle that feed on grass are the suppliers of ALA. EPA and DHA can be found mainly in fish (in particular, oily fish such as salmon, mackerel, herring, and sardine). That is why the two are called "marine omega 3." Our body mainly uses ALA for calories. Omega-3 fat can be turned into EPA or DHA, but it doesn't work in the other way.

Omega-3 fat is important because first, it forms cell membrane throughout our body. In particular, it is the main material that makes up the eyes, the brain, and the cell membrane of spermatids. Second, they become the precursor to be the starting point of hormone production. Third, omega-3 fat inducing hormone conducts coagulation, contraction, and easing of artery wall and controls inflammation. Fourth, it is helpful to the prevention and treatment of cardiac disease and stroke. Omega-3 fat is especially good at preventing cardiac disease, and the reason Eskimos have low incidence rate of cardiac disease even though they are on a high-fat diet is that the omega-3 fat prevents cardiac disease. It prevents heart attack and sudden cardiac death, and this was confirmed again by a massive random research conducted in Italy.

Pregnant women or those who have plans to have a child should eat omega-3 fat every day. Omega-3 fat plays a very important role in forming the fetus' brain and other nerve parts after insemination. Therefore, it is good to cook fish, walnut, and linseed with canola or soybean oil.

4. Trans fat: when vegetable oil is burned with hydrogen and small pieces of nickel, it is "partially hardened." That is, hydrogen combines with some carbons that are in a double bond and change them into a singular combination. At the same time, some of the double bonds that are left is twisted, turning into a linear shape. This gives a new physicochemical characteristic to the fat. In the process, liquid vegetable oil is solidified, and the representative cases are margarine and vegetable shortening. They are easy to be stored and transported and so can be used in place of butter and lard (solidified animal fat) in baking. Even if it is less solidified, the liquid form doesn't go bad as fast as the vegetable oil. However, it is the main culprit that causes cardiac disease.

We need to be sure of what roles fat components in the blood do. Fat is the main source of energy for cells, and they make up fat cells that store energy. Fat also reduces outside shock by covering important organs and protects them and works as insulator. Chemically, cholesterol can't be called fat, but they are essential to forming covers that are around the cell membrane and neurons. Lastly, fat is the precursor of many hormones that are produced in our body.

In order to work in the body, fat has to come out of the digestion system to move toward cells. However, it doesn't blend with like oil and water. Therefore, our body wraps it up with protein so it can flow in our blood, which are small particles called, "lipoprotein (fat+protein)." The particles have in them some cholesterol to stabilize themselves.

Lipoprotein (fat+protein) can be categorized according to the ratio of fat and protein that make up the particle. The ones that have less fat and much protein are heavy and have greater density. On the other hand, the particles with much fat and less protein are light and have less density. Protein not only protects fat from water but also works as signs that show the body to send the particles to specific parts. The most important "fat+protein" that is related to cardiac disease is HDL, LDL, and VLDL, which is very light in density, made up of neutral fat.

In other words, cholesterol that is regarded as one type of fat is known to be the material that causes arteriosclerosis, the main culprit of adult disease. However, it isn't only bad material. Rather, it is a necessary element that our body has to have, and it is in various foods that we take in, including meat and eggs. When we take food that has cholesterol, the amount of cholesterol in the blood increases. Foods with much unsaturated fat also increase the level of cholesterol in the blood, as the unsaturated fat turns into cholesterol in the liver. Cholesterol combines with various types of "fat+proteins" and moves in the blood. Among them, LDL forms "low-density cholesterol" by combining with cholesterol. "Low-density cholesterol" plays the main role in causing arteriosclerosis by moving cholesterol into our body (bad cholesterol). However, HDL combines with cholesterol to form "high-density cholesterol," and it gets rid of cholesterol in our blood to prevent arteriosclerosis (good cholesterol). Bad cholesterol is concentrated in foods such as hamburger, pizza, red meat, and pork belly.

The level of cholesterol in the blood tells how much LDL and HDL are circulating in the blood. The total level of cholesterol that is desirable is less than 200 mg per 1 dl (one tenth of 1 l). The level of cholesterol on the margin is 200–239 mg/dl (considering total cholesterol), and high cholesterol level is more than 240 mg/dl. For instance, the high level of cholesterol in blood means that you kept a bad diet and life habits for a long term.

In this case, health diet that can be found in our everyday life as social medicine is very important. In particular, saturated fat forms the basis of health diet and is in charge of a lion's portion of the day's calorie. It is also proven to be good for long-term health. The following are the good effects of the saturated fat:

First, saturated fat can maintain the level of HDL cholesterol and lower the level of LDL, which is called as the "bad cholesterol."

Second, the increase of another form of fat, neutral, that roams around in blood (it has a close relationship with cardiac disease) can be prevented. The increase of neutral fat occurs when you are on a high-carbohydrate diet.

Third, the incidence of irregular heart pulse and the main reason for sudden heart failure can be lowered.

Fourth, the tendency of clots within the artery that prevents the flow of bloods can be lowered.

Based on the consistent evidence that came out from various fat-related researches until now, I give the following conclusions:

First, the more saturated fat you take, the more incidence of heart disease.
Second, good fat can improve the cholesterol problem.
Third, the more good fat there is, the less heart disease.
Forth, replacing saturated fat with unsaturated fat can save life.
Fifth, special attention is required for trans fat.
Sixth, there is weak link between dietary fat and cancer.
Seventh, liquid vegetable oil should be used in place of saturated fat or trans fat. It
    is not advised to use alternative fat that is yet to be proven or fake food (written
    as milk serum protein).

Carbohydrate

Carbohydrate usually doesn't get much spotlight compared to the healthy foods such as fruits and vegetables. However, carbohydrate is an important element that is related to major source of energy, the increase and maintenance of weight, great influence on diabetes, and occurrence and prevention of heart disease.

First, most of energy that we need comes from carbohydrate in grain, vegetable, and fruits. However, considering the phrase, "For the Best Health via SM Therapy," it is important to get carbohydrate from foreign grain, such as bread made from whole grain, brown rice, noodles, kasha (a kind of soup with oats, barley, and sorghum that is Russian and Eastern Europe cuisine), quinoa (South American grain), oats, and bulgur (a kind of wheat) that are not cracked.

Carbohydrate can be divided into simple carbohydrate and complex carbohydrate. Nutrition-wise, the former is a "bad kid" and the latter a "good kid." However, more useful ways to categorize carbohydrate is by GI, or glycemic index (the impact of carbohydrate on blood glucose), and by whether the carbohydrate is from a whole or cracked grain.

Recently, David Jenkins, a nutritionist of Toronto University, and his colleagues compared other carbohydrates with white bread and what impact they had on blood glucose. Through their study, the conventional wisdom that the complex carbohydrate is good and the simple carbohydrate is bad turned out to be false. Blood glucose indexes developed can be called a lineup of carbohydrates, and the higher blood glucose index the food has, the faster and stronger impact the food has on the level of blood glucose and insulin.

For instance, if the score 100 is the standard of the pure glucose that is digested fast, the blood glucose level of 55 is low. Surprisingly, cornflakes that can be thought of as a complex carbohydrate have an index of 80, which is higher than ice cream (61) and Snickers bar (68), both of which are simple carbohydrates. Their index is even lower than that of white bread, a representative complex carbohydrate of index 70. Foods that have high blood glucose levels rapidly increase the blood glucose level, boosting energyfacilitation (this is one reason why diabetes patients have to bring glucose refinement with them when they travel or exercise). However, as it can lower blood glucose level much faster, it can stimulate the feeling of hunger. On the other hand, foods with low blood glucose levels emit glucose slowly and make feel you full for a longer period of time. It is helpful to preventing diabetes.

The effect of eating based on the index of blood glucose and insulin depends both on the quantity of carbohydrate and blood glucose level. That is why a new concept of "blood glucose load" was introduced. Multiplying the quantity of carbohydrate in the food with the blood glucose level of the carbohydrate equals "blood glucose load." "Blood glucose load" signifies the impact of food on the biochemical reactions better than the quantity of carbohydrate or blood glucose index. For instance, some diet books warn intake of carrot, which has a high blood glucose level. However, carrot is mostly composed of moisture, and it is good food that has little amount of carbohydrate. It is also important to consider other nutrients that are in foods. Therefore, the blood glucose index can be useful in determining what to eat, but it can't be the sole standard. Along with fruits and vegetables, grain that is a little bit processed or that is not processed at all can provide much fiber, vitamin, minerals, and active vegetable chemical substances.

Simple carbohydrate is a kind of sugar, and examples include glucose, fruit sugar, and galactose. For instance, sugar is a combination of one particle of glucose and one particle of fruit sugar. The sugar in the milk (lactose) is the combination of glucose and galactose, one particle of each. The positive aspect of simple carbohydrate is that it provides our body with energy. However, recently, it is pointed out as the cause of constipation, hindering the movements in the stomach and lowering the stomach functions by feeding harmful germs in the stomach. When stomach functions are degraded, it impacts lowered functioning of the brain and other organs all around the body. Therefore, simple carbohydrate is looked upon as dangerous as red meat, to our health. Simple carbohydrate and red meat is on the top of the health diet pyramid, which means you should take as little as possible.

Complex carbohydrate is a long chain of sugar. Many kinds of complex carbohydrates are in foods we eat, and most of them are starch, which is a long chain of glucose particles. Fortunately, the digestion system in our body can decompose complex carbohydrates such as starch into sugar, which is the ingredient. However, most others pass the stomach and small intestine in their original form. Indigestible carbohydrates are called "cellulose." Taking cellulose is very important, and the following is the reasons we should take in enough fiber that includes cellulose. First, cellulose bundles up cholesterol and help them to be emitted through the small intestine. Second, it increases the amount of feces in the small intestine and helps regular defecation. Third, it is a good element in fighting cardiac disease, colorectal cancer, diabetes, obesity, high blood pressure, and more.

In short, most fibers are included in plants, and they are composed of various carbohydrates that can't be digested or are partly digested. The fibers that can wash our stomach clean are included much in the following: whole grain, bran, oats, barley, beans, pea, root vegetables, cabbage, fruits (peel and flesh), seeds of fruits and vegetables (eatable seeds such as in the strawberry), lettuce, citrus fruits, apple, ripe banana, and nuts and seeds. The total fiber amount that is written on the product is the result of dietary fiber and added fiber during the making process combined. The fiber amount needed for a man and woman a day are 38 g and 25 g, respectively. It is equivalent to three servings of barley rice, 4.2 kg of sweet potato, 1 kg each for cabbage and carrot, 850 g of kimchi, six apples, and five pears. This shows us that most people don't get enough fiber a day.

Just like fat, carbohydrate can increase weight. White bread, potatoes, noodles, and white rice also highly increase the level of blood glucose and insulin levels in the blood (it is a hormone that is made in a specialcell in the pancreas, and it guides the glucose to muscles or to the insides of other cells). Fat, protein, grain, and fruit or vegetables whose carbohydrates are absorbed slowly don't increase much blood glucose level.

Adult diabetes is called the type 2 diabetes nowadays. The main cause of the disease is overproduction of insulin, made by the constant stimulation in the pancreas. When there is lack of exercise, results can be more fatal. The mechanism of the disease goes like this. It is a problem that more and more today people are faced with. First, there is an "insulin resistance" in the body, where the organs form a group to the signal of the insulin and "open up the door for glucose." The resistance maintains the level of blood glucose high for a long time and makes the pancreas to additionally produce insulin in order to get glucose into the cells. In the process, the specialcellsthat produce insulin are worn out, just like a pump that is not maintained well, despite running all day. As a result, the production of insulin can be stopped, and it can induce type 2 diabetes, which is diabetes that is not dependent on insulin.

There are four elements that contribute to the resistance of insulin. First, an obese body finds it hard to control glucose when it is further away from healthy BMI (body mass index, it is weight divided by the squaring of one's height, kg/square meter; 20–24 is normal, and above 30 is obesity). Second is lack of exercise. The less you move, the lower the ratio of muscle becomes in proportion to body fat. This can be true even if you have an average weight. Through regular exercise, the muscle cells can process insulin and glucose very effectively. However, it is different for fat cells. The less amount of muscle we have in the body, the harder it is to process glucose in the body. Third is dietary fat. It also contributes to insulin resistance to some point. The resistance becomes greater when less polyunsaturated fat and much trans fat is taken. Fourth is genetics. Insulin resistance is more frequently found in Indians, people living on the Pacific Islands, and Asians than Europeans. However, those who have a genetic cause for insulin resistance can become healthy when they engage in weight control, active movements of the body, and good diet.

Moreover, insulin resistance is not only related to blood glucose but also to high blood pressure and hyperlipidemia (hypertriglyceridemia), lowered HDL, heart disease, and some cancer. That is why my book emphasizes "health diet, health exercise, and health stressor" all at the same time. They have to go hand in hand. At the same time, the importance of social medicine therapy to catch "three birds" can never be emphasized more. Health diet recommends less refined carbohydrate, more good fat, and more carbohydrates from whole grain food.

✻ Eggs: until recently, eggs were highlighted as "perfect food." However, it lost popularity after reports that the cholesterol in the eggs is related to cardiac disease. More than 200 mg of cholesterol in the yolk of an egg is more than two-thirds of the recommended cholesterol a day, and people thought we should eat eggs only once in a while. In fact, egg consumption per person plummeted from 400 to 250 a year.

However, the dangers of eating eggs are not as stark as some reports say. According to one study, adding additional 200 mg of cholesterol only increased a slight amount of cholesterol in the blood. Theoretically speaking, it was only a 10 % increase of contracting cardiac disease. However, there are numerous good sides to eggs. An egg has very low amount of saturated fat and includes much good nutrition such as protein, some polyunsaturated fat, folic acid, vitamin B complex, and vitamin D. Therefore, it is hard to predict that egg can contribute to cardiac disease for its cholesterol content.

Furthermore, every person has a different reaction to the cholesterol in foods. There are people who are directly impacted in their blood cholesterol level by the amount of cholesterol in the food. However, there are people who digest much of the cholesterol and show little difference in their levels after taking in cholesterol. Eggs have relatively little effect on the LDL, which is bad cholesterol. There are no reports that people who eat more eggs suffer from more cases of heart attack than those who don't, either.

According to a comprehensive research on 120,000 people (1999), we don't have to be too careful to eat eggs. After years of follow-up study, the incidence rates of healthy people contracting cardiac disease and stroke, who ate one egg every day, wasn't higher than the people who ate less than one egg a week. However, there was a slight correlation between people with diabetes who ate eggs and the contraction of cardiac disease.

If you had to choose among one egg, one doughnut fried with trans fat, and bagel made with refined flour, egg would be the best option, and it would be more recommendable if it was cooked with unsaturated fat.

Protein

Most of our hair and skin is made up of protein. Protein forms a very long and complex chain, composed of 20 basic components. It isn't stored away as fat, so should be provided with amino acids every day. Essential amino acid can't be synthesized in the body and can't be turned into from other amino acids.

Dietary protein, which is called the "perfect protein," means that it has all the necessary amino acids needed to make a new protein. "Imperfect protein" means that one or more essential amino acids are deficient. In this respect, meat, poultry, fish, egg, and milk products are mostly included in the perfect protein. Vegetable protein is mostly imperfect protein. Therefore, vegetarians should take in food that can be complementary, such as rice and bean, peanut butter and bread, and tofu and brown rice.

People living in today's affluent society don't suffer from protein deficiency, as it's very easy to take it. Usually, taking 0.8 g of protein per 1 kg of your weight is advised. It has been well known that animal and vegetable protein has almost the same impact on our health.

The problem is in what "wrapping state" protein is provided. Beef is a good supplier of animal protein and saturated fat. If you like beef, you should opt for lean meat that includes little fat. Chicken, turkey, and fish can be a better option, and vegetable protein such as bean, nuts, and whole grains can be the best option. They have little saturated fat content and much cellulose. If you like milk and dairy products, it would be better to choose low-fat or no-fat products rather than whole milk. High-protein foods with little saturated fat will be helpful not only to the slim waistline but to the heart.

The more protein you take, the more calcium is emitted out of the body. It's because more calcium is needed when you take more protein, as acid related to the digestion of the protein should be neutralized. In this case, the storage of calcium in our body, the bones, are summoned. For instance, in a study of health condition of the nurses, those who took more than 95 g (25 % of the recommendation a day) of protein a day saw their wrist joint break more easily than the women who took less than 68 g (15 % of the recommendation a day).

In particular, bean protein is a good alternative to animal protein. However, as we don't know what impact bean protein has on breast cancer and memory loss, it is advised to take not too much bean products. Twice to four times of eating bean products such as tofu and soybean milk a week is recommended. When the intake of carbohydrate is lowered and protein is increased, the level of neutral fat in the blood is decreased and HDL index go higher. It can contribute to the lowering of cardiovascular diseases such as heart attack or stroke.

As a result, an ordinary meal can meet the intake of the minimum protein requirements a day. If most of the protein you take is supplied by vegetable products, then taking beans, nuts, whole grains, and vegetables together is advised.

※ Nuts: despite conventional wisdom, nuts have ample protein and other nutrients. For instance, 28 g of almond, walnut, peanut, and pistachio have 8 g of protein, which is equivalent to protein in a glass of milk. There is a significant amount of fat in it too, but most are unsaturated fat that decreases the bad cholesterol LDL levels and increases the good cholesterol HDL levels.

It seems that the omega-3 fatty acids, which is called alpha-linoleic acid, prevent blood clots and reduce chances of arrhythmia. Arginine the amino acid, sufficient in nuts, is an essential element that makes an important molecule named nitric oxide. It eases the contracted blood vessels and facilitates the flow of blood. It makes platelet to make the blood less sticky and reduces the formation of blood clot in the blood.

Nuts are good foods that also include vitamin E, folic acid, potassium, cellulose, and other vegetable nutrients. It is advised to eat nuts rather than potato chips, cookies, or chocolates for snack.

Fruits and Vegetables

"Eat a lot of fresh fruits and vegetables" is an advice that transcends time. These are some of the good sides of eating fruits and vegetables:

- Lowers the rate of heart failure and stroke contraction
- Decreases blood pressure
- Prevents constipation and diverticulitis and painful stomach-related diseases
- Prevents aging-related diseases such as cataract (where the lens of the eyes become opaque) and macular degeneration (a major cause of eyesight loss for senior citizens aged more than 65)
- Delays or prevents memory loss and degeneration of mind activities
- Gives feeling of full by less calories and can impact weight control
- Decorates peoples' diet and is good for reviving taste

However, the aforementioned effects can be from the substances from vegetables or the interactions between those materials. Until now, only a handful of the effects of fruits and vegetables have been known, and some of them are based on uncertain facts. Most vegetable chemical substances (phytochemicals, chemicals made from vegetables) are not yet discovered or named, and they are excluded from the evaluation as they are yet to be scientifically examined.

It may be theoretically possible to produce a magic medicine (pill) that has all the good effects of fruits and vegetables. For instance, let's say all the minerals, cellulose, vitamins, antiaging materials, and vegetable hormones are put into one pill. But then, the pill would have to be very big, and no one would know how much of the good nutrients should be put in proportionately. What I want to say is that the benefits of fruits and vegetables lie in the combination of materials that interact with each other. Let's take carotenoid for example, an antiaging coloring. When we eat tomatoes or carrots, the various carotenoids in them get into the different cells and into the different parts in the cells. That is how it can have an antiaging effect on the various cells to be spread to the whole body.

Apart from the complex effect issue, the biggest weakness of pill is that it doesn't look and taste good. The good smell of cooked corn, the sweetness of tomatoes, the crispy bites of apples, and the bright green colors of broccoli and soybeans can't be felt in pills. What about the smooth silky skin and the savory taste of avocado? Therefore, it is desirable to eat good-looking, good-tasting fruits and vegetables to take in vegetable chemicals.

What we call "vegetables" are really "fruits." In this book, I will use the word "fruit" for foods that are used for making sweet dessert and snacks and "vegetable" for the food that is used for salads and meals. As for general categorization of fruits and vegetables, I referred to the "family" of plants.

1. Crucifer (Cruciferae): the name "crucifer" was given as the plant comes out in the form of a small cross. Crucifer include broccoli, baby cabbage, cabbage, cauliflower, horseradish, mustard, Chinese cabbage, kale, leaf mustard, white radish, turnip, shepherd's purse, etc. Crucifers provide chemicals such as isothiocyanates, indoles, thiocyanates, and nitriles that can prevent cancer.

2. Cucurbitaceae: cucumber, gourd, watermelon, oriental melon, melon, and pumpkin are included.
3. Legumen: alfalfa, kidney bean, pea, and soybeans are included. Beans have ample folic acid, cellulose, and substances that oppress proteoclastic enzyme. They all protect our body from heart disease and cancer.
4. Liliaceae: asparagus, chive, garlic, green onion, and onion are included. The vegetables include various sulfur compounds that prevent cancer. In particular, they have much allicin and diallyl sulfate.
5. Rutaceae: citron, tangerine, trifoliate orange, lemon, lime, and orange are included. There are ample vitamin C, limonene (substances in the peel of orange and lemon), and coumarin in the citrus fruits. They showed anticancer effects in animal experiments.
6. Nightshade: eggplant, pepper, potato, bell pepper, and tomatoes are included. Tomato has a lot of lycopene, which is a type of antiaging element. It is good for preventing prostate cancer and other cancers.
7. Apiaceous: carrot, water parsley, celery, and *Peucedanum terebinthaceum* are included. Carrots are good suppliers of beta-carotene, and our body uses beta-carotene to make vitamin A. Beta-carotene and carotenoid showed that the related materials can prevent some cancer and cardiac disease and can be helpful to maintaining memory in the later days.

There is evidence that specific fruits and vegetables have anticancer effects toward specific cancers. The examples are as follows. First, taking crucifer vegetables such as broccoli is related to lowering the incidence of bladder cancer. Second, folic acid has protection effects on colorectal cancer and rectal cancer. Third, lycopene in tomatoes works to prevent prostate cancer. For instance, in a study that tracked people who worked in health field, men who took tomatoes, tomato sauce, and tomato juice several times a week had a significantly lower rate of contracting or being diagnosed with a proceeded prostate cancer than men who ate them 1–2 times a week.

Fiber is in fruits and vegetables and can't be digested by humans. Those include cellulose, pectin, and gums. Fiber has two types, soluble and insoluble. Both pass the digestion system, hardly being damaged or altered. The difference between the two is that soluble fiber melts by small intestine fluid and that the insoluble fiber doesn't.

Soluble fiber is sufficient in soybean families, apple, citrus fruits, oats, other grains, and seeds. When they pass by the small intestine, they form jellylike material that is sticky. It attracts bile acid that has much cholesterol and emits it through constipation. The more cholesterol is emitted, the lower the blood cholesterol level gets, and the dangers of cardiac disease and other circulatory system are diminished.

Insoluble fiber comes from cell membrane of plants. Its main ingredient is cellulose, and it can't be decomposed in the human digestion system or by the fluid from the small intestine. It is shaped in a long chain of glucose molecules. The insoluble fiber, without changing its characteristics, takes with it some of the undigested food that is in the small intestine as it passes by. As foods going through the digestion tube moves faster, the time the body is exposed to toxic agents or carcinogenic materials of food can be reduced. Furthermore, as the insoluble fiber slowly drags the partially digested food from the small intestine, absorption of sugar and starch is delayed. This can slow down the rapid increase of the blood glucose and insulin levels that occur after we eat food, which can easily change into glucose. It can also prevent dramatic increase of neutral fat, which are particles that move fat from the small intestine to the parts of the body. When the level of insulin and neutral fat remain steadily high, the incidence rate of heart failure is increased, and it can also raise dangers of type 2 diabetes.

Among various fruit juices, grapefruit juice should be distinguished by others. Grapefruit juice decreases absorption of fexofenadine, an allergy medicine named "Allegra"; digoxin, a medicine for congestive heart failure; losartan, which controls blood pressure; and an anticancer medicine vinblastine. In some drugs, it can change the metabolism and increase blood concentration, sometimes to a very dangerous level. The following are some of those drugs: felodipine, which treats high blood pressure named Plendil; nifedipine, named "Procardia"; calcium antagonists nisoldipine, named "Sular"; epilepsy treatment carbamazepine, named "Carbatrol" and "Tegretol"; widely used treatment for hyperlipidemia; lovastatin, named "Mevacor"; atorvastatin, named "Lipitor"; simvastatin, named "Zocor"; and the immune suppressants that are taken by those who underwent organ transplant, cyclosporine, and lastly, buspirone to cure alcohol poisoning, depression, panic disorder, and various other diseases. An element in the grapefruit juice can become the cause for kidney stone.

Identifying the good sides of fruits and vegetables can be very challenging, as vegetables contain various nutritious elements. For instance, the Best boy tomato (a type of tomato) has different chemical components according to the soil it grows on, the amount of moisture, the harmful insects it has to endure, the degree of its ripeness when harvested, and in what condition it was stored. Moreover, nutrition provided differs on how it was processed and cooked.

Recently, the US FDA allowed food manufacturers to signify or advertise that bean protein can "lower the risk of cardiac disease" on the wrappings (note that it says not the cardiac disease itself, but the "risk" of cardiac disease). It's because isoflavones, a ketene found in the bean, can mimic or hinder estrogen, the female hormone. Another compound group, vegetable phytosterols, can have an impact on the absorption and metabolism of cholesterol. The vegetable chemicals detox harmful toxic agents; help enzymes that fight against cancer, infection, or the destruction of cells; and help other enzymes that heal cell destruction. In short, fruits and vegetables are a sort of "anticancer cocktail." Furthermore, they are good suppliers of potassium, magnesium, and other elements, and they are essential minerals that our body needs in order to undertake various important tasks.

As a result, for optimal health, we should eat more diverse fruits and vegetables. For instance, take more than five times a day, each from the following list of the fruits and vegetables. Eating them in their season is recommended as they are fresher. Just remember that tomatoes are better to be cooked. When taken in raw, the lycopene (a strong anticancer material that reduces the incidence of various cancers) that is firmly combined in the inside of cell membrane can be hard for our body to take in. By cooking the tomatoes, their cell membrane can be crumbled down and oil can melt the lycopene, so they can move through blood.

- Dark green vegetables
- Yellow or orange fruits and vegetables
- Red fruits and vegetables
- Beans and soybean families
- Citrus fruits

Vitamins

It's not an exaggeration to say that we are living in a world of vitamins. Vitamins have never been loved by so many people as nowadays. Historically speaking, the first vegetable chemical found by humans are what today's vitamins are. Vitamins are compounds that have carbons, which are needed in trace amounts to maintain our body and facilitate metabolism. Vitamins were discovered and defined as deficiencies such as rickets (lack of vitamin D), pellagra (lack of niacin), and beriberi (lack of thiamine) were studied. It seems that people have taken in sufficient amount of vitamins throughout the years as such conditions have become very rare. Now, there are criticisms on vitamin supplements, accusing they amount to nothing more than making our urine "nutritious."

However, new studies found out that increasing the amount of vitamins in some foods and supplements can promote our health in the long term. It was in folic acid that the relationship between vitamins and deficiency diseases were revealed. Lack of folic acid directly led to inherent defections such as spina bifida and anencephaly. Such diseases, called neural tube defections, occur when the hard pipes that form the spine or protect the spine or the tissues that develop into the brain don't grow normally in the first 28 days of pregnancy. Spina bifida can induce other conditions including paralysis. Patients of anencephaly are born with most of the brain absent and without spinal cord. Most infants of anencephaly are stillborn and live only for a very short period of time even if they are born. Globally, about 300,000 babies are born with defections in the neural tube annually.

The average intake of folic acid that is recommended for now has increased by 100 micro gram than the past for childbearing women, amounting to 400 micro gram per day. The increased intake of folic acid is lowering the number of births with neural tube defections. For instance, about 4000 births were reported to have neural tube defections in 1995–1996. However, after folic acid was promoted, the number fell to 3000 in just 2 years.

These days, the word "antioxidant" includes not only vitamins C and E and carotenoid that are related to beta-carotene. It also includes minerals such as selenium and magnesium that are needed for the functioning of enzymes that fight off free radical. (Free radical is also called active oxygen or harmful oxygen. Free radical is made when fat or carbohydrate is burned, and as it is unstable in electronically, it seeks to take electrons from anything that is near it and the cell is damaged in the process. When free radical is accumulated, it can impact cancer, arthritis, cataract, loss of memory, and aging.) Antioxidants actively studied nowadays include glutathione, coenzyme Q10, lipoic acid, flavonoid, phenols, and vegetable estrogen.

An antioxidant has its unique chemical process and biological characteristics. Therefore, each antioxidant has different roles, and they work as a part of an intricate network. For instance, beta-carotene lies vertically on cell membrane, and it is stuck outside of the surface of a cell like a little flag. Lycopene is hidden in the center of the cell membrane, and other carotenoids and antioxidants are situated on the inside or outside of the cells.

Therefore, we can get very useful information when we understand the chemical process. It means that one single antioxidant can't do what others can do together. That is, one antioxidant can't do the job of fruits and vegetables that have various antioxidants in them, where effects are produced through their multiple and complex interactions. In short, eating fruits and vegetables is a very good way to maintain the fiber, minerals, heart, and blood vessels in a healthy manner and to obtain antioxidants (those that are not yet discovered are included as well).

1. Vitamin A: vitamin A helps cells' maintenance, which covers the inner surface of the body. It also increases the production and activity of white cells and directly helps reformation of bones. It aids growth and differentiation of cells, a process where cells undergo division and characterization. It can be one way that vitamin A prevents healthy cells from turning into cancer cells and the cancer cells to be divided and spread. Too much vitamin A can prevent the good effects of vitamin D helpful to the bones and the muscles, which also soothes cancer cells. It results in lowered bone density, increases fraction of the pelvis and other bones and the incidence rate of cancer. Therefore, the amount of vitamin A taken as supplement should not go over 2000 IU a day. Foods that have vitamin A are liver, fish liver, eggs, and milk products. Provitamin A, which turns into vitamin A once in the body, includes carrot, pumpkin, red and green bell pepper, spinach, kale, and various green vegetables.

2. Carotenoid: it is a big categorization of vegetable coloring. First, beta-carotene is the coloring that marks the peculiar orange color in carrots and sweet potatoes. Second, lycopene results in red in tomatoes and watermelons. Third, the only carotenoids that are in the human retina include lutein and zeaxanthin, beta-cryptoxanthin, and other alpha-carotene. The six types of carotenoid are only a part of the 500 of them that are known. Carotenoid mainly has two important functions. Some of them turn into vitamin A, and the others work as a strong antioxidant. After 20 long years of research, it was found out that lutein and zeaxanthin are important in preventing macular degeneration and cataract.

3. Vitamin C: vitamin C conducts its special role in controlling inflammation. It also helps collagen formation. Collagen is necessary in making healthy bones, tendon, teeth, gum, and blood vessels. It takes part in making various hormones

and chemical transmitters that are used in the brain and neurons. Vitamin C is a potential antioxidant that can nullify free radical and oxidants found in the body. The amount of vitamin C that is found generally in multivitamin supplements can be helpful to easing symptoms on the onset of cold, but I don't support overconsumption of vitamin C.

In the USA, the recommended intake amount of vitamin C per day is 75 mg for women and 90 mg for men (in Korea, it is 100 mg for both). The DRI reports warns against the overconsumption of vitamin C, which is more than 2000 mg a day. When the concentration of vitamin C is very high, it can turn into free radical from antioxidants. Vitamin C can be found much in citrus fruits, strawberry, bell pepper, tomato, broccoli, and spinach.

4. Vitamin E: vitamin E was referred to as the anticancer drug for its antioxidation effects. However, most research didn't find its good effects, and only a handful of them reported it can lower the risk of colorectal and prostate cancer. Up to 1000 mg of vitamin E a day (1500 IU for natural vitamin E) is safe. When taken too much, a rare eye syndrome of pigmentary degeneration of the retina (or retinitis pigmentosa) can be worsened. Vitamin E can lessen the coagulation ability of blood, so patients taking anticoagulant should speak to the doctor before taking vitamin E supplements.

5. B6, B12, and folic acid in the vitamin B complex: there are eight in total in the vitamin B complex. They are thiamin, niacin, riboflavin, pantothenic acid, biotin, B, B, and folic acid. They play the supporting role in our body. They help various enzymes get living energy from carbohydrates and fat, decompose amino acids, and move nutrients that have oxygen and energy in them to every corner of our body. Here I would like to focus on B6, B12, and folic acid. There is new evidence that the three can play an important role in decreasing cardiac disease and cancer.

Nowadays, high levels of homocysteine (a breakdown product of protein that can be a cause for the clotting of blood vessels, which can lead to arteriosclerosis when accumulated in the body) are regarded as a risk factor for cardiac disease. Vitamins can be a good player in this process. The three B6, B12, and folic acid recycle homocysteine and turn it into harmless amino acid. The mechanism is shown in the figure below. A diet lacking more than one of the three can increase homocysteine levels and can escalate the risk of contracting cardiac disease (the relationship between homocysteine and cardiac disease is not yet established and still remains a theory). Therefore, I stress that taking B6, B12, and folic acid is a way to preventing cardiac disease (Fig. 3.1).

Now the recommended intake of the three per day stands 400 micro gram for folic acid, 1.3–1.7 mg for vitamin B6, and 2.4 microgram for vitamin B12 (in Korea, it's 400 micro gram for folic acid, 1.4 mg for vitamin B6 (1.5 mg for man), and 2.4 micro gram for vitamin B12 respectively, in the case of 15 years and older). Only a handful of US adults get the amounts through food.

(i) Vitamin B6 (pyridoxine): this vitamin is a combination of six related compounds. Most of them work in the synthesis and the decomposition of amino acid, which is a component of protein. When lacking, it can lead to

Fig. 3.1 Homocysteine and the three vitamin B complexes (Source: Walter C. Willett, *Eat, Drink, and Be Healthy: The Harvard Medical School Guide to Healthy Eating* (2009), p. 302)

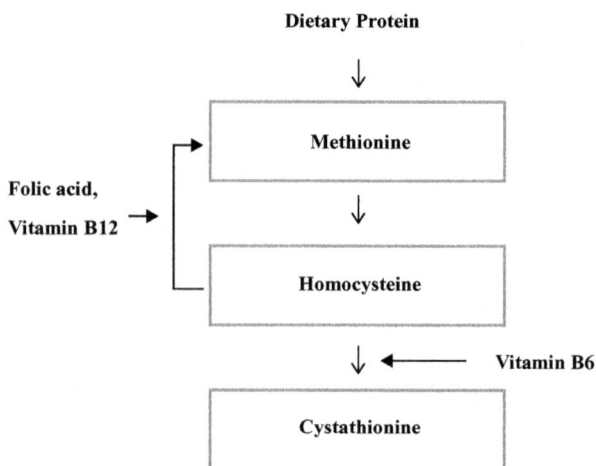

dermatitis, anemia, depression, and convulsion and can cause heart disease. One type of vitamin B6 helps tryptophan, an amino acid, to be turned into serotonin (an important neurotransmitter that is used in the brain and nervous system). Therefore, it has been tested as medicine for depression, attention deficit disorder, and problems related to serotonin. Meat, nuts, and beans provide vitamin B6. However, if vitamin B6 is overconsumed only by supplements a day up to 250 mg, it can cause neural damage.

(ii) Vitamin B12 (cyanocobalamin): in the early twentieth century, pernicious anemia was a fatal disease. The three researchers who received the Nobel Prize in 1934 found out that liver extracts are effective in treating pernicious anemia. It was because the liver had large amounts of vitamin B12 that was essential for producing red blood cells. Nowadays there aren't many cases of pernicious anemia, but the lack of vitamin B12 results in failure of memory, dementia, myatrophy, loss of appetite, and numbness of limbs. As seen in the mechanism on the picture above, it can lead to an accumulation of homocysteine. The vitamin is found only in animal food, so vegetarians have a tendency to have deficiency of vitamin B12. Until the age of 50, enough amount of B12 is accumulated in the body, so several years can pass without problems even if the absorption ability from food is lowered.

Infectious enteritis or AIDS patients have difficulty absorbing vitamin B12 from food. Excessive drinking also hinders the function of the vitamin. Furthermore, antacid; colchicine, the medicine for gout; and various drugs such as Dilantin, an anticonvulsant, hinder the function of the vitamin. Currently, the recommended daily intake of vitamin B12 stands at 2.4 micro gram and it can be supplied mainly by liver. Twenty eight grams of liver can provide 23 micro gram of vitamin B12. Other sources include tuna, yogurt, cottage cheese, and egg.

(iii) Folic acid: folic acid helps the fetus' spine development, and if the pregnant woman takes too little amounts of folic acid, the baby has a high possibility of being born with spina bifida or anencephaly. Folic acid is a helper in eradicating homocysteine, and it can play its part in preventing heart disease. It also takes part in cell division, preventing cancer. If you take much folic acid, it can decrease the risk of colorectal and breast cancer. Alcohol hinders the absorption of folic acid and slows down the folic acid that is circulating in the body. Taking in more folic acid than recommended can lower the risk.

There are many other foods that provide folic acid than liver. They are beans (lens bean and black bean), spinach, pasta, and orange juice. Breakfast cereal includes 120 micro gram of folic acid per dish, and some things include as much as 400 micro gram, which is the recommended daily intake.

6. Vitamin D (cholecalciferol): strictly speaking, vitamin D is not a vitamin but a hormone that is made in the skin. Vitamin D is produced by ultraviolet rays. As for nutrients used physiologically, vitamin D2 (ergocalciferol) and vitamin D5 (cholecalciferol) are popular. D5 is more stable and effective than D2, as D2 is easily decomposable when left in the air. Therefore, when we say vitamin D, we usually refer to vitamin D5.

The sunlight on our skin turns a material that is related to cholesterol into a precursor of vitamin D. The process first takes place in the liver and is facilitated by the kidney, heart, immune system, breast, and prostate cells. There are little foods which contain vitamin D. The fat-soluble vitamin is ample in fish such as salmon, mackerel, sardine, and Japanese bluefish. Breakfast cereals that have high amounts of vitamin and eggs that are from the chicken that ate vitamin D-contained feeds are included.

In particular, vitamin D is important in maintaining physiological functions of the body. As it makes bones and prevents fractures just like calcium, it should be taken seriously. Vitamin D helps calcium and phosphorus' absorption as they pass through the digestion tube. It signals kidney so that the minerals are reabsorbed rather than emitted through urine. It also represses destruction of bones and facilitates formation of bones. It is desirable to take vitamin D than calcium, in order to prevent or diminish the case of wrist and pelvis fracture in the elderly days. Furthermore, vitamin D sends a signal to the muscle cells and orders them to make protein, preventing falls through strengthened muscle (the number one accident to be avoided for the elderly is tripping). It can lower the incidence rate of cancer (just like a blanket that can put out a small fire, it can repress newly made cancer cells) and strengthen the heart (it also plays a role in the blood vessel clotting process called atherosclerosis) and makes blood pressure to remain normal. It also prevents multiple sclerosis (it occurs when the immune system attacks nerve protective membranes by mistake).

In terms of evolution, we can presume that natural selection (adaptation of evolutionary process) made people to have a lighter skin color as they moved northward from Africa, to get more vitamin D from the less sunlight. People who can get enough sunlight even for several minutes every day can make ample amount of vitamin D. However, those living over northern latitude of 40 don't have enough ultraviolet rays to make vitamin D in winter. The deeper skin color you have, the less ability you have to turn sunlight into vitamin D. A research on the US citizens revealed that African-American population had about half of the vitamin D amount compared to the Caucasian population. In the case of Scandinavian people with very white skin, their vitamin D levels are very low, so they take oily fish including liver to supplement vitamin D. Diet nowadays that ignores such tradition is causing damages to the health. People who work all day in the office and don't have free time to take a 15-min walk out in the sun, who can't move freely due to arthritis or other chronic disease, and those in the nursing home can't make enough vitamin D. Currently, about 8–9 people in their 50s and more can't take the recommended daily intake of vitamin D.

Results show that 800–1000 IU is needed a day to take the benefit of vitamin D. Almost all multivitamins have 400 IU of vitamin D, so it's no use taking two pills to get double the effect. Rather, the amount vitamin A (retinol) will be doubled, and vitamin D can't do its work. Some calcium supplements have 220 IU of vitamin D and 500 mg of calcium. Women can take one multivitamin and one calcium supplement together. As for men, overconsumption of calcium can be related to fatal prostate cancer, so I propose taking general multivitamin and a special vitamin D supplement. The best way is to find a multivitamin supplement that offers 800–1000 IU of vitamin D.

7. Vitamin K: it is a fat-soluble vitamin and helps make 6 vitamins out of 13 needed for blood coagulation. Some of the protein here helps make bones, so vitamin K is related not only to blood coagulation but to maintaining health.

   Many people believe that adults take enough vitamin K, as it is found in various foods. However, a recent study on the US citizens' meal proved them wrong. Most young people don't take green vegetables, so they don't get the right amount of vitamin K (recommended amount for men is 120 micro gram and 90 micro gram for women a day).

8. Calcium: no one knows how much calcium is needed per day for adults, as there are so many controversies on its role in our body. Currently, the recommended amount for an adult per day is 1000 mg until ages 50 and 1200 mg for 50 and older, but the amount is more than needed.

   Calcium, the component of bones and teeth, affects various mechanisms in our body. They include heart pulse, blood coagulation, contraction and relaxation of muscle, neurotransmitter process, controlling penetrability of cell membranes, and absorption of vitamin B2. It can also decrease the incidence rate of colorectal cancer and lower blood pressure. Lack of calcium can be a cause for osteoporosis, cancer, high blood pressure, and arteriosclerosis and is presumed to be the cause for dementia of the Alzheimer's type. There is no evidence that overconsumption of calcium can prevent fracture. Rather, recent reports show that excessive intake of calcium increases the incidence rate of prostate cancer fatal to men and ovarian cancer for women. Therefore, we should take heed when taking calcium.

Calcium in meat acidifies our body. When the metabolite of meat, which is acid, is thrown away in the form of urine from the kidney, calcium in the bone is used to neutralize it as alkaline calcium. Therefore, the more meat is consumed, the more calcium is emitted through urine, and it raises the risk of osteoporosis. Lack of calcium doesn't affect our body in the short term, but when there is a steady loss of calcium, bone density is lowered, and children may suffer from growth problems and osteoporosis. It can induce osteomalacia for adults.

The absorption rate of calcium is determined by gastric acid, so it is different for each person. The calcium that is ionized by gastric acid is absorbed in the duodenum by vitamin D. Calcium carbonate only has 4 % of absorption rate, but citric acid calcium and malic acid calcium (already ionized) can dissolve easily. Therefore, people with small amounts of gastric acid can increase the absorption rate up to 45 %. After mid-life, when the gastric acid begins to be diminished, it is good to take citric acid calcium. Magnesium is needed to absorb calcium, so products made up of 2:1 of calcium and magnesium can be easily absorbed through the wall of the small intestine. However, calcium and iron supplements should be taken by intervals, not at the same time. Calcium hydroxide combines with calcium in the stomach and forms calcium salts that is insoluble and sometimes hinders the absorption of calcium (Kim Hye-Yun and Lee Yung-Keun 2013c).

Milk and dairy products are not the best ways of getting calcium, so if you have to take more calcium, it's better to take calcium supplements. Dairy products are an option, not a must as in the past. Calcium supplements don't have additional calorie or saturated fat, and it's much cheaper than taking dairy products several times a day. Calcium supplement will be more useful if it contains vitamin D.

※ Hormones: estrogen and testosterone strengthen bones. Estrogen is called a female hormone and testosterone a male hormone, but both genders make the two hormones in their body. The two hormones produce new bone and maintain it in strong condition throughout our lives. In the case of women, the sex hormone sharply decreases after menopause, while the process is slow for men.

"Alternative hormone therapy" which mixes estrogen and progestin used to be an important remedy to prevent women's osteoporosis. It was known to control facial blushing caused by menopause and to prevent cardiac disease. However, the "Woman Health Initiative" supported by the US federal government reported that incidence rate of breast cancer in women who conducted alternative hormone therapy increased sharply. Risks of cardiac disease and stroke increased as well, and the therapy was called off.

9. Iron: too little iron in the body makes it harder for red blood cells to carry oxygen from the lung to organs in the body. Face loses color and people become mentally dull. Iron deficiency hinders growth and development of children and damages the thinking ability, and it accounts for 20 % of mothers' death when giving birth. Women on their period should take in ample amount of iron by meal. The elderly population is prone to contract anemia when they lack iron.

It can cause loss of memory and cardiovascular disease, and in severe cases, it can damage memory and thinking ability, can lessen the ability to take care of oneself and his/her bodily functions, and can cause depression.

Meat is a good supplier of iron. However, it has much calories, saturated fat, and cholesterol as well. Furthermore, our body can't control the absorption of iron from meat, unlike iron from grain, vegetables, fruits, and supplements.

The daily recommended intake of iron is 8 mg for men and 18 mg for women before menopause and 8 mg after the menopause. Generally, a meal that consists of green vegetables, bean, and the right amount of poultry and red meat can provide enough iron, so there is no need to worry. Whatever gender you are, it is not advisable to take more iron than the recommended iron amount in the multivitamin or mineral supplements. If necessary, talk to your doctor and undergo an iron test and take the supplements according to the prescription.

10. Magnesium: magnesium is an essential element that is needed for hundreds of biological processes in our body. Every cell in our body including the cells in the heart, muscle, and generative organs depends on it. The daily recommended intake for men stands at 420 mg and at 320 mg for women (in Korea it's 350 mg and 280 mg for men and women, respectively). Most people consume less magnesium than needed.

Magnesium controls the calcium amount that goes into cells and prevents the contraction of blood vessels. It also weakens the heart muscles from contracting violently and lowers blood pressure. That's why it's called the "calcium channel blocker" or a cure to treat high blood pressure. Deficiency in magnesium can be a problem for people who take diuretic (a type of medicine that cures high blood pressure) and who drink heavily. Diabetes accelerates the loss of magnesium, and it goes the same for caffeine drinks. When magnesium lacks, even small activities can be tiring, and it can cause abnormal cardiac pulse. In other words, lack of magnesium can contract blood vessels and muscle, which leads to high blood pressure, followed by a contraction in the cerebrovascular area that causes migraine and difficulty of blood circulation. When muscles are contracted by lack of magnesium, cramps occur easily. Tremors below the eyes occur and wrick in the hind of the neck and shoulders can take place. Moreover, menstrual pain often takes place, and asthma can occur due to contraction of the bronchial tubes.

A preference for chocolate can come from lack of magnesium, and desire for sweet things is diminished when magnesium is supplied. People with constipation will have less trouble in the bathroom when magnesium is taken. Mental activities consume a lot of magnesium, so it is not a stretch to say that most people under stress in the modern society suffer from the lack of magnesium. Alcohol emits magnesium through urine, so alcoholics are open to osteoporosis and cardiac disease by lack of magnesium (Kim Hye-Yun and Lee Yung-Keun 2013d).

If you consume much fruits, vegetables, and whole grain, food alone can get enough magnesium requirements. Multivitamins and mineral supplements usually have about 100 mg of magnesium, and it can help fill up the gap.

11. Potassium: potassiumis positive ion particle (the particle that has the "+" electricity) that is the greatest in number in the cells in our body. Our body strictly controls concentration of potassium, and problems arise when it's lacking or too much.

    When the level of potassium is lowered, you feel tired easily and the cardiac pulse is accelerated (especially those with cardiac disease). It can also cause convulsion or pain in the muscle. Too little potassium and too much sodium can cause high blood pressure. Adults are recommended to take 5 g of potassium a day, but most Americans don't get it enough. A low level of potassium is especially bad for people who take diuretic to control high blood pressure and who drink caffeine drinks such as coffee. The diuretic and caffeine increase the amount of potassium emitted through urine. Foods we eat or potassium salt (the salt where sodium is replaced with potassium), or taking in additional potassium through supplements, can lower blood pressure. This in turn can lower the risk of stroke, which is caused by the blocking of blood flow to the brain. Banana has much potassium, and apricot, jujube, kidney bean, orange, and spinach are also good.

    The best way to take adequate amounts of potassium is to eat much fruits and vegetables. Additionally, potassium salt can be very helpful to high blood pressure patients who are on diuretic and those who drink much coffee. Asking the doctor before taking potassium supplements is needed as it can have an impact on the kidney.

12. Sodium: most people tend to take in more sodium than necessary as processed foods have much salt in them (one-third of salt is sodium). For instance, one bag of fries of Burger King contains more than 1000 mg of salt, and more than half of the recommended daily intake of salt is in one cup of pasta sauce.

    The daily value of sodium on the food label stands at 2300 mg, but it is less than 1000 mg for general people. The amount is less than a half of a small cooking spoon. Americans consume 3500–4000 mg of sodium a day.

    If there is excessive sodium intake, it is emitted from our body before it can do actual harm, but not always. Excessive sodium pulls water from cells and increases blood pressure. In particular, it's true for those who are genetically more sensitive to salt. Scholars agree that too much salt induce high blood pressure, but there are controversies whether cutting the intake of sodium can lower blood pressure. Those who are diagnosed with high blood pressure are advised to cut sodium intake. Quitting smoking and doing exercise are recommended as well.

    The effective way to maintain a low blood pressure is to lose weight, exercise, and take in much fruits and vegetables that have much potassium. At the same time, low-salt diet (avoiding food that has much sodium in it) is recommended. It is desirable to avoid food with much salt or canned food and processed food.

13. Selenium: selenium, a metal, is a potential antioxidant, but it can't directly work as one, as there aren't enough in our body. Selenium is combined to the active parts of various enzymes that decompose peroxides, which are potential

oxidants made in our body. Until now, there is no sure evidence that selenium supplements prevent cancer.

Up to 400 micro gram of selenium is safe per day, but it's not certain whether we need more.

14. Zinc: zinc performs an important role, maintaining condition of our immune system. It works as an antioxidant, increases eye sight, and is needed for blood coagulation, healing of wounds, and development of sperm. In particular, zinc represses the enzyme called aromatase, which turns male hormone into a female hormone, and thereby is helpful to the antiaging of reproductive functions. In the USA, the daily value of zinc for men stands at 11 mg and 8 mg for women (in Korea, it's adjusted to men at 9 mg and 8 mg for women, ages 30–49). However, there is no evidence that taking in less zinc is problematic to the health.

Pregnant women and mothers who breastfeed need additional zinc, and the same is for children. In various researches, it is proved that lack of nutrients deters brain development and sports ability and is a cause for hyperactivity and problems related to attention. Some suggest that it can partially be related to lack of zinc.

Senior population also has to take in additional zinc. Senior citizens tend to take less zinc than the younger generation and often have problems in taking zinc from food. If they are on medication (especially diuretic that fights high blood pressure), it can emit zinc more easily out of the body. Fiber and potassium consumed can combine with zinc and can't be absorbed in digestive organs. Furthermore, heavy drinkers, patients of Crohn's disease and ulcerative colitis and those with chronic infections may need additional zinc.

Red meat is the main supplier of zinc. Poultry is also good. Vegetarians tend to lack zinc in their meal, but it doesn't seem to be a problem. There is no way we can consume too much zinc through food. The overconsumption of zinc can arise easily, and the symptoms of overconsumption occur when it goes over the daily value of 15 mg. It diminishes the functions of the immune system and delays healing from wounds. It also raises problems in the tasting and hearing senses and induces loss of hair and skin problems. In particular, overconsumption of zinc can increase the risk of prostate cancer.

Taking multivitamins is like signing up for the best "nutrition-wise insurance," taking cost into account. Most people have five kinds of vitamins they can't get enough through meals. They are folic acid, vitamin B6, vitamin B12, and vitamin D and E. Multivitamins are more effective when they have less vitamin A (less than 2000 IU) and more beta-carotene. It is advised to take vitamin D additionally. Generally, multivitamins offer 400 IU, and it is about half of the daily value necessary for good health. Therefore, the rest 400–600 IU should be supplemented by potassium, vitamin D compounds, and vitamin D tablets or capsules. Some drug companies are making pills that replace vitamin A with beta-carotene and contain an adequate amount of vitamin D. Consumers should take the supplements by carefully reading the labels.

Up to date, the studies on vitamin intake are yet to reach an agreement. Scientific knowledge on vitamins is advancing, so it's wise to wait until there is ample evidence. However, it would be better to take what you can rather than wait for a long time until all the good sides of vitamins are known perfectly.

Alcohol

Alcohol is related to the one-third of car accidents, and excessive drinking can be the major cause of "preventable" death. Alcohol can cause liver disease, various cancers, high blood pressure, and hemorrhagic stroke (cerebral hemorrhage) and steadily weakens the heart and muscle. Drinking with people can be elating, but too much alcohol can cause problems.

However, adequate amount of alcohol can be useful sometimes. A glass of drink before meals can help digestion, and it can relax our mind after a long, stressful day. Hanging out with friends and drinking can be a social booster. The physical and mental effects improve our health and well-being. Drinking alcohol increases HDL levels, which is a protective form of cholesterol. It blocks artery of the heart, neck, and brain, which is helpful to decreasing blood clots which ultimately cause heart failures and stroke. There is stark evidence that proper drinking prevents cardiac disease and ischemic stroke, and more studies show that it also prevents diabetes and gallstone.

However, even drinking appropriate amounts of alcohol can be a bit dangerous to both men and women. Alcohol hinders sleep and prevents clear judgment. Drinking a lot can interact with various medicines such as acetaminophen (a major ingredient of Tylenol), antidepressants, anticonvulsants, painkillers, and sedatives. Alcohol is toxic, and more so if there is a family history.

Pregnant women, those recovering from fetus alcohol addiction, liver ailment patients, and those who are on one or more medication that interacts with alcohol can't enjoy any benefits but only potential threats. Then who would benefit from drinking every day? A 60-year-old man who have high cholesterol levels and a family history where his father died at the age of 61 by heart failure (on the premise that he isn't an alcoholic) can enjoy benefits of a glass of alcohol a day, which far outweighs the potential risks. That is, alcohol in this case can work as a protective tool against cardiac disease. The risk-benefit calculation becomes a little bit tricky for a 60-year-old woman who has a sister suffering from breast cancer. The number of women who die from cardiac disease is more than ten times than that of death by breast cancer. Women are more afraid of contracting breast cancer than cardiac disease (death by breast cancer tends to occur in younger age groups than in cardiac disease), so this has to be taken into account.

"French paradox" came about from the study that adequate drinking can prevent heart failure and cardiac disease. French people take high-fat meals traditionally, but they have a low incidence rate of cardiac disease. Some research pointed to wine's good effects, and it is greatly supported by the wine industry. However, wine alone can't explain the low incidence rate of cardiac disease among the French. The Mediterranean-style meals in the southern part of France and other factors can be contributors. Recent studies show that any drink that contains alcohol can be beneficial as well.

Therefore, drinking habits are regarded as more important than the type of alcohol drinks. If you don't drink, it's not necessary to start by force. One glass a day by three times a week is more desirable than 3–4 glasses a day in a week.

Coffee and Tea

1. Coffee: many people like coffee for its energy-boosting effect and a little bit of head trip by caffeine. However, too much coffee can shake your body or give you a nervous breakdown or insomnia. Caffeine consumers who are addicted (by habit) tend to suffer from a strong headache if they skip their morning coffee. Espresso, French presses, and other coffee that don't go through the paper filter can slightly increase cholesterol levels. Other heavy drinkers of coffee have a higher possibility of contracting osteoporosis or fracture.

    Despite these downsides, drinking adequate amount of coffee can be safe, and it has several good effects:

    – Coffee lowers the possibility of kidney stone.
    – It lowers the possibility of gallstone.
    – It reduces risks of type 2 diabetes mellitus.
    – It diminishes suicide rates.

2. Tea: in 2737 BC, Shen Nung discovered the way to make tea through vegetable leaf. The black tea favored by Westerners is made by adding spice after the leaf withers. Green tea leaf, however, is dried after the leaf is steamed, so the polyphenol in the green leaf (it is a second metabolite that some of the carbohydrates are turned into when the green plant photosynthesizes. It is an antiaging and cancer-suppressing material that kills free radical) can be kept intact. Taking 300 mg of green tea extract a day is good for health. Some of the good sides of coffee also apply to tea. They include working as a stimulant for physical and mental health, lowering the risks of kidney stone and gallstone.

However, flavonoids (vegetable coloring) in tea are still disputed, so the good effects of tea up to date is nothing more concrete than giving a relief at the end of the day.

As the first step in catching the "three birds," it is desirable to combine various healthy lifestyle patterns and eating habits such as the Mediterranean-style meals mentioned in the book. Health diet is one of the most representative social medicines. Based on the various and concrete social therapies of health diet, I advise you to "eat enough breakfast, an adequate amount of lunch, and small portions of dinner."

3.2.1.2 Therapy of Social Medicine Derived from Health Exercise

Health exercise can be applied to all age groups. However, it can be more beneficial to senior citizens as we live in an aging society. In reality, more than 50 % of the senior population suffers from chronic disease. As for the healthy silver population, they need functional abilities necessary in daily life to maintain a dependent life.

It is known that effective exercise can prevent cardiovascular disease. Exercise not only has the effect of lowering traditional risk factors. The role of nitric oxide

(NO) is being emphasized. Nitric oxide makes it possible for the blood vessel to adapt functionally and structurally, thereby relaxing blood vessels. When you exercise, oxygen usage rate in the body goes up. Oxygen combined with hemoglobin is separated to flow into the tissues according to demand. The hemoglobin, which is separated from oxygen, becomes the catalyst that turns the precursor of nitric oxide into nitric oxide. The nitric oxide produced can be potential treatment for cardiac infarction, stroke, high blood pressure, and stomach ulcer. In short, the dynamic whole-body exercise promotes the production and transference of nitric oxide, and the good effects of exercise can remain.

Regular exercise improves fat in the blood in an ideal way. Exercise facilitates a fat-decomposing enzyme called lipoprotein lipase, and it gives positive stimulus through other fat metabolism enzymes so they can bear good results. When a lipid metabolism patient engages in regular exercise, he/she can benefit from various results such as increased cardiovascular endurance, decreased blood pressure and pulse, increased high-density cholesterol in the blood, diminished neutral fat, increased muscle strength, muscular endurance and flexibility, and lessened body fat. The more exercise the patient does, the bigger effect he/she can enjoy.

According to a 20-year-long study that was conducted by the Harvard University on 17,000 people, those who had a habit of exercising enjoyed longer life. The following is the results (Gong In-deok and Ye Byeong-il 2012b):

1. People who engage in light exercise often has greater life expectancy than those who don't.
2. Regular exercise can offset lessened life expectancy by smoking and overweight.
3. People with high blood pressure can benefit halved mortality rate when they engage in regular exercise.
4. Walking 16 km a week decreases 20 % of mortality rate than people who don't.
5. People with family history of early death can prolong life when they do regular exercise.
6. Active lifestyle including exercise prevents complications from cardiovascular disease.

The following is the guideline of health exercise with which you can alter your physical condition. With health exercise, you will be able to catch the "three birds," which are disease prevention, antiaging, and longevity. First, increase the time you move your body rather than sitting down. Second, start with a medium-hard exercise and avoid strenuous exercise. Third, the amount of exercise should be increased step by step. Fourth, perform muscle exercise together so that loss of muscle is diminished and engage in a variety of exercise. Fifth, do exercise according to your condition, and participate in group exercise with members with similar exercise skills. Lastly, manage the factors for chronic disease and prepare for damage.

Let's look at the reports by the American College of Sports Medicine and American Heart Association in 2007 on the basic recommendations for senior citizens for physical activities. Aerobic exercise should be conducted at least 5 times a week in medium intensity or at least 3 times a week in a slight strong intensity as in the case of healthy adults. Intensity of the exercise should be in line with personal ability. At least 10 min of exercise with minimum intensity of 50–60 % to maximum 70–80 %, with more than 30 min a day, is recommended.

Considering the facts, I attuned the social navigation to the characteristics of health exercise to catch the "three birds." Development of core muscle (it plays an important role in balancing the body and maintaining posture. When weakened, it can cause injuries in the body. It refers to the muscles that are located in the stomach, back, and pelvis) is the most important. It connects hip-body-stomach and focuses on the practical functions of the body such as "actions and movements." It is a more desirable target than the so-called slim "S-line" focused on muscles or "six-pack."

The three principles of health exercise are (1) balance and harmony of the body through core muscle, (2) stabilized posture, (3) and how to make the right posture. The five types of exercise include aerobic exercise, muscle strength, balance, posture, and flexibility. In particular, the seven HETs (Health Exercise Test) stressed in the balance exercise is useful in providing people with ways to catch the "three birds" in this aging society.

Aerobic Exercise

Aerobic exercise is needed for our body to contain enough oxygen and use it in the right time. In short, when our ability to deliver oxygen, which came into the body through breathing, to every corner of the body is improved, antioxidation and anti-aging skills will be improved.

Aerobic exercise should be conducted steadily for a limited period of time (more than 2 min) by increasing pulse and breathing. Walking, swimming, bicycling, and mountain climbing are representative exercises that mainly use legs. After the age of 40, strenuous exercise (e.g., jogging and running) can cause arthralgia or damages in the lower part of the body and is not recommended. In fact, health exercise refers to an ideal exercise conducted more than 30 min at a time almost every day, including a day's rest to restore stamina. However, resting for 2 days straight is not recommended.

As in Table 3.2 below, aerobic exercise should start from an easy one (step 1) and move upward (step 3). Begin with a low-intensity exercise of 5–10 min a day to the level where the pulse goes up to 100–120. As for endurance exercise, it should be increased steadily with the aim of more than 15–20 min. If your aim is to work out for 30 min, 10 min should be set aside for other types of exercise (Morley and Colberg 2008b).

1. Step 1 – walking: generally, people in the modern society take in 2500–3000 kcal a day by food. Natural consumption by metabolism takes away only about 1500 kcal, so the rest should be spent by extra movements or engaging in exercise, which is hard as the lifestyle is changing into doing less exercise. The first, easy step of aerobic exercise is "walking 10,000 steps."

Table 3.2 Aerobic exercise by intensity

Light exercise (step 1)	Walking slowly (below 3 km/h), trimming the garden (cutting grass, watering), housework (washing dishes), walking or kicking legs in the swimming pool with buoyancy belt on, sitting down without leaning, hitting Frisbee by pushing, playing golf while moving in a cart (* but most of these activities are too low-intensity activities to be included in the real exercise program once physical condition is improved)
Medium exercise (step 2)	Swimming, bicycling (outdoors), riding a fixed bike, gardening work (cutting grass, raking, hoeing), walking with power on the level ground, moping, playing golf without moving in a cart and moving with the club in hand, tennis (doubles), volleyball, rowing, water aerobics, chair movement, and dancing
Strenuous exercise (step 3)	Climbing stairs or hill, clearing away snow, quickly climbing hills on a bicycle, tennis (singles), going to and from a swimming pool lane, cross-country skiing, downhill skiing, mountain climbing, jogging, running, and most sports (soccer, basketball)

Source: *The Science of Staying Young*, 2009, p. 81

The following are several ways to keep this as everyday habit. First, remember BMW. It stands for bus (B), metro (M), and walking (W). Second is 1-2-3 exercise. This exercise is promoted in the "Korea Walking Federation (www.walking.kr)." 1 stands for walking at least the distance of one station, 2 for walking at least up to 2 km, and 3 for climbing the stairs for at least to the third floor. Not engaging in exercise becomes the cause for chronic diseases such as diabetes, obesity, and metabolic syndrome.

When walking, it is better to move your arms actively rather than walking only with legs. Drinking water can be good when thirsty, but it is more desirable to drink it occasionally little by little before getting too much thirsty. Regularly repeating walking and taking rests, 50 min and 10 min each, is recommended. To get benefit out of exercise, it is good to walk more than 30 min a day every day, without taking a rest. You should wear comfortable shoes, so that soaring feet shouldn't hinder walking (Gong In-Duk and Ye Byung-Il 2012c).

2. Step 2 – interval training: when the step 1 aerobic exercise is completed, it is advised to upgrade your goal, which is to conduct interval training. Interval training is a very hard exercise, but it is less boring as it is not about engaging in exercise with the same intensity. Relatively in a short period of time, you can experience the same effect and exercise amount as done in long hours. In interval exercise, you work out in a higher intensity than you're adapted to, so the oxygen usage ability of the muscle can be improved as well.

Interval training is composed of 5–10 min of pre-exercise. Next, 3 min of exercise similar to step 1 (standard of 50–70 % of pulse) should be performed. After 3 min comes 1 min of exercise in the level of step 2, at the 80–90 % of pulse (Table 3.3).

In the beginning of the exercise, prolong the rest period. When adjusted, the time gap between the exercise and rest should be narrowed down. In the early days, make sure the intensity gap of exercises between the two periods is not too wide, but steadily enlarge the gap as time flows. This method is useful when you

Table 3.3 Time arrangement in interval training

Phase of exercise	Pre-exercise	Rest period	Exercise period	Rest period	Exercise period	Rest period	Wrap-up exercise
Time	5 min	3 min	1 min	3 min	1 min	3 min	5 min
Pulse	40–60 %	50–70 %	80–90 %	50–70 %	80–90 %	50–70 %	40–60 %

Table 3.4 Time arrangement in jumping up training

Phase of exercise	Pre-exercise	Aerobic period	High-intensity period	Aerobic period	Wrap-up exercise
Time	5 min	Pulse	1–3 min	Pulse	5 min
Pulse	40–60 %	60–70 %	85–100 %	80–90 %	40–60 %

exercise outdoors, where landscapes are composed of uphill and downhill. Step 2 exercise should be mixed with step 1 exercise. Step 2 exercise should be conducted once a week with step 1 exercise or alternate with it day by day (Song Yung-Kyu 2011a).

3. Step 3 – jumping up from the floor: step 3 exercise is an aerobic exercise that can also improve flexibility. As it is strenuous exercise, patients with cardiovascular disease or metabolism symptoms should be careful. Once a week or twice a month is recommended.

   After pre-exercise, engage in pulse 60–70 % of intensity. Slowly increase intensity to reach more than 85 % and maintain the status for a minute. Steadily lower the intensity to 60–70 % and do the wrap-up exercise (Table 3.4).

   By alternating between the high-intensity exercises, flexibility and muscle strength can be improved, and much energy can be consumed. However, it should be conducted according to one's physical strength and condition, and exercise schedule should be adjusted to your daily physical condition. If the exercise gives you fatigue and it lasts until the day after, the intensity of the exercise should be lowered or you should wait until you're more prepared (Song Yung-Kyu 2011b).

Muscle Exercise

Muscles in our body are divided into three parts. First, there is entrail muscle, which is the muscle in the inner organ. Second is the myocardium of the heart muscle, and third is skeletal muscle, which is on the bones and conducts outer activities and exercise. The red muscle, which is often called as flesh, has color red due to myoglobin that stores oxygen. Red muscle has higher content of myoglobin in the muscle fiber than the white muscle and therefore has much oxygen. The red muscle fiber is very important in conducting aerobic exercise for long periods of time.

Slow-twitch muscle fiber is also called slow muscle fibers, and although it contracts slowly, it is good for long periods of exercise and activity as it rarely feels fatigue. Energy that moves slow muscle fibers is mostly carbohydrate and fat. Long duration of exercise, where slow muscle fibers are used, is good in weight control and improving cardiovascular functions.

However, white muscle fiber has low oxygen, that is, low myoglobin content, and can't be used for more than several minutes. Therefore, it gets tired easily, and fat is not burned when white muscle is used. However, white muscle fiber can let out greater force rapidly compared to the red muscle fiber. White muscle fiber can contract quickly and is suitable for doing rapid movements and letting out great force right away. That is why it's called fast-twitch muscle fiber. Energy in the fast-twitch muscle fiber is muscle glycogen and chemical fuel, and they are stored in the muscle. The stored amount is limited, so it's hard to be sustained for a long time and induce feelings of fatigue easily.

Mostly, people have 55 % of red muscle fiber and 45 % of white muscle fiber. As for long-distance marathon runners, 80 % of their muscle is red muscle fiber. However, 100 m-distance marathoners have up to 70 % of white muscle fiber. The ratio is almost inherent, and that's why people say marathoners are born with the ability.

Aging process eats away muscle, and the white muscle fiber diminishes more and faster. In order to strengthen white muscle, exercising in a speedy manner under strong intensity is needed, with great force. Letting out large force in a second is called "flexibility" or "power." (Song Yung-Kyu 2011c).

In muscle exercise, muscle burns oxygen and sugar when it contracts. The waste is carbon dioxide. Through the detox mechanism of our body, it melts in the blood as carbon and moves around the body, and when it enters the lung, it turns into gas and is emitted through breath. However, if you engage in more powerful anaerobic exercise, another waste, lactic acid, is produced. Anaerobic exercise burn sugar faster than oxygen is taken in, so energy consumption gets abnormally greater. When the situation persists (when you don't have the time for detox mechanism), muscle pain arises in the body and prevents the body from engaging in any more exercise. When the exercise is stopped, our body immediately goes into detox mechanism and lets out lactic acid, and this is how the natural healing power (NHP) of our bodyworks (Lee Yung-Keun and Choi Joon-Yung 2011c).

In fact, for the last several decades, lactic acid was thought of as waste from the process that limits metabolism. However, new studies show that lactic acid is not a mere waste but a substrate that produces blood sugar in the exercise. Lactic acid is also reported to provide energy necessary for skeletal muscles and the heart (Brooks 1986a, b; Hargreaves 1995), and this is how the mechanism goes. A limited amount of lactic acid that is produced from the skeletal muscles in exercise is delivered to the liver through blood. Then lactic acid in the liver is turned into glucose through glucose birth process. New glucose is emitted through blood and is taken back to the skeletal muscles to be used as energy source in exercise. The process where lactic acid is turned into glucose from the muscle and the liver is called "Cori cycle." Lactic acid circulates through "lactic acid transport" in our body while we exercise and has various benefits, in the order of importance: (1) exercise muscle, (2) the liver and kidney and (3) the heart (Powers and Howley 2008).

Taking enough protein can help us sustain physical strength in the aging process. The component of protein is amino acid. When the aging process takes place, we need more protein to form, maintain, and restore body protein structure such as muscle. For instance, adults over 50 years old need at least 1.1 g of protein per kilogram of his weight. However, about 0.8 g is sufficient for those who are under the age of 50. It is also known that a specific amino acids' compound is important to maintain muscle strength. For instance, athletes such as weightlifting players need creatine supplements along with muscle exercise to boost physical strength. In the same sense, leucine, found in the milk serum protein of milk, is an essential amino acid for muscle so should be taken adequately.

Stress is needed for the growth of the muscle. Here, let's look at weight training, an exercise too boost muscle strength and muscle endurance, and squat jump for promoting flexibility:

1. Weight training: weight training is imposing heavy weight on the muscle to enlarge the size of muscle fiber and to induce biochemical changes in the muscle so that it's easier to let out muscle strength and muscle endurance. Three types of muscle contractions are accompanied. First, isotonic contraction is an active contraction where power is produced as muscle length is shortened. Second, isometric contraction refers to the slow contraction where the length of the muscle stays the same when power is let out. Third is isokinetic contraction, where the length of the muscle is shortened and is done at the same speed throughout the entire process of the exercise. The method of exercise differs on what type of muscle contraction you use. Most people are acquainted with weight training by isotonic contraction (active contraction).

    The total sum of tension produced in the muscle contraction process, that is, the amount of power that the muscle can let out at one time, is called "muscular strength." Muscular strength is proportionate to the number of muscle fiber that is mobilized in the contraction of the muscle, as well as the cross size of the muscle fiber. It is determined by the frequency of immediate impulse that stimulates muscle fiber. Muscle fiber is governed by motor nerve, and the composition of muscle fiber that is mobilized with one motor nerve is called "motor unit." According to the type of exercise, motor nerve lets out muscular power by determining the mobilized motor unit and the type and number of muscle fiber. Therefore, muscular strength is highly influenced by the development of motor nerve and muscle fiber.

    Therefore, increased muscular strength needs activation of nervous system and hypertrophy of muscle fiber. In the early days of muscle training, the nervous system is activated to increase frequency of stimulus and the number of exercise unit that is mobilized, promoting interaction between muscles. In the middle of muscle training, hypertrophy is produced through combination tissue and thickness of muscle fiber, which increases muscle strength. Then how to boost and strengthen muscle strength? You can use barbell, dumbbell, and weight tools, which use outside resistance of weight as load. Others include using an elastic body such as rubber tube and spring, using a training partner's weight as load, and using resistance of outside environment such as sandy beach, up/downhill, and climbing stairs.

Muscle endurance enables you to keep exercising for a long time. It is based on the storage status of energy source and the development stage of slow muscle fiber and energy carrier system. To develop muscle endurance, the number of slow muscle fiber that has high content of myoglobin and muscle glycogen storage amount should be increased by low-intensive training. In addition, the number of capillary vessels and their bores should be enlarged to respond effectively when moving oxygen. Moreover, lactic acid and carbon dioxide, emitted when exercising, should be rapidly eradicated.

In short, the purpose of weight training is to improve muscle strength and muscle endurance. Generally, people engage in weight training as a way of body building, which is to promote health and to look fit. The following Table 3.5 is the major sports of weight training and the muscles they focus on growing (Kim Jae-Ho et al. 2004a).

2. Squat jump: it is an exercise to improve flexibility and to make you agile. The following is the detailed ways of exercising:

   1. Stand with the feet at shoulders' length. Straighten your back and put both of your hands on the hind of the neck.
   2. Bend your knees and hips so thighs can be in parallel with the ground. Then immediately straighten your legs and jump as high as you can.
   3. After landing, take 1–2 s of rest and repeat the cycle. It is good to do the exercise about two to three times a week regularly (Song Yung-Kyu 2011d).

BalanceExercise

If the focus is on the individual muscles in muscle and muscle strength exercise, it may not be suitable for the entire body. As you age, exercise amount and moving distance lessen, and the ability of the joints are decreased. In this case, the harmony of the entire body is important, which is an essential part of preventing injuries. Only focusing on muscle exercise with the hope of restoring the healthy and energetic past is not preferable. It is more important to make a physical condition so you can do the things that you were able to do, rather than making your body full of muscle.

When limbs move, the backbone and pelvis strike a balance and move together. The basic force of the body is called "mobility" and "stability." Mobility enables us to stretch our arms and to bend our legs. Stability can maintain and strike a balance of the body when doing the actions. Therefore, both mobility and stability are needed for daily life (Song Yung-Kyu 2011e).

The Health Exercise Test, or "HET," is composed of seven components. It is not newly developed and was developed by the renowned trainer Gray Cook, who

Table 3.5 Major sports of weight training and strengthened muscle

	Sports	Improved muscle	Main parts
Wrist exercise	1. Wrist curl	1. Palmar muscle, radial flexor of wrist	1. Arm (fore)
	2. Wrist abduction	2. Extensor carpi radialis longus muscle, extensor carpi radialis brevis muscle	2. Wrist (side)
Upper-part exercise	3. Two-hand curl	3. Biceps brachii, antebrachial muscles	3. Arm (fore)
	4. Concentration curl	4. Biceps brachii, antebrachial muscles	4. Arm (fore)
	5. French press	5. Deltoids, musculus triceps brachii, pectoralis major muscle	5. Shoulder
	6. Standing press	6. Deltoids, musculus triceps brachii, pectoralis major muscle	6. Shoulder
	7. Alternate press	7. Trapezius muscle, deltoids, Musculus triceps brachii	7. Shoulder
	8. Back press	8. Deltoids, trapezius muscle, pectoralis major muscle	8. Shoulder
	9. Bench press	9. Pectoralis major muscle, musculus triceps brachii, deltoid	9. Chest
	10. Lateral raise	10. Pectoralis major muscle, deltoids	10. Chest
	11. Straight-arm pullover	11. Pectoralis major muscle, latissimus dorsi muscle	11. Chest
Back and stomach exercise	12. Sit-up	12. Musculus rectus abdominis, outer musculus rectus abdominis	12. Stomach
	13. Side bend	13. External oblique, musculus rectus abdominis	13. Flank
	14. Bend over	14. Gluteus maximus, intrinsic muscles of back	14. Back
	15. Bend over rowing	15. Intrinsic muscles of the back, gluteus maximus, deltoids, trapezius muscle	15. Back, shoulder
Lower-part exercise	16. Squat	16. Quadriceps muscle of the thigh, intrinsic muscles of the back, gluteus maximus	16. Legs
	17. Leg extension	17. Musculus rectus femoris, midvastus, musculus vastus lateralis	17. Legs
	18. Leg press	18. Quadriceps muscle of the thigh, gluteus maximus	18. Legs
	19. Leg curl	19. Biceps femoris	19. Legs

Source: *Health and Exercise*, 2004, p. 178

developed FMS (Functional Movement Screening) in 2001 by analyzing the functions of our body by looking at the bodily movements. The following is quoted from his seven components:

[7 HETs]

1. Deep squat: your hips go down as far as they can in a sitting position in deep squat. Generally, squat is the "king of the muscle strength improving exercise." It is maintaining body weight by one leg, and you repeat standing up and sitting down in the position. As you need to keep balance, the muscles are developed evenly than any other exercise. If you have a weak hip muscle, you will twist your body. In the case of deep squat, the knees and the hip joints should bend well, and the ankles should be able to feel whether the center of weight changes or not and to sustain it. The waist shouldn't lose balance, and if the muscles in the hips, the waist, or the thigh are not flexible, it will be impossible to maintain a good position and you will end up bending over. To seat deeply in this exercise, you need the mobility of the arms and legs, along with the stability of the pelvis and the core muscles, and the ability to control the changing position. The following is a detailed exercise tip:

   1. Grab the stick with both hands, and point the tip of the feet to the front. Put your feet in shoulders' length.
   2. Straighten your elbows over your head as you raise the stick.
   3. Slowly sit deeply, and don't let the knees go over the tip of the feet. Maintain a straightened position of the chest.

   In this case, the chest should be in parallel with the shinbone (shin) as you sit down, and the thighbone should be situated below the knees. The knees should be put over the feet in a way that is not on the inside or the outside, and the feet shouldn't turn whether inside or outside. The feet should then be glued to the ground. When performing the exercise, the back should be straightened and the arms and chest should be in parallel. It is score 2 when only the back of the heels are in the air. When there are other shortcomings, the score is 1 and 0 if you feel any pain in doing the exercise.

2. Hurdle step: it is an action where you go over a barrier by striking a balance with one leg. Various parts in your body should move together, and you should be able to control the actions. In order not to twist the posture, you need the stability of the pelvis and the core muscle. The ability to evenly disperse your weight as you move with one leg is needed. The following is the detailed way of exercising:

   1. Use a hurdle that is slightly lower (2–3 cm) than your knees.
   2. Start with both your feet right next to each other. Put the stick on your shoulder when grabbing.
   3. Straighten your back and raise your legs over the hurdle.
   4. Do the same exercise with the other leg as well.

   The main point of this exercise is to move the upper and the lower part of your body in a line. When a movement in the waist shoves the stick on the shoulder, it is score 2, 1 if the feet trips over the hurdle, and 0 if you feel pain in performing the exercise.

3. Inline lunge: it is a sitting-down position with the feet in a line. The ability to decelerate your actions is essential. The action calls for a high sense of stability,

so the ability to disperse your weight, to maintain balance, and to move the feet under your control is needed. The following is the detailed way of exercising:

1. Put your feet in a line, one at the front and the other at the back.
2. The distance between the two feet should be close so that when you bend the knees, the hind knee touches the back heel of the front feet.
3. Hold the stick behind your back, and straighten your chest.
4. Bend your hind knee so as to touch the ground.
5. Do the same exercise with the other feet as well.

   This action calls for special balance. It is a way to see the stability of the most joints in the lower part of your body from the ankle to the hip joint. There shouldn't be any movement in the upper body, and the position of the feet should remain unchanged. The hind knee should touch on the floor, and the body shouldn't sway to the left or to the right. When the waist is bent or the knees don't touch the ground or when the body sways to either side, the score is 2. It is 1 if you almost lose all balance and 0 if you feel pain in conducting the exercise.

4. Shoulder joint mobility: as aging process kicks in, it gets harder to make large movements. However, different from knees or elbows, shoulders can move in various directions, so the mobility and the stability of the shoulders can be maintained when you promote flexibility in all directions. In particular, movements can occur in various directions from the shoulder joint, such as internal version, abdominal version, introversion, extroversion, and bending. Therefore, it's not only about the ability of shoulder movement. Various parts in the chest such as the thoracic area and thorax should participate in the movement. The following is the detailed exercise method:

   1. Put your thumb in the inner part of the palm and curl other fingers into a fist.
   2. Touch both your hands behind your back.
   3. Do it once again with the other thumb.

   In this exercise, the shorter the distance between the rocks, the better mobility you have. When the mobility of the thoracic area decreases and the shoulder girdle can't move on the shoulder in a stable manner, or when there is a problem in the position of a round shoulder, the mobility of the shoulder joint can be lowered. If the actions on both parts are different, observe it steadily, and engage in exercise where you can improve the stability of the core muscles in the right position. If the rock of your hand is situated from a rock-length distance, or in the distance of 1.5 times, the score is 2. If it's over then it is 1 and 0 if you feel pain doing the exercise.

5. Raising legs: raising your legs in the lying position seems like you're only bending the hip joint of your legs. However, to do the action correctly, you need a stable pelvis, back, and abdomen so that other parts aren't engaged when you raise your legs. You need flexibility of the hamstring muscle (it is femoral muscle and refers to the four muscles on the front, the back, and the inner part) and the iliopsoas muscle (it is the combination of psoas major and iliacus (the muscle that is situated near the groin of the leg near the floor)). The following is the detailed exercise method:

1. As you lie down, the hands should face upward and the arms should be placed on the sides of the body.
2. The tip of the feet should be pushed to the body, and the legs should be raised as high as you can.
3. Take heed that the waist and the hips don't move.
4. Do the same exercise for both legs.

In order to conduct the exercise well, the muscles in the hips, the waist, and the hamstring shouldn't limit the movements. When you raise your legs, the functions should be controlled easily. If the ankle bone of the ankle is placed between the knees and the anterior superior iliac spine, or ASIS, the score is 1. It is 0 if you feel any pain conducting the movements.

6. Push up (for body stabilization): push up is a representative exercise that uses your weight. Here, you put your hands at a higher point than general push up, so the stability of the body can be evaluated. If the hips or the waist is twisted or is bent too much, the core muscles in body are not doing their job. The following is the detailed exercise method:

1. Perform it as in general push up. As for men, the point of the hands in the beginning should start from the top of the head. As for women, it should start from the jaw.
2. Lift up your body and try not to bend the waist and hips.

In doing the exercise, the easier position for you to perform becomes the barometer of the stability of the core muscles. If you can lift your body without lagging position of the waist and hips, it will be score 2, 1 if there are changes in the position, and 0 if you feel pain in conducting the exercise.

7. Turn stability: it is a test to see if the stability of the shoulder girdle, which manages the pelvis, the core muscles, and the movements of the shoulders, is controlled when you move both the upper and lower part of your body as you crouch on all fours. It includes a variety of movements that include bending and twisting, going beyond simply bending and stretching. It is a complex exercise that is higher level than general movements. The following is the detailed movements:

1. Put your knees and palms on the floor, and crouch on all fours.
2. Stretch one arm and a leg so they can be in parallel with the body.
3. If the arms and leg on the same part can't be used, stretch one arm and the other leg.
4. Bring in the elbow and the knee that were stretched to the body so they can touch each other.
5. Do the same exercise with the other arm and leg as well.

It is hard to maintain balance and position when you raise the arm and the leg (on the same side) and engage in stretching and bending exercise. If you can perform the action flawlessly (score 3), it means you can move and control the center balance of your body even in an unstable position. If you lose balance or your knees and elbows can't touch each other (score 2), use the arm and leg on the other side. If you can't do this (score 1), the stability of your body and core muscle is diminished, as well as the stability and the mobility of the shoulder girdle and hip joint. If pain occurs in doing the action, it is score 0 (Song Yung-Kyu 2011f).

Posture

If your body loses balance when you engage in aerobic or muscle strengthexercise, it will not be a good sight and it will be inefficient as you move about in your daily life, and you will feel easily tired. The reason many people sit with their back slouched in the chair or with their legs twisted is because the position is easier to make, as it uses less muscles. However, the "comfortable" postures make us use less of our muscles, weaken them, and gradually destruct the form of our body. When the posture of the body is deformed and twisted, functions of a healthy body are degraded and will have limited exercise effects. As you can see, posture affects the function of the body and the appearance, so it should be checked periodically.

Recent research reports that the more time you sit down, the more danger there is to cardiovascular diseases ("aging of the blood vessel") and you get to die early due to the gradually reducing life span. The muscles you use when you stand up or move aren't used anymore when you sit down. Hip muscle is a glaring example. With time, the muscle amount decreases and the hips become lagging, and the place where the muscle used to be is replaced by fat. When hip muscle decreases, the body looks bent. The changed location of the pelvis moves and flattens the lumbar, the hind part of the spine, and it hinders hip muscle development.

※ Hip exercise (raising the legs in lie-down position): the basic exercise of the hips is to raise your legs in lie-down position. Generally, exercise for hip muscle is to stretch your legs to the back of the body (one direction). However, the hip muscles don't work in one direction, so it is good to move the muscle in multiple directions. This exercise is recommended for curing most leg-related diseases or recovering from injuries.

It is to raise your leg in each direction and is performed in lie-down with the face up or down. When doing the exercise, legs should be stretched far out. The actions shouldn't be rushed. About 2–3 times a week, 12–20 times at a time are recommended (Song Yung-Kyu 2011g).

Flexibility Exercise

Flexibility refers to the ability where the joints and the muscles can move to their fullest. It depends on the elasticity of the muscle and the developmental status of the joint and tendon. When flexibility is practiced at an early age, it can be maintained throughout the old ages, but if not, the ability can be significantly diminished even at an early age. Being flexible means you can be good at exercise. It is more meaningful as you can prevent injuries and can eliminate a great cause for pain, even in later life.

Therefore, flexibility prevents exercise disorder and injuries and is used as a barometer for youth. It is the most important factor in daily life exercise. However strong your muscle is, if you are not flexible, you can't use the great physical strength. When contraction of the muscle or damage in the tendon hurts flexibility, it can cause injuries or pain and can even bring out abnormal posture.

There are two major reasons of flexibility degradation. First is the lack of effort to maintain or increase flexibility from childhood. Second is the lack of elasticity of the muscle due to the aging process and abnormality in the muscle due to the wrong body movements and injuries. If you don't engage in activities much, contraction force is produced in the combination tissue and makes the muscle shorter and weaker.

In short, flexibility is the ability to move freely in the range of normal joint movement. As people age, people tend to see less flexibility. However, we need confidence to claim victory with health exercise. Here, let's look at the factors that affect flexibility and then look into the stretching techniques that increase flexibility.

Muscles in our body can be categorized into two groups. The first group is the muscle group of which the life span is shortened when you don't exercise or when strenuous exercise is performed without basic exercise. The second group is another muscle group that elongates as it weakens. In the case of muscle contraction, found in people who rarely engage in physical activities, the contracted muscle group should be normalized first before engaging in balancing exercise, rather than strengthening the weakened muscle group. For instance, it occurs frequently for people who play the tennis or golf without basic exercise. A person who can't sit comfortably on the floor also suffers from contraction of the thigh muscles. Even if you have good physical health and flexibility, lack of balance on both sides of the body will cause abnormality in either side (Sul Joon-Hee 2012).

3.2.1.3 The Characteristics of StretchingExercise

Flexibility can be improved through stretching exercise. The good sides of the exercise are as follows: (1) it eases muscle tension, (2) it improves the cooperation of the body, (3) it prevents injuries such as the wrench of muscles, (4) it is possible to perform strong movements in various sports, (5) it increases the awakening of the level of the body by communication between body and mind, (6) it helps the flow of blood circulation, (7) and lastly, it makes you comfortable.

1. Active stretching: active stretching utilizing elasticity is a traditional method. It is to give rebound to stretch the tissues that are combined with the muscle or to shake the body in every direction. The repeated contraction of the agonist is used to bring about rapid contraction of the antagonist. (Agonist is a muscle group that is in charge of the action when we bend and stretch the limbs. In flexion exercise, flexor muscle becomes the agonist, and extensor muscle takes the place in extension exercise. Antagonist muscle numbers up to 1 trillion and has contrast workings such as the flexor muscle and extensor muscle of the limbs.) The twists and the pulling in the exercise increase the moving extent of the joints. The method can enlarge the muscle quickly, but if the stimulus is greater than expansibility of the tissue, it can cause injury or muscle pain.

2. Passive stretching: the slow and passive stretching method is to stretch the muscle around the joint and the combining tissues at the extreme of the joint workings. The method quickly adapts to the location where the active part of the muscle spindles (a spinning wheel-shaped organ that checks contraction degree of the striped muscle) is elongated, so the force of the muscle to come back to its original state decreases. This diminishes reactive contraction of the muscle, and by slowly stretching the targeted muscle and tissue, it is to prolong the time you feel a little pulling of the muscle. The biggest advantage of the passive stretching is there is a less likelihood of the dangers in the tissue or break of muscle pain that can occur in active stretching.

3.2.1.4   The Guidelines of Stretching Exercise

1. Type of exercise: perform stretching exercise to increase flexibility by maintaining the same posture for some time. Here, you shouldn't give a rebound to the muscle and tendon but slowly stretch them. Include exercising the body parts such as the face, neck, shoulders, arms, flank, waist, back, hips, legs, and ankles. First, perform 6–8 exercises per muscle and joint. When you get accustomed, gradually increase the types of exercise.
2. Exercise time: first, slowly move to make an extended posture (where your joints are stretched). Maintain the posture for 6 s and gradually give overload to the muscle group. To boost flexibility, maintain the extended posture for up to about 30 s. Stretch some more to the extent that you feel some pain in the muscle. It is important to keep the muscles warm (muscle temperature), so make sure the rest time between the sets don't go over 1 min. The entire exercise time should be 5 min in the beginning. It should be extended up to 10–15 min.
3. Frequency of exercise: to boost flexibility, stretching exercise should be performed at least 3–4 times a week or everyday if possible. The effect can be felt after at least 4 weeks of exercise. To maintain flexibility, the exercise should be conducted at least 1–2 times a week. It is desirable to do the stretching before and after main exercise or when doing your daily chores.
4. Breathing and counting: don't stop breathing and keep it natural. Taking a deep breath and starting the stretching and letting out breaths as you extend is one way. Count seconds silently in each exercise. In this case, you can maintain tension for a limited amount of time. When you feel accustomed at counting, do the stretching by feeling (not actually counting out aloud).
5. Attention: don't do the stretching exercise if it gives you much pain. Injuries may arise when you stretch waist muscles, so be especially careful. For the first 2–3 weeks, it is wise to avoid excessive stretching.
6. Tips: if you engage in fast walking or jogging in slow steps before stretching, it can increase "muscle temperature" and you can safely enjoy the stretching exercise. Rebound actions can cause not only extension but also contraction of the muscle, so it can result in inefficiency of stretching and muscle pain. Lastly, doing the exercise with a rhythmical music can boost exercise effect (Kim Jae-Ho et al. 2004b).

Exercise and Weather

Weather plays an important role in exercise, and you should be careful when doing exercise in hot weather. Exercise too burdensome on the body should be avoided, so don't sweat too much or persist in exercise by ignoring pain. You sweat in exercising because the skin has to emit heat through sweat. The heat emitted from our body turns into heat necessary for going out, so it cools down the skin. Therefore, when blood vessels are enlarged to control temperature, and sweat is emitted through the skin, the body is likely to suffer from lack of moisture.

Dehydration significantly decreases the effect of aerobic exercise and mental functions. When it is not corrected immediately, you can lose consciousness or can suffer from lowered neurological function. When more than 3 % of the weight is dehydrated, the risks for heat dehydration or heatstroke are increased. Various symptoms such as skeletal muscle spasm, which is caused by the loss of electrolyte apart from water, can occur.

Therefore, while it is important to drink water when you are thirsty, it is more desirable to make yourself not thirsty. Water and sports drinks can both supplement moisture, but the soft drinks containing much carbon dioxide and glucose don't help much to quench the thirst, though helpful in elating the spirits. Electrolyte and salt go out with sweat, so 1–2 g of salt per liter of water should be taken in along with electrolyte.

In summary, our body's adaption abilities can be hurt when you exercise suddenly in a hot weather. Therefore, exercise amount should be gradually increased. On the first day, 20 min of exercise in the shade is good, followed by 20 min of rest. In the duration of 2 weeks, the amount of exercise and time should be increased gradually. Early in the morning or at night, rather than afternoon hours, is better for exercise as the temperature is lower (Gong In-Duk and Ye Byung-Il 2012d).

> When four weeks pass after strenuous exercise, capillaries that used to be situated side by side in the muscles, due to exercise, go back to the level of pre-exercising. The capillaries were organized tightly side by side so they could effectively provide oxygen to the muscle upon immediate demand. When you stop exercising, capillaries diminish, and the oxygen usage rate of the body also goes down. Even if the muscles were made through strenuous exercise, five months of rest would make all muscles disappear.
>
> The characteristics of the muscle also change. The trait of the so-called red and white muscles change, and you feel fatigue easily, and efficiency of movements is lowered. Not only the figure of the body change, but also the vitality of the body is lost. If you engage in fewer activities than normal level, the fat from internal organs that is situated in the depths of the abdomen rapidly increases. In a study, people who used to walk as much as 10,000 steps were asked to walk within 1,500 steps for two weeks. In the short period, the increased fat of internal organs was a striking 7 %. If three weeks pass in this state, the sensitivity towards insulin also diminishes.
>
> In just the period of one month, moving less than before or not engaging in exercise can create in-depth changes. When we think about this in "body age," you gain fat easily and the ability to use necessary nutrients and oxygen is lowered. The muscle content in the body is decreased, so the body becomes "aged." Even if you exercised hard, it's just an instant before you go back to the old self. (Song Yung-Kyu 2011h)

Youth never lasts forever, and the same goes for muscles. When you lie down 1 day, it's similar to adding 1 year to your age. We learned through social medicine therapy derived from health exercise that we can overcome hot weather and move our body freely, overcoming the weight and gravity that pushes us down every single minute. We can conduct health exercise regularly in our everyday life and correct our behaviors. It is wise to keep holding to belief that we can catch the "three birds" with one stone.

3.2.1.5 Therapy of Social Medicine Derived from Health Stressor

People living through infinite competition in the modern society are burned out and are becoming magnets to various diseases. Stress is like a shadow to the city people. Stress is a process where life shows non-special responses to stress it experiences. It puts people in the state of disease, and the following three are the major methods of stress' working. First, stress comes through the autonomic nervous system, followed by the endocrine system and immune system. One of the representative ways among these are through the autonomic nervous system, and indigestion is a glaring case (Gong In-Duk and Ye Byung-Il 2012e). The various responses in the heart are expressed through the body via the autonomic nervous system, and that's why mind and body are reflected in each other like the other side of the coin.

Generally, feelings are temporary and don't last long and don't have fatal effect on the body. However, if certain feelings are expressed chronically, such as feeling depressed (depression), it has an impact on various bodily functions and even destroys metabolism. Therefore, chronic stress is the main culprit that drives various conditions such as aging, depression, arthritis, and diabetes. The following is the detailed mechanism.

First, when there is a chronic stress, the steroid coming out of the body can't follow up with the demanding amount. Furthermore, a hormone organ called adrenal gland, which produces steroid, feels tired and the production of the steroid decreases or stops. In this case, the transfer from omega 6 to arachidonic acid can't be repressed, and type 2 of PG (prostaglandin, a substance that induces inflammation in the body which acts differently in each tissue) is produced. As a response, white bloodcells and immune cells are activated and make much free radical in cells, which results in inflammation in our body (Lee Yung-Keun and Choi Joon-Yung 2011d).

In short, along with toxic materials that come from the outside, free radical inevitably produced from the metabolism of the body, the incorrect diet and the fatigue from overwork, and chronic stress cause much free radical that destroys our body. The main culprit that deters our health is chronic stress, but there is no silver bullet to tackle the condition (using drugs to get away from stress is not helpful, and it is like locking yourself up in a prison called, "addiction." The warning from epigenetics is it can pass down the stress genes to your children). The core issue and target of the social medicine therapy derived from health stressor is to discover ways to make a "healthy mind" through diminishing or eliminating chronic stress.

Health Exercise Makes Healthy Mind

In the old saying it goes, "a sound mind in a sound body." This is proven true as almost all exercise can induce the secretion of endorphin (endorphin is a peptide that is similar to morphine which is repeatedly extracted from hypothalamus and posterior pituitary of an animal's brain. It combines in a unique way with the acceptor of narcotic painkillers such as morphine and is a natural painkiller that is not addictive. The effect of endorphin is 200 times stronger than morphine, and it isn't produced automatically in the body but is related to the status of the heart). When we exercise, we are rewarded with feelings of relaxation, confidence, and positive attitude. This is used in the secretion of endorphin, and this is called "runner's high" (happiness that is felt when more than 30 min of medium-intensive exercise continues).

In short, health exercise not only reduces chronic stress but also increases a sense of balance. By maintaining a healthy state of the body, you can be more satisfied with yourself. As strength and vitality are restored, anxiety, depression, tension of the muscle and jaw joints, expressionless face, neck pain, diarrhea, fast heartbeat, hastiness, chronic fatigue, indigestion, and sleep disorder begin to fade away (Shrand and Devine 2013a). Now you can see that the relationship between health exercise and the secretion of endorphin can't be separated. Health exercise makes endorphin in our body, and just like "invisible hands," the workings of the endorphin bring a healthy mind.

Furthermore, the phrase "move your body" doesn't only stick to health exercise. In health stressor aspect, we should increase the amount we sleep, laugh, socialize with people, and spend time out in the nature so that chronic stress doesn't make itself a home in our body. For instance, the ordinary days can be categorized into good days and bad days, and the latter can be made into a good one when we do some extra work for our health. Let's look at the examples below:

> Adding 30 minutes of sleeping time or one hour of social activity can be a barometer that separates a good day from an ordinary day. Changing a little part of our daily life can increase the quality of life greatly. Surprisingly, a small difference in the sleeping hours can make you much more pleasant the next day. People who had a good day had 7.1 hours of good sleep the other night on average. On the other hand, people who went through a difficult day had 6.6 hours of sleep on average. It was only 30 minutes that set apart a good day and a bad day. The amount of time spent on social activities is another factor that distinguishes a good day from a bad day. Those who had a better day than the rest spent 1.4 hours more on social activities than others. (Tom Rath and Jim Harter 2010b)

An interesting fact was revealed regarding health exercise recently. There is a movement called "green movement," and it is described in a thesis in the online edition of *Environmental Science and Technology* (Mar. 25, 2010). Barton and Pretty of Essex University in the UK argued that a small amount of exercise every day can improve our health. When exercise was conducted for 5 min a day, it was argued to help improve peoples' mood, self-evaluation, and mental health. "Green movement" here refers to doing activities out in the nature. In this study, the ways of measuring how much you were exposed to nature was introduced for the first time.

About 1252 people from various age groups participated in the study, and they did ten outdoor activities including gardening, walking, bicycling, boarding, fishing, horseback riding, and farming. The results showed that the activities helped them a lot in improving their mentalhealth.

In "green movement," the effect gets stronger even if you increase either exercise intensity or time. The effects of exercise continued as well, as it took some time for the effects of the exercise to wear out. This was even so when people stopped exercising the moment they saw the effects took place. Lastly, the exercise effect was greater when people worked out places near water, for instance, a lake or a pond, rather than working out indoors or on dry ground. Therefore, we can see that doing exercise out in the wild is more effective. "The exercise environment offers a good health service" (Gong In-Duk and Ye Byung-Il 2012f). So keep in mind that a light exercise that includes running around your neighborhood is the surest way to start off with health exercise, which can eliminate acute and chronic stress and help maintain a healthy mind.

A Healthy Brain Makes a Healthy Mind

As I mentioned earlier, the stimulus of stress produces subjective physiological events in each individual through the brain. It means all people have different feelings resulting from stress stimulus, even if the stimulus is similar. Therefore, people can reach a healthy mind by training their brain (prefrontal training). According to psychology professor Mihaly Csikszentmihalyi at Chicago University, it is good to be in the "flow" to achieve your goals, with ways that are suitable for your lifestyle. If you do this, you can overcome stress, make a healthy mind, but also awaken the potential you have inside of you. By discovering "a creative self," he says you can find your extreme happiness (Hwang Nong-Moon 2007).

1. Relaxation response: it was the research on practitioners of transcendental meditation that made medical experts recognize mind and body are intertwined and that mind can actually control the body. The meditation practitioners who took part in the research had lower blood pressures than average people, and they believed it was the result of their meditation.

   Herbert Benson of Harvard University measured the usual blood pressure, metabolism, heartbeat, brain wave and breathing of the practitioners. Then, he measured the same categories after making them go through a 20-min meditation. The results were impressive. Just by "changing the thinking patterns," the metabolism, the breathing, and the heartbeat of the practitioners decreased, and their brain waves slowed down. It was a totally different response from the stress reaction, and Dr. Benson called it "the relaxation response."

   It took several decades for the relaxation response to be accepted in the medical world. Now, it is regarded as one of the strongest tools to fight chronic stress. After follow-up research that tracked Benson's research for long a time, it was revealed that relaxation response not only got rid of the anxiety and depression through relieving stress but also decreased blood pressure and chances of cardiac disease. It was also helpful to weight management and relieving pain and asthma.

From molecule-biochemical perspective, relaxation response makes the parasympathetic (nervous) system to reorganize the stress hormone and can fix chronic stress cycle. It is due to the increased levels of nitrous oxide, as our body produces it more when it is relaxed (nitrous oxide, or N_2O, is a combination of one oxygen atom and two nitrogen atoms and is known as the so-called laughing gas that makes you feel good and laugh when you drink it). In short, you can make a healthy mind through relaxation response by training the prefrontal. It doesn't cost you anything, and it's just sad that not many people know the importance of prefrontal (Shrand and Devine 2013b).

In short, our distraught heart can be controlled with a focused mind ("mind control or mind unification"). You should also remember that there are many ways to overcome chronic stress by exercising relaxation response, other than meditation. Experts say that abdominal breathing (diaphragm breathing) and repeating prayers, Qigong, t'ai chi chuan, yoga, gradual muscle relaxation method, jogging, sewing, and many more ways can spark relaxation responses. The common ground of these activities is they make you focus on one thing at a time. We already know from experience that if we engage wholeheartedly in love, movies, or reciting poetry or do activities with passion and focus, there is no room for stress. However, t'ai chi chuan, yoga, and Qigong require training in order to prevent wounds and learn the techniques. These techniques are good to remain active in your senior years, and it gives much benefit to you in relaxation response. Anyone can drive out stress with a "healthy brain," which is made complete by the prefrontal training:

1. Sit down in a comfortable position without making any sounds.
2. Close your eyes.
3. Start relaxing your muscles in the following order: the feet, legs, thighs, stomach, shoulders, head, and neck. A little bit of a practice is needed. Think that even a small amount of stimulus felt in the muscles is relaxed. Don't get stuck in this stage, or it may give more stress to you.
4. Repeat the words, phrases, or prayers that you selected in a small voice as you breathe out. Breathe slowly and naturally.
5. Don't think about how well you're concentrating on the words or phrases that you selected. It is natural for other thoughts to hinder you in the early stages of the technique. You might even find yourself thinking, "What am I doing now?" When other thoughts keep coming up, just tell yourself in your heart. "Now I'm thinking about other thoughts. Let me go back to the words or phrases that I selected."
6. At first, do the training for about a minute or two. Start increasing the time span as you move on. Later, perform the training for about 10–20 min.
7. After you finish, open your eyes and embrace the world. The colors seem more vivid and the sounds more clear. The world is at peace. Just enjoy the moments and look on.

8. Don't stand up right away. Remember that the amount of nitrous oxide in your body increased and that your blood pressure went down. Sit still for another minute and let other thoughts come to you.

9. Practice the technique for about once to twice a day. Set a comfortable time for you in your day and do it steadily. Practice is very important (Shrand and Devine 2013c).

If you want to go deeper into the relaxation stage, or if you have difficulty imagining in creative ways (patients who haven't gone to a place where they felt relaxed), I suggest the following techniques:

1. Select a quiet place where you can sit down or lie down.
2. Be in a comfortable position.
3. Breathe in and out. This can take even minutes.
4. Close your eyes and keep on breathing. Focus on your breaths.
5. You don't have to try and fight other thoughts. Those thoughts are natural ones.
6. Just look at the thoughts and let them pass.
7. The 1st stage of travel: pack up your things. This means imagining that you're putting in some necessary things in a bag, in a baggage or in a suitcase. You can also put in comfortable pillows, blanket, and sunglasses. You don't need to bring your shoes. But if you want, you can imagine yourself putting your shoes away in the shoe case.
8. The 2nd stage of travel: now imagine you're opening the door and getting in the car, after putting the luggage in the trunk. If you want, you don't have to drive.
9. The 3rd stage of travel: you are driving your car to the destination. As you drive toward the bridge and breathe, your muscles are more relaxed.
10. The 4th stage of travel: you are driving on the bridge, trying to get to the comfortable place on the other side of the bridge. When you get there, your car slows down.
11. The 5th stage of travel: you get off the car and take a look around. You are now at your destination.
12. The 6th stage of travel: imagine yourself in a safe and comfortable place, such as a beach, a resort, or a cabin in a forest. Wherever you go, there are comfortable beds, sofas, and chairs, the most convenient ones on this planet that you can think of. This place is solely for you, where you can be relaxed.
13. The 7th stage of travel: unpack your luggage and take out your blanket and pillow. Change into comfortable clothes and imagine you're putting on your sunglasses. Try to picture yourself looking at your other self in a bed, on a sofa, or on a chair. You have found just the right place to relax yourself.
14. If you're ready to go, do the exercises in reverse. Pack your things and end your imagination by taking out your shoes from the shoe case of your home (Shrand and Devine 2013d)

2. Being awake: we all have experiences where we are embarrassed because we're not solely concentrating on the present. For instance, you find yourself getting

off the elevator to see that you've landed on the wrong floor. You might even catch yourself going into the direction that you're accustomed to, rather than the destination you should be headed toward. These things happen because you thought of something else. That is, you weren't "awake" at the moment. "Being awake" or "staying at present" is to keep from thinking about other things but to focus on one thing at a time.

Modern society calls us to have a multitasking ability, to do two or more different things at once, and it can cause more stress to our brain. Therefore, to overcome chronic stress, we should get rid of multitasking habit and try to "be awake." "Being awake" (or taking care of your mind) is regarded as one of the good meditation techniques to eliminating stress. Experts refer to this as "MBSR (mindfulness-based stress reduction)."

Recently, a researcher compared the before and after of a group of people who participated in a meditation program (being awake). He had an MRI scan of the brains of the participants and found out that the gray matter of hippocampus, which is in charge of memory, learning, and thinking, increased.

Hippocampus, which is in the limbic system, is highly related to memory, and it combines short-term memory with the long-term memory. A quick judgment on what is threatening and what can be beneficial to us is made by the hippocampus, and it plays a very important role in our survival. By practicing "being awake," the connection between the limbic system and prefrontal can be strengthened. When we use prefrontal in our awaken state, we can memorize more effectively, and it decreases stress. The damaged brain areas in the early onset of the Alzheimer's disease is hippocampus, and the results are loss of memory, diminished ability of storing up new data, and loss of ability to receive new information (Shrand and Devine 2013e).

In short, "being awake" makes you think about being wide awake. It is the state of healthy brain which stops you from being overwhelmed by worries, fear, distracted, anxiety, and depression, which are all warning signals of chronic stress. "Being awake" is not about waiting for the next moment but about living this moment, "right now," and experiencing relaxation. Through practicing various techniques of "being awake," and training your brain, you can reach a healthy mind with a healthy brain.

Let me introduce "stop, see, and listen," which is a simple technique to practice "being awake." It is to stop at your walk intentionally and to see and listen. When we "stop," we get the chance to see what's happening now and here around us. When we "see," we can lead the world around us to come into our inner world. When we stop, we can take a look around us in a peaceful and considerate way and listen carefully to what others are saying. It's when we stop and see that we feel what others are going through, what they are speaking about, and how to help them. Furthermore, we make others realize that they are valuable and precious beings by concentrating our focus on them. The stress and cortisol levels are lowered, and the secretion of oxytocin is increased (Shrand and Devine 2013f). When you are "awake," the stress of other people including you can be decreased, and so it is desirable for us to stop, see, and listen in our life.

SHS Makes a Healthy Mind

People try their best to look good, so we keep clean, put on makeups, and wear good clothes. When we feel that we are not valued from others, we tend to get stressed out easily, and this applies to all human beings.

When we socialize with people, we share our thoughts with others and reaffirm our status in the society and feel valued. Human beings inherently have SHS in them based on reciprocity. Therefore, people share loving feelings and help out and, in the process, form various relationships. According to various researches, people who have a healthy, satisfying relationship with their friends and family are happier than people who don't. The happier you are, the more reminded you are of the fact that there are people around you whom you can lend a shoulder to cry on. Due to this recognition, these people can withstand stressful situations and have better overall health conditions than those who don't (Shrand and Devine 2013g).

So it is also true that people who don't have good relationships with their family and friends are less healthy than people who do. Lack of valuable relationships and social cohesion are often pointed to as major causes of death. In aging society, lone deaths of a single family or of senior citizens who live alone are becoming social problems.

Scholars have another idea about emotional bond's shielding role from stress. They studied the influence of hormones such as oxytocin (which is secreted from the posterior pituitary and has nicknames such as "bond hormone" or "embracing hormone"). It is secreted from the brain when humans engage in specific forms of interactions. When mothers hugged their babies or were near them, the oxytocin levels of the mothers increased. Couples who had oxytocin agent sprayed on their noses had easier time solving their conflicts as well. Cortisol secretion of the couples also decreased, and it seems to hint that they were less stressed out, were less angry, and have better relationships (Shrand and Devine 2013h).

The essential function of relationships is love shared among people based on SHS. Just like the phrase, "Pleasure doubles when shared, and pain halves when shared," it becomes easier to bear pain when we share stress by socialization process. Therefore, take effort to have good relationships with people. Relationships are like "a net of love," so it's wise to take to the heart that "quality" of the relationships are more important than their "quantity."

Make "Healthy Mind" by Enjoying Lavender Fragrance

This means that you should enjoy life, with a mental space of your own. Recently, researchers in Japan found out for the first time that specific fragrances change genetic activities and chemical traits of blood, thereby decreasing stress. The researchers exposed laboratory rats to stressful situations and measured immune cell activities. Then, they selected some from the group to smell linalool fragrance (a chemical substance that is emitted naturally from lemon, mango, lavender, and various other flowers and herbal plants). As a result, only the stress levels of mice which smelled linalool came back to normal. Smelling linalool decreased the activities of more than 100 genes as well, which are known to overreact when under stress. This discovery highlighted the importance of aromatherapy, and I believe products that target specific genes to relieve stress will come out on the market in the near future (Shrand and Devine 2013i).

Normally, people live about their lives without much problem. However, in cases where they are faced with troubles that break peace in the family, such as the death of their spouse (100), divorce (73), or separation (65), their health is deterred due to the stress. It's also true for spending time in prison (63), hearing about the death of a close friend (63), the sudden contraction of disease or having injuries (53), being fired (47), or being retired (44) also raises stress levels, which have an impact on the overall health condition (the numbers in the blank are "Holmes and Rahe Stress Scale," and the higher the number is, the more negative impact it has on our health). This is the result of various researches and it shows that stress has a negative impact on almost all body systems.

We should realize that the origin of our stress is mostly "everyday things" and "challenges regarding our psychology." Research shows that chronic stress is the main culprit of deterioration of health, and the SM therapy derived from health stressor in the book naturally focused on how we can overcome chronic stress. However, as I said, understanding mind, brain, and body is needed in order to conquer stress. By using social navigation to tackle this, we first focused on healthy mind. In a healthy brain that overcomes stress, N_2O plays the main role which is secreted in relaxation response in a static state such as meditation. However, in the case of a dynamic state, for instance, when jogging, the brain is very much dependent on endorphin that is secreted in a runner's high state. Such responses were believed to exist however little they were. In this part, such responses were newly defined as "health stressor response," clearly shown in the interactions among mind, brain, and body.

Even in a state of chronic stress, our brain can maintain a healthy mind through health stressor response, according to the condition of the body (dynamic or static). If you are in a situation where you feel chronic stress, how we overcome the difficulties are based on how we move our body, that is, on our determination and will.

We should take pride in ourselves as being health prosumers. It is good to have meditation time, or to run around the neighborhood, or to have a chat with your friends. If you can move your body in various ways, there is hope that you can maintain a sense of healthy and peaceful mind, where you can get out of the vicious cycle of chronic stress.

3.2.2 SM Therapy that Originated from Complementary Alternative Medicine

Some of the contents here are quoted and summarized from *Complementary Alternative Medicine* (2004), which is one of the important books published by Jeon Se-Il.

3.2.2.1   SM Therapy from Pro-Western Medicine CAM

Chiropractic Therapy

Chiropractic therapy is a manipulation therapy that uses hands to relieve various symptoms such as pain and to improve the condition of the entire body. It is done by correcting a crooked spine or backbone. Here, "manipulation therapy" refers to spine realignment, and the therapy is based on the theory that various diseases can be cured by realigning the crooked spine. It is one of the most popular therapies in the USA, and it is as famous as the acupuncture in Korea.

The therapy was made by Daniel Palmer in 1895. Palmer, a Canadian, was amused by osteopathy and magnetic therapy when he moved to the USA. The magnetic therapy increases the "flow of magnetic power" by stroking a patients' body. The therapy was already in use by natural therapists and some doctors then. Palmer learned the therapy and opened up a treatment room in the state of Iowa in the 1880s. One day in 1895, he met the security guard of the building he was in, who lost his hearing abilities after spraining his back 17 years ago. After examination, he found out that one of his bones in the spine was out of place, and put it back in the right place with the massage of his hands. Suddenly, the guard was restored of his hearing abilities, and it was how the chiropractic therapy was born.

According to his theory, humans have enough "treatment potential" where he can maintain a perfect state of health. Perfect health is directly related to the normal functions of the neuro-system. The spine is the lifeline of the neuro-system, so the spine should be taken care of in order to maintain health. Therefore, the therapy is very effective in treating the imbalance of the body.

He believed abnormal alignment of the spine presses the spinal nerves that come out of the spine to be delivered to all parts of the body. When this causes damage to the flow of the usual nerve, he thought that it can have an impact on the normal functions of the muscle, breathing, pulse, digestion, and immune system. Therefore, he argued that correcting the alignment of the spine would eliminate oppression of the nerve, and health will be restored. He emphasized that the spine is not just a hard structure to protect the nerves that comes down from the brain. He said it was a special part of our body made up of 33 bones. He added all joints in the spine had to take their places at all times to maintain flexibility. He believed that all diseases in the body are caused by subluxation, which is the state of crooked spine.

At the "Palmer Chiropractic Research Institute," which he established back in 1897, he taught theories about realigning subluxation (twisting manipulation that included massaging or pressing). Five years later, the first ever 15 chiropractic experts graduated from there. One of them is his son Joshua, and he developed chiropractic for 50 years since then.

Most diseases are the subjects of the therapy. The therapy mainly focuses on the following conditions: pain, headache, tension of the muscle, digestion system problems (duodenal ulcer), nocturnal enuresis of children, abnormal bleeding in the womb resulting from backache, facial muscles of facial paralysis patients, Erb's paralysis of infants (where you can't use your arms as the upper limb nerves are pressed), nervous disorder of diabetes, nervous syndrome related to the problems of the muscles and joints of the feet, shoulder pain, carpal tunnel syndrome, the cervical vertebral disk, damaged muscle and neuro-system due to electric shock, headache resulting from an abnormal alignment of neck bones, and backache of pregnant women.

Chiropractic experts use different manipulation methods. One group is called the originals. They sometimes use manipulation of stretching, where the joint is pulled so hard that there is a clicking sound. At the same time, manipulation of gentle touch is also used, where there are no such sounds. Another group mostly uses therapeutic modalities when conducting the manipulation. Heat, cold, ultrasound and electrical stimulation nutrition are included.

Just like other therapies, chiropractic therapy can have side effects. The pain can be added when the tissues with degenerative changes are damaged. Disk bulging can be made worse to a condition of ruptured herniation. When receiving the chiropractic therapy, major arteries connected to the brain can be damaged, and there are reports of fatal injuries related to this. Therefore, it is necessary for the patients with problems in the blood vessel to consult the doctor before receiving the therapy. The manipulation of the lower spine can result in complications such as abnormal functions of the bladder, muscle contraction of the lower parts and rectum, and fertility disorders.

A degree of DC (Doctor of Chiropractics) is given upon the graduation of chiropractic universities. The therapy is so popular that patients come to receive it, even without the recommendation from doctors. It is becoming widely known around the world, and the population receiving chiropractic therapy in Korea is on a steady increase.

Podiatric Medicine

It's our feet that made us human beings. The creation and destruction of civilization was made possible by human hands. It was due to feet that humans were able to use their hands freely. In short, walking upright, which freed human hands, was the reason we could utilize such high intelligence.

One of the stark characteristics of our feet is that it can make us stand comfortably for quite a long time. Our feet form an arch with the alignments of their bones and muscle structure. Even with two legs, we humans can stand balanced and move and run for long periods time. With the arch of the feet, people can walk on flat and steep hills and shifty sandy ground and change directions rapidly when running in a fast speed.

In order to run fast, the centroid used to be located in the front of the feet in previous generations. However, modern people who walk and run less and who live in a more sophisticated society tend to have the centroid closer to the heels. For example, according to a research in 1960, the centroid when you stand with two feet side by side used to be located about 47 % more to the front from the heels. Twenty years later in 1980, it was 40 % and 33 % in 2000.

The importance of feet as the foundation of health is very critical. You should prevent yourself from going to the doctor's every time you feel a little sick. In some countries including the USA and Australia, there is a system of "feet doctor." The feet doctors are all bachelors who mastered 4 years of studying at college and spent another 4 years studying about feet. The degree they receive is DPM (Doctor of Podiatry Medicine).

The following are the conditions treated in the therapy. Moles, corn, and callus come about on the sole and annoy many people. In this case, corn can be melted by certain drugs or can be taken out with a simple operation. Tinkering with your shoes to make it comfortable is another way.

Patients with "hallux valgus" frequently visit the feet doctors, too. Those with hallux valgus have the outside parts of their big toe swollen red, and it is bent toward inside. It gets so close to the second toe that it produces severe pain. This occurs often in middle-aged women and in senior citizens. It is very painful when you wear high heels.

Feet doctors can also cure various other diseases such as fasciitis (the inflammation that occurs on the muscle membrane that covers the sole), Morton neuroma (the disease that makes you leap with pain with a small lump in the peripheral nerves. The space between the third and the fourth toe usually hurts), lipping (a phenomenon of aging where a part of your bone pricks out of the skin), rheumatoid arthritis, and gout (inflammation of the toes when there is too much uric acid in the blood). Feet doctors can be useful when you have injuries in your ankles or toes as well. Nowadays, experts in Korea are widely spreading feet medicine.

Chelation Therapy

Chelation therapy is eliminating toxic materials and wastes from the metabolism process from the blood. The word "chele" is derived from the Greek word "pincers" (the big foot of a crab). This is how the chelation process works. When the amino acid compound EDTA (ethylenediaminetetraacetic acid) touches materials such as lead, iron, copper, calcium, magnesium, ion, plutonium, and manganese, which has positron, EDTA snatches off the materials just like the pincer and lets it out of the body after going through the kidney.

According to a research conducted by double blind study in 1989, about 88 % of the participants showed increased blood amount in the brain blood vessel and peripheral blood vessel after ten times of chelation therapy. There are reports that through chelation therapy, 50 % saw the arrhythmia in their hearts improve, and it was an increased memorizing ability for those with amnesia and lessened loss of eyesight related to blood vessel conditions. Patients who couldn't walk well due to pain caused by infarction of peripheral vasoconstriction could walk normally, and cancer patients' death rate decreased. It also had preventative effects on iron toxicosis and could get rid of snake or spider poison.

In the USA, chelation therapy is said to decrease the necessity of cardiovascular operations to a large extent. The final product of oxygen metabolism in the body is free radical, and it becomes harmful when it combines with metal such as copper. Chelation therapy gets rid of the metal, and so it is helpful to prevent and fight conditions such as cancer, chronic adult disease, chronic fatigue syndrome, and degenerative aging related to free radical. However, many parts of the chelation therapy are yet to be proven, and its effect should be closely monitored. There are even some risky aspects to it, let alone the high cost. So in reality, it is not yet fully accepted by the public.

Hypnotic Therapy

Hypnosis is to make physiological changes (such as in temperature and pulse) that is uncontrollable by our will in ordinary life. It is to pull humans into an extreme state of conscious concentration. There are records that hypnosis was used in treatments in ancient Egypt, Greece, Persia, and India by monks. American Indians are believed to have treated pain through hypnosis. It was a German doctor named Franz Anton Mesmer who started to use the therapy in earnest in the late 1700s.

Mesmer argued that various nerve disorders can be cured through hypnosis. At first, the therapy was called "Mesmerism" after his name. Later, an ophthalmologist named James Braid in the UK called it "hypnosis," taking the Greek word "hypnos," which means "sleep."

Just before anesthesia was introduced, some doctors found out that hypnosis can lessen patients' pain during the operation, even without tying them or giving them alcohol. Sigmund Freud frequently used hypnosis at first but distanced himself from it in the 1890s as he focused more on his psychology analysis theory. Nowadays, hypnosis is developing into a professional field with its own standing.

It was in 1955 when hypnosis was approved as formal medicine in the UK. Hypnosis that used to be in the boundaries of traditional (Western) medicine was confined mainly to relaxation of the mind, pain, and anesthesia. When hypnosis began to be used in larger swaths, going over the current institutional boundaries, it was regarded as an alternative, complementary medicine (CAM).

Successful hypnosis should have the following conditions: first, the good rapport formation between the hypnotist and the person being hypnotized; second, a comfortable environment, free of distraction, and third, the will of the patient that he wants to be hypnotized. He should be able to understand that hypnosis is not about "surrender of control" but simply an "advanced form of relaxation."

It is not yet known how hypnosis takes effect in our body. We can only presume that it activates the nervous routes of the brain, which secretes natural opium such as endorphin. Endorphin in turn changes various subjective symptoms such as our action, senses of pain, etc., by working in our immune system. There are several objective phenomena that can be observed. It can induce breathing and relaxation response of the patient. It can also produce "positive thinking and behavior" of the patients, which can increase the "sense of well-being." To some extent, activities of the autonomic nerve can be controlled intentionally, such as the temperatures of our hands and feet and the speed of the pulse. Lastly, it can decrease our sensitivity toward stress.

The following are some of the conditions that are the objects of hypnosis experts nowadays:

1. Pain: headache, face-ache, sciatic neuralgia, arthritis, collum sprain, menstrual pain, and tennis elbow
2. Anesthesia: metrectomy, hernia, breast biopsy, hemorrhoids, C-section, burns, thyroid ablation, appendicitis ablation, carpal tunnel release, pacemaker insertion, amputations of extremities, and tooth extraction
3. Stress reduction and improvements of symptoms related to stress: insomnia, asthma, irritable bowel syndrome, allergic reactions, phobia, anxiety disorder, obsessive-compulsive neurosis, hysteria, and nausea vomiting
4. Before-life therapy: when the memories are regressed under hypnosis, the memories in our unconscious can be tracked. A psychiatrist Brain L. Weiss of the USA observed that memories from other dimensions can be retrieved when you overturn the mental clock of the patient to travel further, even before he was born. He called the memories, "memories of before life." Before-life therapy utilizes medical information learned from the patients' before life to cure their current disease. Before-life therapy is controversial in traditional medicine.
5. Others: people suffering from morning sickness, childbirth, obesity, nocturnal enuresis, and moles and paralyzed patients also use hypnotic therapy. One of the side effects can be a "posthypnotic effect," where the allusion that the patient received in the hypnotized state seems like real even after being awake. Other conditions such as posthypnotic amnesia can occur naturally or by allusion of the expert. In rare cases, memory can be greatly improved, which goes over the normal range. The positive effects of hypnotic therapy are good for treatment, but the negative ones can be harmful to mind and body, and patients should take heed.

Enzyme Therapy

Enzymes are special proteins that work as catalysts in the biochemical reactions in the body. It plays the most important role in the digestion process of food. Enzymes don't produce reactions but just facilitate the process. In order for the enzymes to play such roles, other enzymes that can help the process are needed. Such coenzymes include nutrients such as vitamins, minerals, and proteins. When enzymes participate in a certain process such as digestion, they should be supplemented immediately.

Each cell in our body has about hundreds and thousands of enzymes, and most of them are provided through food. Enzymes that decompose the food we eat, such as protein, fat, and carbohydrate, are made in various parts of the boy. The most important ones are generally made in the pancreas. If the pancreas is damaged due to injuries or inflammation, the important enzymes are not made enough, so fat, protein, and carbohydrate taken in are emitted out of the body through the stomach, without being digested. In this case, nutrients can't be taken in, and the nutrition state gets in bad condition.

Pancreatic enzyme and plant enzyme are used in the enzyme therapy. The latter is used to strengthen the functions of the digestive system, and the former is used to make both the digestive and the immune functions stronger. There are records of ecologist John Beard of the UK, who treated cancer patients by injecting pancreas extracts in 1902. Other cases are multiple sclerosis, cancer, and virus infection.

Enzyme experts say that enzymes dissolve the surface of cancer cells and can penetrate not only white blood cells but also other cells in the immune system. Even anticancer drugs are said to penetrate into the cancer cells to destroy them. Enzymes can kill various types of viruses such as AIDS virus. Enzymes digest the surface protein of the virus so that the natural defense mechanism of our body can kill them easily.

Under the theory that enzymes are also good for healthy people, similar additives to protease, amylase, and lactase, which are enzymes made in the body, are used. Taking in much enzyme can take the burden off of the pancreas, and it can be maintained in a healthier and more effective state.

Plant enzymes help the pancreas in another way. Digestion starts from the stomach, and hydrochloric acid and gastrin, a digestive enzyme, work on the food taken in. Pancreas digestive enzymes don't exist in the stomach, so they don't take part in the process. However, plant enzymes ample in vegetables, fruits, nuts, and seeds can work when the plant is still in the stomach and helps its digestion. In the predigestive stage, enzymes in the pancreas set everything ready so that the food can be digested more easily when it goes down the duodenum. Therefore, pancreas with less workload can take more rest and, thereby, become healthier.

Also, cellulose, a special digestion enzyme of plants that decompose fiber is used. Cellulose can't be produced inside our body and should be taken by eating vegetables. If you only eat cooked food and don't take plant enzyme supplements, you can't enjoy the benefits of predigesting from the stomach. Low-temperature sterilization, canned food, using microwave, and dish that involve cooking in over 50 °C all decrease the effects of plant enzymes. Plant enzymes are used not only in digestion diseases, sore throat, seasonal allergies, ulcer, and candida but also in promoting health conditions of healthy people.

Applied Kinesiology

The creator of applied kinesiology is George Goodheart D.C., who was the doctor of chiropractic in the USA. In 1964, he discovered that some people who sit in abnormal positions have functional muscle disabilities, even without problems in the skeletal system. The theory of applied kinesiology states that abnormal position of the body is the root of many diseases. It argues that hormone, blood, nerves, and lymph all relate muscle with the inner organs, and muscle functions not only reflect the physical, emotional health but also determine them. By finding the weakness of specific muscles, applied kinesiology argues that the imbalanced state of our organs or endocrine gland can be found. In short, the "muscle-gland-organ link" is very important in diagnosis and treatment of disease.

Muscle testing is the most important factor of clinical test. Muscles with contradictory functions should be checked. For instance, biceps located in the front of the arms should be contracted when we bend our arms. At the same time, triceps, in the behind, should be relaxed. When the movements of the elbow are not good, we need to find out if spasm or weakness prevents muscles from contracting or relaxing. Applied kinesiology emphasizes the correlation between muscles and organs, based on the theory that a particular muscle is closely related to another specific organ.

One of the aspects of applied kinesiology that can be used clinically is that specific vitamins or nutrients can be very helpful in checking the status of patients. For instance, let's say a test is conducted to see what components are good for a patient who has weak deltoid. When you touch certain components on the patient's tongue, some components will make the deltoid stronger, and it can be observed at the site. Experts argue that when certain components touch the tongue, they stimulate specific parts of the brain, and the stimulus can change the tension of the muscle. That is why applied kinesiology experts say that when a muscle shows a weak response, it's not due to the muscle but because of other hidden abnormalities. By looking into the strong and weak responses of the muscle, various types of allergies, deficiencies, the intoxicated state, and sensitivity to food can be found out.

Applied kinesiology is a highly professionalized field. Interpreting the results of the complex tests correctly can lead to good treatment. Therefore, applied kinesiology should be conducted by skilled experts of the field. The reason the therapy is not conducted widely is because there is a lack information on how correct and reproducible it is.

Craniosacral Therapy

Among the manipulation therapy that falls into the category of physical therapy, craniosacral therapy involves massaging the cranial bone and the sacral bone to overturn conditions. There are eight cranial bones and five sacral bones that cover the brain. In infancy, the copula of the bones is not yet fixed, and they move when you touch. However, they become almost firmly fixed as we age. The foundation of the therapy goes like this. Experts of craniosacral therapy can detect "slight movements" of the copula, and by this, they can see the responses that follow the pressure changes of the cerebrospinal fluid.

The cerebrospinal fluid that flows through the brain and spinal cord is about 120–150 cc in amount. In average, about 500 cc comes out from the blood vessels a day and the same amount is reabsorbed to flow into the blood vessels. When the cerebrospinal fluid comes out from the blood vessel, the pressure of the fluid goes up and down when it's reabsorbed. The rhythm of secretion and reabsorption of the fluid repeats about 6–10 times a minute. A skilled craniosacral therapy expert can detect the rhythm. When there is a glaring limitation of the cranial sacral bones and joints' movement in some parts, experts presume that the limitations of the joints' movement and a certain disease have a correlation. Therefore, conditions can be overturned when limited joint movements are treated.

The following is several ways of the therapy: first, stimulating the adjoining parts of the skull; second, stimulating the brain; and third, using the reflex response. Conditions that can be treated through craniosacral therapy include various chronic pains, headaches, TMJ syndrome, anxieties, stress-related symptoms, epilepsy, cerebral palsy, tinnitus, high and low blood pressure, sinus infection, impotence, asthma, vomiting, constipation, hearing difficulty, etc.

Iridology

Our eyes have black and white parts, and the latter is called, iris. The word refers to the "goddess of rainbow" from the Greek mythology. Iridology was created by a Hungarian doctor named Ignatz von Peczeley, in the late 1800s. When he was twelve, he was very surprised to find two big yellow eyes staring at him, as he was walking in the forest. Suddenly, a large owl was grabbing at his arm and attacking him. He couldn't move his arms freely, and only by breaking the owl's leg he could be set free. In that fearful moment, he saw that there is a black line in the owl's eyes. He took the owl home and treated it and it became healthy. He saw that the black line in the owl's eyes had turned white. He remembered the change of the owl's eyes for a long time. Even after he became a doctor, he saw similar changes in his patients' eyes. He was certain that the iris of the eyes reflect the state of our inner organs. He made a complicated chart of the correlation and established a new cure in 1881. The book went through some corrections, but it's still in use.

He argued that a disease in an organ brings out "slight inflammation" changes of a certain part in the iris, and the change results in the shape and color transformation of the iris tissue. Strangely, the coloring of the iris has peripheral nerves, and it is closely related to sympathetic nerves. That's why it responses relatively well to stress and inflammation.

The left iris represents the left part of our body and the right iris, the right part. The 12 o'clock part of the iris is related to our head, 6 o'clock to legs, 2 o'clock to thyroid, and 8 o'clock to the intestines. If we have liver problems, the color of the 8 o'clock part changes. If it's an acute syndrome, the color turns into a lighter one, but darker when it's chronic. If you have inflammation in an organ, the iris related to the part will get white lines or snow-like dots. When the inflammation turns chronic, the color tends to turn into black. When the lines or dots that occurred out of nowhere turn darker, it may mean that the disease would be long lasting. When fine, white lines start to appear in distorted shapes on the darkened iris part, it is a sign of recovery. If the patient has anemia, the margins of the iris will look unclear, not showing the clear and distinct black color.

The good sides of iridology is that it shows the condition of your overall body, it doesn't use needles or knives, it can be easily learned, it can prevent disease, and its test can be done in a short period time. As a result, iridology can be applied in public health.

Neurolinguistic Therapy, NLP

The ultimate goal of neurolinguistic therapy, or NLP, is to "change the current unhealthy condition of your body by reprogramming your faith about curing your disease." It is a therapy that involves both mind and body, which is a mix of psychotherapy and imaging.

Neurolinguistic therapy has all three concepts of thinking, behavior, and program. N (neuro) means nerve, but in a broader sense, it includes the brain and the thinking and the workings of your mind. L (linguistic) is about linguistic expressions or images. The therapy argues that thinking influences our behavior and vice versa. With this, the therapy programs or reprograms our thinking, language, and behavior so that our mind and body can work in the way we want them to.

Neurolinguistic therapy is related to the Korean saying, "Be careful what you ask for." When we keep on repeating certain phrases, they are written deep in our brain, and ultimately, our body changes to fulfill the phrases. In this sense, it's related to the so-called, self-fulfilling prophesy. Language reflects our unconscious and how our inner world recognizes the problems we face. A doctor in Florida, USA, argues that the most important factor in peoples' health is "how people recognize their identity." It's very true for those who have chronic syndromes. For instance, patients with diabetes or high blood pressure often say: "I'm having diabetes" or "I have high blood pressure." These patients make it sound like they are the diseases by identifying themselves with the condition. Experts of NLP first make the patients understand that they are not disease and try to separate the patient from the disease. Their main role is for the patient to "regain their own self." In short, their role is to persuade the patient, who thinks that he is the disease itself, into thinking that he is "suffering" from the disease. It is giving the patients their true identity back.

As you can see, the goal of NLP is to change the perspective of the patient in how he sees his emotional or physical conditions. NLP experts not only analyze the words and phrases used by the patient to explain his symptom but also the expression, body language, and change of facial color and moisture of the lips and eyes. By doing so, experts redesign the minds and the mental imaging of the patient. By language usage, behavior correction, and imaging, they change the negative outlook into a positive mindset.

NLP was created by John Grinder, a linguistics professor at the University of California, and a psychology student named, Richard Bandler, in the early 1970s. They concentrated their research on several celebrities who were highly evaluated by being successful in various fields at the same time. Their subjects of research were Fritz Perls, who is called the father of gestalt therapy; Virginia Satir, a family psychology therapist; Milton Erickson, a hypnotist and a doctor; and Gregory Bateson, who is an anthropologist and also the author of dialogue theory. The thinking process, the language pattern, and the behavioral pattern of the four people were closely looked into. As a result, the two creators of NLP discovered important behavioral, psychological factors that led these people to success worked in unconscious and intuitive way and that the renowned people didn't know what had led them to such success. The analysis of their speaking attitude, the highs and lows of their voice, their word choice, the attitude, the body language, and the movements of their eyes when they speak told them that there is a very strong relationship between body language and the way you talk.

Based on such information, Grinder and Bandler started to build on their experiences by helping people dealing with psychology problems. They asked various questions to the patients and observed how the patients behaved as they answered. The patients' eye movements, the bodyposture, the highs and lows of the voice, and the breathing are all unconscious factors that reflect the emotional status of the patients. The factors were applied to the diagnosis and the treatment of the patients. When the unconscious problems were revealed, experts induced the patients to adapt to a new pattern that will benefit them. By doing so, Grinder and Bandler devised, produced, and distributed a detailed method to systematically analyze a person's language, thinking, and behavior.

The therapy is being widely distributed around the world at a rapid pace. The conditions that have shown great improvements include allergies, arthritis, migraine, various phobias, the Parkinson's disease, cancer, and AIDS. If the therapy is applied along with acupuncture, Oriental medicine, homeopathy, and diet, it can be more effective. Some experts presume that NLP will become highly popular in the future, but more studies are needed for confirmation.

Reconstruction Therapy

Reconstruction therapy includes injecting specific materials that stimulate the growth of the combination tissues in order to strengthen the injured or weakened tendon or sinew. The physiological common ground of tendon, sinew, cartilage, and bones is that these tissues have incomplete blood circulation. So when tissues are injured, the curing process relatively slows down. For instance, when the tendon is prolonged and the joints are destabilized due to the injury, our body forms lipping (some parts of the bones grow like thorns) to complement it. Due to the formation of lipping, the friction of the joints gets worse, the pain increases, and the movements of the joints decrease. To cut off the initial problems of the chain response, the damaged tissues have to be stabilized right away. The sclerosis and the proliferation of the tissue play the stabilizing role. That's why the reconstruction therapy is called "sclerotherapy" or "prolotherapy."

The injections that are used in the reconstruction therapy are sodium morrhuate (materials extracted from cod-liver oil), glucose, glycerin, phenol, and minerals. The specific materials stimulate the increase of the combination tissues and harden them. When stimulating injections are put into the body, an extraordinary effect is brought about in 6 times. In most cases, about 10–15 times of treatment is required.

Experts of reconstruction therapy argue that the success rate of curing backache stands at about 92 % (in particular the functional backache) and that there are no side effects. The disease that can be cured by the therapy include: degenerative arthritis, pains in the back and neck, the damaged tendon and cartilage, degenerative disk conditions, migraine, inflammation of bursa, carpal tunnel syndrome (numbing of hands), damaged Achilles tendon, tennis elbow, damaged muscles surrounding the shoulders, bunion, and other musculoskeletal conditions. It is forecast that the reconstruction therapy will be spread around the world rapidly as it will be applied in the sports medicine.

Cell Therapy

Generally, cell therapy includes transfusion and bone-marrow transplantation that are used in traditional medicine. However, in the area of alternative, complementary medicine, which is a new approach, it includes injecting live cells extracted from the organs, the fetus, or the embryo of animals to facilitate the curing process of the body, to repress the aging process, and to cure the degenerative diseases.

The first person who started the cell therapy was Paul Niehans, a doctor from Switzerland. In 1931, Niehans was conducting a thyroid operation on a female patient. By mistake, he damaged her parathyroid, which was located very close to her thyroid. The parathyroid produces a hormone that controls calcium levels in our blood, and our body starts to shake when the calcium levels go down much. So his patient stared to shake her body. Niehans was planning to transplant the parathyroid of cattle, but as it was urgent, he ground the parathyroid tissues and mixed it with saline solution before injecting it into her body. Then surprisingly, her shaking stopped, and her parathyroid continued to function normally later.

By his amazing experience, Niehans discovered that the damaged organs can be restored only by transplanting healthy animal cells and not the entire organ or tissue. Later, Niehans conducted the cell therapy to thousands of people. Many renowned people were included in the list, such as Winston Churchill, Pope Pius XII, Japanese Emperor Hirohito, President Eisenhower, President de Gaulle, Onassis the king of ships, royal family members including the British family, and other rich people.

In cell therapy, animal embryonic cells and the human organ and fetus cells are used. In most cases, sheep cells are used, but the popularity of pig cells is increasing for their similarities with human cells. To minimize the concern of infection and adverse reaction of our body, fresh cells are freeze-drying in the sterilization process, and ultrafiltration is used to eliminate protein that may cause adverse reaction on the surface of the cell.

Interestingly, cells have particular receptors. It means that when adrenal cells are injected, it goes to the adrenal, kidney cells to the kidney, sex gland cells to the sex gland, and liver cells to the liver. Cell therapy is used in the following circumstances: preventing aging, increasing anticancer ability, promoting strong immune system, and fertility. It can also cure arthritis, cardiac disease, menopause symptoms, menstrual pain, infertility, herpes, chronic bronchitis, geromorphism, epilepsy, weak mentality, arteriosclerosis, Down syndrome, Parkinson's disease, liver infection, and skin problems. Cell therapy is popular in Europe, but it is yet to be generalized in the USA as there are fears that it lacks scientific evidence.

Biofeedback Therapy

Nerves in our body are distinguished in two parts on whether they can be moved by our will or not. First, there is somatic sensory nerve (sensory-exercise nerve included), where arms and legs can be moved freely. Second, there is autonomic nerve (sympathetic-parasympathetic nerve included), such as pulse and body temperature that can move on its own.

In the late 1960s, Dr. Barbara Brown and Elmer Green of the USA observed that Yogi, the meditation expert, could control his brain waves. It became the momentum where the concept of biofeedback began to spread. Biofeedback refers to the input the signals coming from the body to the body again.

If you can see for yourself how tense your muscle is, when you want to flex it, it will be helpful when you do muscle relaxation training. There is a gadget where you attach small electrodes on the skin. According to the tension of the muscle, you can hear the sounds, strong or weak. You can also see the tension by the brightness of the light and the needle that points to numbers. For instance, if your muscle is entirely relaxed, you won't hear any sounds nor see any light and the needle would point to 0.

As you can see, EMG biofeedback uses the electronic signal from the muscle. It can also observe the amount of sweat coming out our body through skin resistance and the severity of the cold hands and feet by measuring temperature. Biofeedback of finger pulse can follow up your anxiety levels and the status of cardiovascular status.

The following conditions are where biofeedback is used in clinical treatment: chronic pain, tension headache, migraine, slight arthritis, stress, insomnia, anxiety, hyperacidity, gastrointestinal ulcer, irritable bowel syndrome, dysphagia, tinnitus, quivering eyelids, fatigue syndrome, cerebral palsy, epilepsy, asthma, Raynaud's disease, cardiac disease, high blood pressure, incontinence, distraction, hyperactivity, muscle reeducation, correction of posture, and kyphosis.

The ultimate goal of biofeedback is to teach the patients to perform the therapy anytime without the help of the machine and once a week is adequate. Some people learn the entire therapy in 3–4 sessions, but most people need 12–20 sessions of training.

Mind-Body Medicine

Mind-body medicine is to recognize the in-depth correlation between the mind and the body and to seek treatment by making the patients take the responsibility for themselves with their innate treatment ability. Various forms of treatment such as vital dynamics, imagery therapy, hypnosis, meditation, and yoga are mobilized together.

"Self" is composed of "materialistic self" and an "unmaterialistic self." The core of materialistic self is the root form that continues in the materialistic world. The root form can be expressed as "gene" in modern science. The root form of materialistic self, which is gene, is the map of self, and it is the factory that makes the components which make up the self.

Our body is a structure made according to the root form. The body is the expression of "Che" (body), and "Sinche" (body) is immersed in the energy field that is called "Jeong" (affection). The materialistic mass that is our body is in a larger container named environment. Environment is in a larger container named Great Nature, and Great Nature in turn, lies in the infinite space. The unmaterialistic self that prevails forever is called "soul."

The expression of soul is "mind." "Simryeong" is immersed in the energy field that is called god. The unmaterialistic self relates with a "different self" that is called "you," and both are in a large container called the human society. Human society is in a larger container called human history, and human history, in turn, exists in everlasting time.

In order for the "Soma" to be healthy, which we generally refer to as body, harmony of the body, body, and "Jeong" (affection) is needed. It has to be harmonized with the environment that surrounds them, and the environment should be harmonized with the Great Nature, and the Great Nature should be in harmony with infinite space. In this context, the term "balance" refers to the "harmony between individual and individual," and "harmony" refers to the "coexistence in the whole."

In order for the "sprit" to be healthy, a harmonious status of spirit, mind, and god is needed. It has to be harmonized with the human society, and the human society has to tune in with the human history where the past and future lie and all of it have to be harmonized with everlasting time.

Being in harmony with everlasting time and infinite space means following the providence of "the absolute." When god, which embraces mind and spirit, respond to others (not self), it is called "consciousness." For "Soma" to be healthy, the consciousness of the individual has to be in harmony with the convention of human society that surrounds it. The consciousness of the human society, in turn, has to be harmonized with the consciousness of human history, which yet again, has to be in harmony with the "absolute consciousness."

Therefore, "spiritual health" means that mind and spirit are in harmony with the consciousness of human society through the works of god, and this in turn, is in harmony with the consciousness of human history. The consciousness of self is referred to as "self-consciousness," and the consciousness of the human society and human history are called as "cosmic consciousness." In this sense, the harmonious state between the self-consciousness and the cosmic consciousness is the healthy state of the spirit. In short, when the mind rediscovers the spirit, and when both have an "attunement" to the cosmic consciousness (following the providence of "the absolute"), it is the state of spiritual health.

Harmony is health, and disharmony is bad health. The body pursues stability of nourish and protect. When our body is healthy, it experiences stability, and if the nourish-protect is too much, it experiences instability. Mind pursues convenience, and when mind works well, we experience comfortable feelings. When mind is out of order, we feel anxious. Society pursues peace. When the society works well, people experience peace, but disharmony and complaint rule when the society is abnormal. Nourish seeks happiness, and we experience happiness when nourish works well but sorrow when it is in an abnormal state.

A new definition of health goes like this: a truly healthy person should have a healthy body and mind and spirit and should be healthy in social sense. Our body can maintain health when we eat, sleep, breathe, and move properly. The actions can be performed properly only when we are healthy. Our mind can maintain health when feelings such as happiness, anger, sadness, anxiety, sorrow, surprise, and fear are in harmony. In turn, a healthy mind can harmonize such feelings. The society is healthy only when there is peace, and peace can be maintained when the society is healthy. Nourish is healthy when it can maintain happiness, and happiness, in turn, can be kept when nourish is healthy.

"Self" has a self-healing mechanism with which it restores the "normal self" from the "abnormal self." Self-healing mechanism can be activated to its maximum only when the self is physically, psychologically, socially, and spiritually healthy. It's also true the other way around. "Self" can be utmost healthy when the self-healing mechanism is at its highest. Moreover, the self-healing mechanism can show its maximum potential when body-body-Jeong (affection) is harmonized with environment and the nature and when mind-nourish-god is in harmony with the society and the history. One element that hinders the self-healing mechanism is "too much or too less of something." Our little desire affects whole treatment and overall health.

Magnetic Field Therapy

The oldest record of magnetic field therapy is reportedly from Gallen of Greece in 200 BC, when he used magnets in his therapy. In the nineteenth century, Louis Pasteur of France observed that wine or other fermented fluid rot even faster when a magnet was put beside it. The most interesting observation and research comes from the scientist Albert Roy Davis of the USA. While he was fishing, he accidentally saw the behavior of the fishing worm and started his research on magnetic power. He put the worms in two separate containers made of thick paper. After some time, he saw that worms in one container were tangled with each other. However, worms in the other container were moving actively, and some of them even broke free from the container. After close observation, he discovered that there was a magnet that happened to be there beside the containers. Its north pole was pointed to the tangled worms, and south pole was directed at the active worms.

Davis did another research, this time with little chickens. He exposed the eggs in the high-intensity magnetic field before hatching. The eggs that were exposed to the south pole hatched faster, and the chicks that came from the eggs grew bigger and faster. They were more rebellious and died sooner. Chicks exposed to the north pole were born later and had small figures. They were passive but lived longer.

Through such observation, scientists nowadays continue their study with the following premise: that the south pole has an asthenia effect on the fertility of the living body and that the north pole has a contraction and calming effect. In small portions, countries around the world, including the medically advanced nations, are already using magnetic fields to diagnosis and treatment. MRI and electromyography also use magnetic field, and conditions such as arthritis, diseases related to inflammation, headache, insomnia, circulatory disease, stress, pain, and even facilitating the agglutination of sprained bones benefit from the magnetic field. It is forecast that the application of magnetic power will be promoted in disease treatment. However, we should take caution that inconsiderate use of the magnetic power may cause serious damage to our body.

Oxygen Therapy

Life is an existence with "nourish" and "P." It has the power to nourish itself and to protect itself. Our body is made up of about 100 trillion cells, and each cell is the basic unit of life. Therefore, our cells do their own type of "nourish and P." The most important elements in the process are oxygen and sugar.

Each organ reacts sensitively to the amount of oxygen and sugar. Brain cells are the most sensitive, and too low or too high levels of sugar or oxygen can make us fall. If oxygen supply is cut for more than 4 min, brain cells all die. Brain cells can't be regenerated once they die.

When heart stops pumping and breathing is stopped, as in the case of a patient suffering from heart attack, the person will die if an "emergency CPR" isn't conducted in 4 min. Breathing is how you take in and out the oxygen, which is called "sum" in Korean. As the breathing (sum) goes in and out through the neck (mok), we call "life" as "moksum." That's why "the person lost his breath" (sum) or "he lost his life" (moksum) all imply that the breathing is cut.

At the same time, it is oxygen that also hinders life. There are various types of oxygen, and how you take it in determines its impact on health. Normal breathing is composed of elementary and secondary breathing. Elementary breathing refers to the process of oxygen exchange in the lung. Secondary breathing is the oxygen exchange in the cells. Asthma, which occurs often in children, and pulmonary emphysema, usually found among the elderly citizen, arise when the elementary breathing isn't performed well. Stress, tension, and anxiety hinder peripheral circulation through capillary, and as a result, it undermines secondary breathing.

The process where oxygen sticks to blood or tissue is called "oxygenation." The process where electrons adhere to or run away from the oxygen atom is called "oxidation." In short, "saturation process" equals elementary breathing, and "oxidation process" equals secondary breathing. In the metabolism process in our body, harmful oxygen is produced and it makes us age and sick. Our body secretes enzymes such as SOD and catalase by itself to kill harmful oxygen. However, secretion is diminished as we near the age of 40, so harmful oxygen finds its way easier to be stored up in our body.

It has been about 100 years since people used oxygen to cure disease. We should take in useful oxygen and eliminate harmful oxygen in order to promote health. The following are ways to maintain our health: (1) quit smoking, (2) do breathing exercise, (3) eat less, (4) work out, (5) eat antioxidant food, (6) engage in positive thinking, (7) do oxygen therapy, etc.

Hyperbaric Oxygen Therapy

Hyperbaric oxygen therapy came around in early twentieth century, but it wasn't until mid-1960s before it was earnestly used. It is practiced in an acrylic container box about 2.2 m long with a diameter of 80 cm. A patient is put into the container on a stretcher in a lying position. After the exit is closed, the pressure is increased to about 2.5 (pressure), and the patient drinks in pure oxygen for about 30 min up to 120 min. Such oxygen with high pressure can be effectively absorbed into the body. After the treatment is over, pressure is slowly lowered to the normal level. The therapy is used in the following conditions: injuries, crash accidents, burn, wounds, gangrene, intoxicated by carbon monoxide, bedsore, edema, restoring dead tissue from chemotherapy, skin transplant, recovering from operation, stroke, peripheral vascular diseases, addiction to drugs and alcohol, multisclerosis, lung disease, low-volume anemia, and cyanosis.

Hydrogen Peroxide Therapy

Hydrogen peroxide is liquid in which 2 hydrogen atoms and 2 oxygen atoms are combined. It has 1 more oxygen atom than the water molecule, which consists of 2 hydrogen atoms and 1 oxygen atom, and therefore it is less stable and can easily induce oxidation. It was back in 1984 by Dr. C.H. Farr when the process of hydrogen peroxide participating in the oxidation in our body was reported for the first time.

The oxidation by hydrogen peroxide is used in treatment of tissues, breathing of cells, growth, immunity, endocrinology, and production of cytokines. It can also directly kill bacteria, viruses, fungi, and parasites.

Conditions or symptoms that can benefit through the hydrogen peroxide therapy are as follows (they have been proved clinically): AIDS, arthritis, cancer, candidiasis, chronic fatigue syndrome, depression, varicose veins, sprains, arteriosclerosis, headache, infectious disease, necrosis, stroke, allergies, asthma, pneumonia, diabetes, simple herpes, herpes zoster, and preventing wound infections.

Ozone Therapy

Oxidation and oxygenation all take part in the ozone therapy. Ozone has 3 oxygen atoms, so it's very unstable and can oxidize other chemicals very easily. Among the 3 oxygen atoms that ozone has, one runs away and the other two becomes normal oxygen molecule and results in the increase of oxygen content in the blood. This is why the oxidation and the oxygenation process occur at the same time. Ozone increases the supply of oxygen in the focal region, facilitates healing of wounds, represses growth of viruses and bacteria, increases the temperature of the regional tissue, and accelerates metabolism of the regional area. The conditions that show clinical effects through ozone include chronic infections, liver inflammation, multi-sclerosis, AIDS, and herpes, and it is also used to boost immunity.

However, there are side effects to using ozone. They include phlebitis, blood circulation disorder, chest pain, loss of breath, dizziness, cough, multicenter trial, arrhythmia, and blister.

Nutritional Supplement

The theoretical background of nutritional supplement goes like this. "When we look at the diet of modern people who often suffer from malnutrition, we can presume that diet alone can't supply ample nutrition to all parts of our body. Nutrition should be supplied that contain vitamins and minerals, so it can cure various diseases, injuries and prolong life. In this way, nutritional supplement can also help maintain physical, mental health and prevent chronic disease."

Osteopathic Medicine

Osteopathic medicine was established by Andrew T. Still in 1874. Its theory is based on the thought that "when our body is in a normal, structural relationship and is equipped with a good environment and nutrition, our body can cure itself from other diseases and addicted state." It is often applied to treat spine and joint-related diseases, arthritis, disorder in the digestive system, and chronic pain. Osteopathic manipulation is stressed as one of its techniques.

Detoxification Therapy

Detoxification therapy refers to eliminating harmful components or toxic agents of the body. Humans are exposed to numerous pollutants and chemical toxic agents from the atmosphere, water, food, and soil. As a result, the immune system and the functions of hormones can be lowered, and you can suffer from neurologic disease, mental conditions, and cancer. In this case, therapies related to fasting, diet, colon, vitamin C, and heat are used to get rid of the toxic agents from the body, and they are called detoxification therapy.

Energy Medicine

Energy medicine is injecting electromagnetic waves into our body to strike a balance among energies so that our body can become normal or healthy. It uses gadgets to measure the various electromagnetism that flow in our body, so that diseases that may occur in the future can be found out.

Orthomolecular Medicine

Orthomolecular medicine refers to maintaining the balance in our body (the balance of molecules in our body) by using the vitamins, minerals, and amino acids that make the best condition of our body. It is argued that the therapy is helpful to curing high blood pressure, cancer, depressed mood, schizophrenia, and other mental disorders.

Environmental Medicine

Environmental medicine studies show health and disease are related to our eating habits and lifestyle. It also explores how dust, fungi, chemical materials, and various foods become the cause for allergies. By thoroughly understanding the correlation among biology, body, and environment, it seeks to promote patients' physical and mental health.

Bodywork

Bodywork uses regional or whole-body massage, deep-tissue manipulation, conscious exercise, and energy balancing to relax tension and promote relaxation to diminish pain and to restore damaged muscle and stimulate blood circulation. By doing so, its ultimate goal is to increase the structure and function of the body and to promote health.

Rolfing

This therapy takes the name of Dr. Ida P. Rolf, who created the Rolfing therapy. The treatment method or skills are not so surprising. It argues that we need to control "vertical gravity" to maintain health, as humans walk on two feet. By using gravity, it stretches the body vertically and strikes a balance in the musculoskeletal (to the right and to the left). In this way, the musculoskeletal system and the health of the entire body can be promoted.

Dream Therapy

Dream therapy believes that dream is a form of self-realization. So remembering the dream and connecting it with the awakened conscious world is important. By acting and training this, it seeks to promote health.

Recreation Therapy

Recreation therapy is to induce treatment through engaging in funny actions, exercise, and behaviors. Some of its techniques are already in active use in rehabilitation medicine. It is to engage patients in treatment with a "willing and delightful" heart, rather than "out of duty" or against one's will. According to the likes and talents of each patient, arts, writing, pottery, music, dancing, exercise, floral arrangement, magic, and gardening can be used.

Magic Therapy

Magic therapy uses magic to induce treatment effects. Magic itself doesn't produce treatment effects. Rather, it seeks to make patients engage in the process to do particular behaviors repeatedly, which can be helpful to treatment. With a voluntary and willing heart, the patients have a pleasing time when learning magic and also a good time teaching the magic to others. In all these times, patients repeat the behaviors (embedded in the magic techniques) that help their treatment.

Neural Therapy

Neural therapy is based on the theory that the injection of the anesthetic can free the flow of energy in our body and normalize the function of our cells. The structure of our body is such that even in a perfect state, injuries can cut the flow of energy in our body. When this happens, anesthetic is injected to the nerve part of the autonomic nervous system, acupuncture locus, wounds, or other tissues so that the flow of energy can't be blocked.

Autogenic Therapy

The therapy was established by a German doctor named Johannes Schultz in the 1930s. It is a psychological therapy to promote the overall health condition by strengthening the relaxation and awareness state of the self, through focusing one's consciousness on his mind and creativity. Here is an example of the autogenic therapy. The doctor gives a self-implication to the patient that "my left arm is heavy." Then the patient's arm can be relaxed. If there is a self-implication that "my left arm is getting hot," the blood circulation of the patient's left arm can be promoted.

Reichian Therapy

Reichian therapy is created by Dr. Wilhelm Reich, who was born in Austria in 1897 and worked in the USA from 1939. It was mostly used to treat disorders in the sexual function. It avoided the tendency to focus on mental analysis or psychology.

Rather, the therapy directly dealt with the physical and mental side and effectively let out sexual and emotional energy that were abnormally repressed.

Guided Imagery

This therapy uses the strength of our mind or imagination. It seeks treatment effects by imagining that the disease is slipping out of our body. For instance, a patient can be induced to imagine that a happy day in the past is happening right now. By uplifting the spirits in this way, physical health can be improved. Or by imagining that a pain, ulcer, or a certain disease in his/her body is getting out of the body, the therapy believes that the patient can be freed from the disease.

Dance Therapy

Dance therapy is to focus on the dance moves of the body to induce physical and psychological changes. It is used to cure physical disorder but is more often used to treat mental disease. Dance moves prick interest, so it is also used as a light exercise to promote cardiopulmonary function.

Biological Dentistry

The therapy focuses that the health of human teeth has a great impact on the overall condition of the body and that chronic, regressive diseases are directly and indirectly related to the teeth problems. It anesthetizes the surrounding areas of teeth, holds a resistance checkup of muscle, or performs meridian massage to eliminate the rotten teeth, infection, addictive materials, and allergy-inducing materials. By correcting the position of dental root or the misalignments of the teeth and jaw, it seeks to treat and prevent diseases in our body.

3.2.2.2   SM Therapy from Pro-Oriental Medicine CAM

Ayurveda Medicine

Ayurveda is a science, religion, and philosophy. Everything that we come across in life is regarded as sacred in Ayurveda. Truth refers to "pure existence" or "the origin of all life" in Ayurveda. Therefore, Ayurveda is a science of truth that is realized in our lives. Ayurveda is a medical system that correlates the universe with human beings. It first began in India and is widely practiced in the country.

Ayurveda is a Sanskrit word meaning "the science of everyday life." "Ayu" means "life" or "daily life" and "Veda" means "knowledge." Ayurveda was first recorded in Veda, which is known as the oldest recordings in human history, and the medical system has been practiced for over 5000 years in India, in the daily lives of Indians.

This is what they teach in Ayurveda. "Every human being has four biological or spiritual instincts, and they are: religious instincts, economic instincts, fertile instincts, and free instincts. In order to satisfy such instincts, you need a balanced health to begin with. Ayurveda helps healthy people to maintain their health and the sick to restore their health. Ayurveda is an everyday science that is both medical and abstract transmundane, and it is the foundation of all therapies. The detailed guidelines of the Ayurveda are devised to promote happiness, health, and creative growth of humans. By studying the teachings of Ayurveda, anyone can learn practical knowledge to cure themselves. By maintaining a balance among all the energies in our body, people can effectively respond to the physical weakness or disease. The founding premise of Ayurveda is that all human beings have the ability to cure disease by themselves."

The common ground between Ayurveda medicine and the Oriental medicine is that both argue "Human beings are small universes" and "Order is equal to health, and disorder is equal to disease." However, the five elements of Oriental medicine has "Mok, Hwa, To, Geum, and Su" (wood, fire, earth, gold, and water), but in Ayurveda there are five elements called "ether (emptiness), air, fire, water, and earth."

In Ayurveda, there are three body conditions, which are Vata (air and sky), Pitta (fire and water), and Kapha (water and earth). The following Table 3.6 includes their characteristics.

There are the arguments of Ayurveda. The three components in our body, the Vata, the Pitta, and the Kapha have to maintain equilibrium, and the three excrement, the urine, feces, and sweat, have to be emitted well. Furthermore, the sensory organs have to function normally, and body, mind, and consciousness should work as a harmonious unity. The diagnosis is very unique, too. Ayurveda steadily looks at the correlation between order and disorder and sees that the process of disease is the response among the three elements and tissues. The condition of disease is regarded as being related to the disharmony of the three elements, and pulse, tongue, face, eyes, fingernails, and lips are observed every day, as symptoms can be expressed through them.

One of the treatment principles of Ayurveda is to eliminate toxic agents in our body and to neutralize them. In most cases, the following treatments are used together. They include: drug treatment, acupuncture, spine pressure, massaging, vomiting therapy, purgative, enema, putting in drugs in the nose, bloodletting, diet, controlling tastes (in India there are six tastes), lifestyle and regularity, yoga, breathing and yoga, and mantra (reciting).

Ayurveda has the philosophy to "control our health through lifestyle." That's why it's a science related to life. The following are some of the methods:

Get up before sunrise. Look at the sunlight. Open your eyes and get rid of urine and feces in your body. Eat slowly. Bathe everyday so as to give a fresh sense to the body. Do the 12 types of breathing training, and the body and the mind will be refreshed. Eat breakfast before 8 a.m. Wash your hands before and after you eat. Take a light walk for 15 minutes

Table 3.6 Ayurveda medicine

Vata	Pitta	Kapha
A skinny body	Not skinny, not fat	A plump body
Visible joints	Small amount of hair	Lots of hair
Cold and dry skin	Hot and sweaty skin	Greasy and cold skin
Active	Precise	Slow and generous
Sensitive	Easily tenses	Relaxed
Lots of energy	Quick to anger	Slow to anger
Always sleeps and eats	Always eats regularly	Slow eating
Imaginative	Knowledgeable	Passionate
Nervous systemdiseases	Gastric ulcer	Obesity
Constipation	Hemorrhoid	Allergies
Positive thinking	Warm and loving	Patience and forgiveness
Intuition	Good at speech	Generosity
Cramp	Contused wound (acne)	High cholesterol
Anxiety	Perfectionism	Slow

after meal. As you eat, try to feel the food and don't talk while eating. Put some sesame oil on your finger and massage your gums. Don't eat for a day a week in order to decrease the toxic agents from the body. Go to sleep before 10 p.m.

Qigong Therapy

It was in the 1950s in China when the word "Qigong" started to be used in the generalized meaning as it is now. Qigong is a regimen that includes not only the moving of your body but also breathing control and mind training. It is body exercise, breathing training, and transcendental meditation combined together.

There are two types of Qigong. One is "Health Qigong" that is related to medical health. The other is "Martial Arts Qigong" to make a strong body. "Health Qigong" takes flexible training, so it's also called a "Soft Qigong." As for the "Martial Arts Qigong," the intensity is higher, so it's called a "Hard Qigong." When ordinary people refer to Qigong, they usually point to "Health Qigong." Health Qigong is divided into two, a health-promoting "Welfare Qigong" and the disease-treating "Treatment Qigong."

In Qigong therapy, there are two types. First is called "open-air treatment." In this case, the therapist doesn't lay his hands on the patient's body but uses his energy or "ki" (energy) to cure the patient. Another is "manipulation technique," where the doctor touches the patient's body and gives a direct stimulus. In the "Soft Qigong," which has the same training techniques as the "Health Qigong," there is one called "Special Ability Qigong" or "IQ Qigong." The goal of it is to cultivate human potential or superpowers.

The detailed way of training Qigong is called, "Gongbeop." It has been with us for the last 3000 years, and there are more than 3000–4000 techniques that have been passed down until today. The examples are Mokgong (rolling your eyes up/down and right/left), Seolgong (relaxing the muscles of your tongue), Jehangong (pulling up your anal muscles), and Sangsangong (imagining certain things when you sleep).

The following are the effects of Qigong on our body. It has a relaxation response where the functions of the sympathetic nerves are decreased. It also has neurological, chemical responses that control the immune abilities. Furthermore, by emitting toxic wastes, the resistance against disease is increased, and the increased efficiency of the metabolism strengthens tissue-regenerating ability. It also controls the laterality of the left and right side of our brain, thereby promoting emotional stability. Controlling the functions of the hypothalamus, pituitary gland, pineal gland, and cerebrospinal fluid can ease pain and help emotional stability. Today, Qigong treatment is used in digestion conditions, asthma, arthritis, insomnia, pain, depression, and anxiety. It's also tested in cardiac disease, cancer, and AIDS to boost patients' strength in fighting rare, incurable diseases.

In China, the infra-tonic QGM is being distributed. Here, the base frequencies refer to sounds that our ears can't hear. The sounds with very high sound wave that we can't hear are called ultrasound, and the sounds that are too low for us to hear are called base frequencies. From the hands of Qigong experts, much high base frequencies, or "Ichaeum" (high level of low-frequency acoustic waves/secondary sound), comes out, and base frequencies' energy brings out treatment effects. Every one of us can emit base frequencies' energy, but from the skillful Qigong experts, the energy is emitted 100 times stronger than ordinary people and about 1000 times more than patients.

In the early 1980s, Dr. Lu Yan Fang of National Electro Acoustics Laboratory, Beijing, China, developed a machine that can emit similar energy as the QGM (8–14 Hz, 70 dB). The machine has been put in use since then, and it is highly effective in curing pain, especially migraine. It's also used to increase blood circulation, relaxing muscles, and treating depression.

Qigong, which is the regimen of Oriental medicine, can be conducted while you stand, walk, sit, or lie down or even when you sit on a wheelchair. That's why it's helpful not only to healthy people who want to promote health and prevent disease. It's also helpful to treating various diseases including the conditions of critical patients. Qigong is also related to training your mind, so it's being widely spread around the world including the USA and Europe.

Naturopathic Medicine

In treating disease, you can either use an artificial therapy where you use manmade materials and machines or use natural materials as they are. Natural therapy, as can be derived from its meaning, refers to using natural materials in treatment. There are two kinds of natural therapies. The first one, a broader concept, is about all folklore therapies that use the usual natural energies. Traditional medicine is also included here. Second is used in a narrow sense, where only experts can practice.

The word naturopathy or naturopathic medicine started to be widely used in its general meaning since the nineteenth century, but philosophical roots go up thousands of years. It includes techniques learned from various wisdoms from a variety of cultures in the ancient world. They include the Ayurveda medicine of India, traditional Chinese medicine, American native medicine, and Hippocratic medicine.

In naturopathic medicine, the following "six principles" are emphasized:

1. Healing power of nature: our body has a strong healing power to heal itself. The role of natural therapists is to mobilize the natural and harmless therapies to activate the natural healing power.
2. Cure causes, not the results: natural therapists don't only provide a simple allopathy but focus on eliminating the cause after narrowing it down. Every condition is regarded as an "expression of body's natural attempt" in terms of physical, mental, psychological, and spiritual perspective.
3. "No harm" first: natural therapists conduct safe and effective natural therapies so that even a little harm isn't induced on the patient's part.
4. "Treat the whole person" (treat the patient in a holistic viewpoint): patients are not dealt partially but are dealt in every aspect including physical, mental, psychological, social, and spiritual ways. The treatment is conducted after evaluating all aspects comprehensively.
5. Natural therapists are teachers: they don't do everything themselves for the patients. Rather, natural therapists encourage patients, explain to them, give them energy, and are just like teachers who teach patients the right things to do.
6. Prevention is the best medicine: natural therapists make it their utmost priority to prevent disease by improving lifestyle habits and giving education to patients.

In natural therapy, two elements are emphasized for affecting people to contract disease. First is how strong the toxic traits of etiological cause (the cause of disease) are. Second is how strong our body is in retaliating to the disease. The greater defense ability we have, the stronger we will be to fend out the etiological cause that would come in to break the harmonious state of our body. Therefore, maintaining and promoting health means "weakening the toxic traits of the intruder and increasing the defense ability of the body." This is how natural therapy looks at disease: "every disease has one common ground, and that is, they are in the body because the body has weak vitality." Therefore, two elementary ways are needed to regain health. The lacking parts should be filled up, and the toxic traits should be emitted out of the body. First, the lacking parts in our body should be filled with pure food, water, thinking, exercise (movements), and peace of mind. Second is a cleaning process and purifying the body free of toxic agents.

Natural therapists argue that patients tend to follow the "law of cure" when you look at the cycle of patients contracting disease and recovering from it. The cycle of the curing process can be put in this way: "as the nutrition level of the body gets higher, body is cleansed and the symptoms of past disease reappear. In this case, the most recent symptoms appear first and then come the symptoms of the diseases that the patients suffered first. As you can see, the first becomes the last, and the last, first." Let's presume that a 45-year-old patient suffers from arthritis. He has a history of contracting sciatic neuralgia, migraine, eczema, and indigestion. In the process of curing his latest condition, arthritis, he may go through the past symptoms one by one.

Patients and therapists have to go on reeducation programs together. In the reeducation process, ways to increase spiritual harmony is practiced, which include improving eating habits, developing daily exercise techniques and putting it into practice every day, letting out toxic agents from the body, and doing meditation, breathing exercise, prayer, and relaxation exercise. To have a successful natural therapy, an active participation has to come from the part of the patients. Patience, steady efforts, and a strong will are needed.

One thing you need to remember when implementing natural therapy is that various ways of therapies don't work the same on every patient. For instance, a patient may need "complementation" and "repair." But if you use the "cleansing technique" on the patient, it may cause unnecessary stress to him. Patients who have relatively good nutrition levels or physical health may experience faster recovering process than the patients who don't. This type of healthier patients will also have easier time emitting toxic agents as well. In this context, "nutrition" is not manmade but has to be a genuine, natural one. In terms of nutrition, the two sides of psychological and spiritual aspects should be dealt with at the same time. Therefore, various types of physical treatments including diet, nutrition, homeopathic medicine and Oriental medicine, acupuncture, exercise treatment, hydrotherapy, manipulation therapy, and electric and sunlight treatments should be utilized.

Natural therapy has been with humans for the longest time as treatment, and humans will know and use the therapy forever. To increase its efficiency and minimize the possible side effects, objective and scientific research should follow.

Aromatherapy

The Origins and Definition of Aromatherapy

In the 1920s, there was a French chemist named Gattefosse who worked in the fragrance industry. When he got a severe burn on his hand, he happened to put his hand in the lavender oil that was beside him. It became the beginning of aromatherapy. To his surprise, the burned skin and pain quickly disappeared, and he was made certain that the lavender oil has treatment and sterilization effects. Later, he tested several other oils and those also had effects on various skin diseases.

Aromatherapy is one branch of herbal medicine therapy which uses medicinal properties that are from various plants' essential oil. The essential oil is extracted from flowers and their roots, leaves, bark of trees, and fruits through the way of steam distillation or cold pressing. The oils have strong scent, and they are highly flammable. An aromatherapy expert, Dr. Kurt Schnaubelt, explains aromatherapy like this: "Some people think aromatherapy is a simple scent-related effect, but the essential oil has specific pharmacological properties. The molecules of the properties are very small (small molecular size) and can penetrate into human tissues easily. That is why the treatment effect is very high."

The Mechanism of Aroma Therapy

1. The pharmacological traits of oil: antibiotic, antiviral, antispasmodic, diuretics, vasodilators, and vasoconstrictors.
2. The functional traits of oil: it works on the adrenals, ovary, and thyroid to energize the organs, detoxify, facilitate the digestive process, treat infection, interact with various branches of the nervous system, modify immune response, and harmonize moods and emotion.

The Physiological Effects of Fragrance

1. Smell is the most sensitive part of our five senses. When there is a certain fragrance or smell in the air, it floats in the air and activates the olfactory sense recipients that are on the ceiling of our nostrils. When we are young, the thin and cotton-like recipients grow new every 30 days, but as we age, the growing speed slows down and they don't grow new when we age. This is why most elderly people can't smell well. When the smell arrives at the nasal cavity in the form of aromatic molecule, it changes into electric signals at the peripheral nerves. The electric information produced then enters the limbic system, which controls our emotions. The limbic system is directly related to the past experiences and emotions within us, but it's also connected to the heart pulse, blood pressure, breathing, memories, level of stress, and balance of hormones. Therefore, oil can be a tool that can bring about physiological or psychological effects in the fastest way. Such elements work in a complex way to influence specific diseases or abnormal conditions.
2. According to a study, aroma oil such as orange, jasmine, and rose has tranquilizing effect and produces brain waves that can induce calmness and sense of well-being. Exotic aroma oil such as basil, black pepper, rosemary, and cardamom produce brain waves that induce heightened energy response.

Ways to Use Aromatherapy

Oil is taken in through inhalation or external application through the skin. It can also be used through ingestion.

1. Diffusor: you disperse the microparticles in the air. It can be used to overturn breathing-related symptoms or to simply have a mood-lifting effect or improve calming quality.
2. External application: oil can be absorbed easily through the skin. One of the convenient ways is bathing, massaging, hot and cold compress, or just rubbing it against the skin. Oils such as rosemary can eliminate toxic agents through rubbing it on the skin. Compression can relieve slight pains, can soothe edema, and can also treat sprains.
3. Internal application: it can be helpful when you wish to relieve a slight condition made by dysfunction or disorder, not a disease in an organ. In this case, supervision from a medical expert is needed.

Indicants of Aromatherapy

1. Bacterial and viral infection: oil has very strong antibiotic effects. Unlike other antibiotics, it doesn't have side effects such as kidney toxicity, anemia, loss of white blood cells, or deafness. It also doesn't kill symbiotic bacteria that live in our stomach.
2. Herpes simplex: lemon and geranium mixed oil, eucalyptus and Bergamo mixed oil, and rose or bee balm oil are suggested to cure herpes. If aromatherapy is applied immediately after the herpes blister comes out, the blister dries in about a day or two. It usually takes 3–5 days to cure the blister completely.
3. Shingles or herpes zoster infection: Dr. Schnaubelt mixed *Ravensara* and *Calophyllum inophyllum* in a 1:1 ratio and found out that it took a week to fight off the infection.
4. Skin conditions: thyme has high antibiotic, and neroli oil is known to have rejuvenating properties, and that is why the two are used frequently in skin management. Rosemary oil helps regeneration of cells and it activates the metabolism of the inner layer of skin. Thyme and rosewood oil are also effective in curing acmes. When bitten by bugs, basil, cinnamon, garlic, lavender, lemon, green onion, sage, savory, and thyme are advised. They have antitoxic and antivenomous properties.
5. Muscular disorders: mixed oil of sage, chamomile, and lavender have a special effect of relieving muscle cramps convulsion.
6. Arthritis: Dr. Hildebret Wagner of Germany reported that clove, cinnamon, and thyme have anti-inflammatory effect and are good for treating arthritis. It is widely known that the oil stimulates adrenal glands and secretes corticoid substances that fight inflammation.
7. Relaxingbody and mind: oil is used to relieve various symptoms related to stress. It is also used to relax mind, to help overturn insomnia, and to cure light indigestion or the churning feelings of the stomach nausea.

Clinical Application of Aroma Oil

1. Eucalyptus

   Antivirus
   Expectorant

2. Everlast

   Tissue regeneration
   Anti-inflammatory
   To prevent bleeding and edema from sports wounds or bruise

3. Geranium

   Antifungal
   Antivirus

4. Lavender

   Burns
   Small injuries
   Insect bites

5. Mandarin

   Uplifts your mood
   Releases anxiety

6. Niaouli

   Represses allergies in the respiratory system
   Vitalizes overactive oily skin
   Helps cure hemorrhoids (when it's not acute)

7. Palmarosa

   Uplifts your mood
   Antiseptic
   Antivirus and treats herpes

8. Peppermint

   Cures nausea or travel sickness
   Helps cure irritable bowel syndrome
   Helps strengthen liver functions

9. Roman Chamomile

   Relieves physical and mentalstress

10. Rosemary

    Activates metabolism of outer layer of the skin
    Increasescell regeneration

11. Spikenard

    Promotes life energy and psyche

12. Tea tree

    Nonirritating antiseptics
    Antibiotic, antivirus, and antimycotic
    Effective in treating festering inflammation and chronic inflammation

Caution

1. Drinking oil extracted from hyssop, sage, thuja, wormwood, mugwort, and tansy
   can bring out toxic side effects in the body.

2. Taking oregano or savory for long periods of time (10–21 days) can hinder liver functions.
3. Most oil is made to be taken in through external senses, not by eating. When clove or cinnamon oil is applied on the skin, allergic responses such as dermatitis can be produced as a side effect in about 5 % of the population. The oil shouldn't be applied near the eyes as well.
4. Peppermint oil can be helpful in curing digestion-related diseases, but it can worsen insomnia.
5. If not used adequately, the aromatherapy can produce side effects in all cases, as many parts of their effects are yet to be proven.

Prospects

Aromatherapy is spreading widely around the world. There are countries like France where the institutions are established so doctors' prescriptions are needed. However, in most countries, it is not yet institutionalized. In the future, aromatherapy will be highlighted as a very important therapy in managing stress.

Transcendental Meditation Therapy

Meditation means that "thinking is deeply engrossed in something." It is a safe and simple way to balance your physical, mental, and emotional self. Meditation has been conducted by people for several thousand years in human history. However, it's only been 30 years since it was researched in scientific sense. There are two types of meditation. One is "concentrative meditation" and the other is "mindful meditation."

Concentrative meditation is to focus our mind on breathing or on a certain image or sound. It is to soothe our mind, to clear our head, and to deepen our understanding. It is similar to looking at a very narrow field with a microscope or a zoom lens of a camera. If someone becomes anxious, fearful, and excited, he/she would take shallow and fast breaths, and his/her breathing will be irregular. However, if he/she has a comfortable and stabilized mind focused on something, his/her breathing will be slow, deep, and regular. That is why when our conscious is focused on breathing, our heart tunes into the rhythm of our breathing.

Mindful meditation is not about focusing your conscious on a small corner. It is rather opening up your conscious and expanding infinitely so that all senses, feelings, images, sounds, and smell are left as they are and to let them flow as they will. In short, it is to leave them alone as they fill up your mind. It is similar to looking through a telescope or the wide-angle lens of a camera.

Let's take an example. Televisions and radios are full of electric waves that come from various stations all around the world. However, the televisions or radios next to us don't show any sounds or images until I tune them into a certain frequency. It's only when the electric wave that traveled far and the radio beside me have the same frequency or cycle that a clear sound comes out. It works the same way in our minds, too. When our conscious is tuned into the same cycle of the conscious of the universe, which fills the space around us, my conscious is able to exchange information with the energy of the universe. The act of getting the cycles tuned is what meditation is.

When it becomes small to extremes, the state becomes nothingness. When it becomes large to extremes, it also becomes nothingness. Therefore, the act of meditation is tuning into the frequency of the nothingness. It is to make our mind to either of the extremes (nothingness), whether small or large. In this case, we can use image as a tool, but sound can also be a tool to better our concentration skills. It is to open your ears to sounds that are too small to hear or that are too big to hear.

As you can see, meditation is about "being completely absorbed in something." Recently, it is highlighted as a clinical treatment that relieves various symptoms related to stress. The goal is to stabilize our mind and to promote concentration. Many parts of it originate from Oriental religions, where the goal is to clear your mind of everything. Indian yoga expert Maharish Maheshi Yogi popularized easy-to-learn meditation skills for Westerners, and the word that describes it is "transcendental meditation or TM." Recently, an Indian-American doctor named Dipak Chopra established a meditation center in San Diego, USA and plays a central role in spreading the meditation techniques by combining it with quantum medicine. Many Westerners think meditation is very personal, quiet, and static (maybe due to the impression they had from Zen meditation), but in Eastern countries, meditation has various active elements such as doing it in groups or combining it with t'ai chi chuan and martial arts. Mind-body medicine such as Qigong, yoga, biofeedback, and induced imagination techniques all have meditative elements in them.

NCCAM or the National Center of Complementary Alternative Medicine reports that studies have shown transcendental meditation increases quality of life, shortens the hospitalization periods of patients, diminishes the health management costs, and increases the average life span of the general public. In concrete medical research, transcendental meditation is reported to have the following effects: decreasing cortisol, the stresshormone, and anxiety, relieving chronic pain, lowering blood pressure and pulse, decreasing the level of cholesterol, and diminishing drug addiction. However, there are also reports about transcendental meditation's side effects. After meditation, some people felt more depressed or confused, and some schizophrenia patients' condition got worse.

Reflexology

Reflexology is based on the theory that when pressure is administered to the specific parts of the body such as the head, palm, soles or ears, as if pricking with our fingertips, the particular organs or endocrine gland connected to the pressure points are stimulated and the functions are increased. In Northeastern Asian countries, where acupuncture takes effect through meridian massage, reflexology has been used for 5000 years. Reflexology is described in the presto wall paintings of Egypt about 4300 years ago and a similar technique was used in ancient India as well. There are records that American Indians also used similar techniques.

Recently, it was by Dr. William Fitzgerald, who lived in Connecticut, USA, shone a new light on the therapy, calling it zone therapy or reflexology in 1913. He discovered that pressing the patients' palm or soles just before the operation spared them pain to some degree. Through long time of observation, he put out the theory that certain parts of our hands and feet are functionally related to the other organs of our body.

"Foot reflexology" is the most widely spread therapy in reflexology. It states that the thumb is related to our brain and the center of our soles to the solar plexus of the stomach and that the heels and the tops of the feet are related to the anus and rectum. Dr. Fitzgerald pioneered the field so it can be given a new meaning, but it was Eunice Ingham, the physical therapist and the massage therapist, who earnestly spread it. He argued that the effects of reflexology go further than just diminishing pain to include curing various physical symptoms. His argument rapidly spread around the world, as it was when acupuncture of the Oriental medicine was introduced in the West.

Currently, reflexology is used in more than 100 symptoms and diseases, such as digestion-related diseases (diarrhea, constipation, and indigestion), stress-related conditions (asthma, migraine, and fatigue syndrome), chronic pains (arthritis, neurogenic pain), allergies, skin diseases, and multisclerosis. Reflexology is used to manage the symptoms, and it doesn't cure the cause of the disease directly, so patients are advised to be checked from the doctor first before getting reflexology.

It takes about 45 min to receive reflexology. In the case of foot reflexology, you put your feet in hot water, massage your feet, or stimulate certain parts with a specially made tool. Reflexology is mostly safe, but in the case of wounds, boil, sprain, phlebothrombosis, phlebitis, and ulcer and in particular for diabetes and arterial occlusion by atherosclerosis, patients can experience serious side effects, and special attention is required.

Touching Therapy

"Touching" includes physical stimuli such as patting the skin, rubbing cheeks together, hugging and piggybacking, and breastfeeding, and as for adults, it includes massaging, kissing, and all other forms of expressing love. Recently, touching is being used as one form of treatment, and it is spreading across the world.

The Oriental meridian massage technique can be one form of touching therapy. In our body, especially in our skin, there are "reactions points" that are sensitive to a physical stimulus, which are called "meridian points." "Reaction line" refers to a line of these reaction points connected together, which is called "meridian massage." When we touch or massage such meridian points or do meridian massage, the "natural healing power" in our body is facilitated. The theory of the Oriental medicine states that it is helpful to preventing and treating disease.

There are reports that massaging immature babies at the hospital makes them grow 50 % faster than other immature babies. Cultures with a lot of hugging and embracing have lower violence rates as well.

About 50 years ago in the Soviet Union, a new technology was developed by the Kirlian couple, which was to photograph the some kind of unkown energy that comes out of our body. This is called "Kirlian photography" and the most amount of energy came out from our fingertips. When the hands of the person who had a strong ray of light coming out touched the hands of the person with less energy, there were improvements of the energy coming out from the latter person's hands. It can be evidence that backs up the effects of touching therapy, but traditional medicine experts argue that accumulated research on the topic should follow.

Zen Dance Therapy

It is a therapy that was made 30 years ago by a Korean doctor named Lee Sun-ok, who observed the healing effects of the Korean traditional "Zen dance." It is one of the mind-bodytherapies that combine TM, abdominal breathing, and dancing movement.

It helps our general health and relieves stress and anxiety. It is also helpful to insomnia, arthritis, joint contracture, and the before and after phase of pregnant women. If there are continued clinical tests and an accumulation of experiences, I believe it has a potential to grow into a fine therapy. It is slowly being distributed around the world.

Yoga

For several centuries in the India, Ayurveda, Tantra, and yoga were the wisdom of life that has been passed down by generations. Among them, yoga refers to combining with the sacredness, that is, the truth. The meaning of the word yoga is "union," and it refers to a complex of physical, mental, and psychological energy. Yoga is one of the longest prevailing health systems known around the world. Through position, breathing, and meditation, yoga is known to have the effects of relieving stress, lowering blood pressure, evening heart pulse, and preventing aging.

Flower Remedies

Flower remedies are ways of getting treatment effects by using flowers. It is to improve the emotional status by directly dealing with the physical and mental aspects. Emotions play various roles on our physical strength. Flower remedies improve negative feelings or strike a balance of stress to recover health effectively.

Here is one of the ways that flower remedy experts use. They pick flowers early in the morning when they still have morning dew on them. Then, they put the flowers into a pot filled with fresh water and expose it out in the sun for about 3 h. They take the flowers out and separate the flower and the small branches. They mix the flower water and brandy in 1:1 ratio and use the formulated concentrate as medicine.

Sound Therapy

Sound therapy includes sound treatment and music treatment. Sound and music play a very important role in our health. Sound therapy is an effective treatment to decrease stress, and it is used in mental and scientific treatments or curing low blood pressure or continuous pain or curing learning disabilities. It is also used to improve exercise and balancing sense and patience.

Horticulture Therapy

Horticulture therapy is to increase patients' confidence and self-esteem by growing flowers and tending to vegetables and plants. Those with mental weakness, emotional instability, or mental disorder can also benefit from horticulture therapy.

Bee Venom Therapy

Bee venom therapy is to get treatment effects by using the bee sting. The meridian point is usually the place selected for bee stings, but not always. The selected skin parts of the body are artificially shot with bee stings, and the effects include diminished pain, overturning of arthritis, and advanced mental health.

Psychic Healing

In psychic healing, patients don't do anything by themselves, but the people known to have special powers conduct special spiritual therapies on the patients to cure their disease.

3.2.2.3 SM Therapy from CAM Combined with Western and Oriental Medicine

Herbal Therapy or Phytotherapy

Herb therapy refers to using parts of plants as medicine, such as leaves, flowers, stems, seeds, fruits, and barks. Herb is the oldest form of therapy that is used by humans, and each culture has their own type of special herbs. The English word "drug" originated from the ancient Netherlands word "Drogge," which refers to "dry." The word takes it form from the old tradition where trees or grass was dried to be used as medicine. About 25 % of all the drugs that are prescribed in the Western medicine are taken from tree or grass. Digitalis (cardiac medicine), reserpine (blood pressure-lowering medicine), colchicine (gout cure), and morphine (painkiller) are good examples.

From 250,000 up to 500,000 plant species live on our planet, and about 5000 among them are used as drugs. Natural products have in them the natural chemical products that produce various physiological responses in our body. Some are very mild to be eaten as food, but others have strong traits such as poison.

The Drug-Like Functions of Natural Drugs

1. Adaptogenic: increases resistance and adaptability to stress and other problems that result from the surrounding environment. It facilitates functions of the adrenal gland.
2. Alterative: it slowly restores the physical condition by increasing health and vitality.
3. Anthelmintic.
4. Anti-inflammatory.
5. Antimicrobial.
6. Antispasmodic.
7. Astringent: it contracts the focal parts when administered in those parts.
8. Bitter: used as medicine that tastes bitter. It is also used as alterative, tonic, or appetite booster.
9. Carminative: it relieves the drum belly (gas filling the stomach) and eliminates pain.
10. Demulcent: it relieves pain on the parts where inflammation or abrasion is.
11. Diuretic.
12. Emmenagogue: stimulates menstruation.
13. Expectorant: promotes sputum expectoration.
14. Hepatic: improves liver functions.
15. Hypotensive.
16. Laxative: gets rid of constipation.
17. Nervine.
18. Increases stimulating works.
19. Increases tonic works.

The Forms of Natural Products

1. Whole herb
2. Teas
3. Capsules and tablets
4. Extracts and tinctures
5. Essential oils
6. Alves, balms, and ointments

The Effects of Natural Products

1. Used in light symptom management: relieves indigestion, cold, influenza, slight pain, constipation, diarrhea, cough, headache, menstrual pain, skin spots, dandruff, and insomnia.

2. Used as treatment for various diseases: used in gastrointestinal conditions such as peptic ulcers, colitis, and irritable bowel syndrome, chronic skin diseases such as eczema and psoriasis, and gynecological conditions such as menstrual irregularity or premenstrual syndrome. It is also used in treating stress-related conditions such as anxiety, breathing difficulties, high blood pressure, allergies, and arthritis.

The Differences Between Oriental Herbal Medicine and Natural Products

1. The prescription of Oriental herbal medicine is based on the Oriental medicine. It is to find out the "8 Gang" of the 12 internal organs and to prescribe according to them. "8 Gang" refers to yin and yang, duplicity, coldness and heat, and false and truth. In terms of sex and quality, sex takes priority in prescription.
2. Finding out the components of herbs and prescribing them to their functions and effects are the beginning of natural products' prescription. For instance, herbs that produce diarrhea are used to cure constipation. In terms of sex and quality, quality takes the priority in prescription.

Prescription of Natural Products

1. Aloe vera: it is mixed with cosmetics for its skin-softening effect. It is often used as laxative. However, caution is needed as electrolyte imbalance can occur when used for a long time to cure constipation.
2. Cayenne: it is used as systemic stimulants. It boosts blood circulation, digestion, and metabolism.
3. Chamomile: it is used in teas and beverages for its fresh fragrance. It helps digestion and has a slight relieving and anti-inflammation effects.
4. Chasteberry: it is a type of strawberry and it helps cure the imbalance of female hormone. It works in the pituitary gland to maintain a balance between estrogen and progesterone.
5. Echinacea: it is a purple, cone-shaped flower and was traditionally used by the North Americans. Recently, it is popular in Germany and European countries. It cures wounds and has anti-inflammation and immunity boosting effects.
6. Ephedra: it has been used in the East to cure respiratory conditions such as asthma for thousands of years. Ephedra contains two types of important plant alkaloids. One is ephedrine and the other is pseudo-ephedrine. Ephedrine has strong contracting traits on peripheral blood vessels, and pseudo-ephedrine expands bronchial tubes. The herb shouldn't be used on patients with high blood pressure, diabetes, and glaucoma.
7. Feverfew: it is a herb that has been used since the ancient Greek and the Roman era to control the periods of young women. Later, the herb was found to have effects of decreasing fever and was widely used. That's why the name became "feverfew," which means that the fever (fever) is lowered (few). Recently, it is also used to cure migraine.

8. Garlic: garlic is one of the most well-known herbs in the world, as it has been used in almost all cultures traditionally. For the last 30 years, some 1000 theses have been reported on garlic. Garlic has antibiotic, antimycotic, and antiviral effects, and it is used in respiratory syndromes such as cough or bronchitis. It is useful to preventing cold or influenza and is used in stomach conditions such as dysentery, ulcer, and arthritis. Recently, it is used in various purposes such as lowering blood pressure, repressing the production of blood clots (anticoagulation), boosting immunity, and preventing several types of cancers.

9. Ginger: it is one of the frequently used herbs in Korean Oriental medicine or the Ayurveda of India. It helps other herbs and also facilitates digestion. It has a strong power in curing nausea and vomiting, so recently it is used to cure motion sickness and soothe the sickness of pregnant women. It is also used as cardiotonic, headache treatments, and burn cures.

10. Ginko: ginko trees appeared on earth about 200 million years ago and is regarded as one of the longest surviving trees in the world. It was since the fifteenth century that it was used as medicine in the East. In the West, it was applied to the research and clinical tests since the 1970s. Based on the study results that improve the blood circulation of peripheral blood vessels, it is widely used in cerebrovascular and cardiac diseases. Related to the blood circulation of peripheral blood vessels, it is also used in intermittent claudication and eye disease.

11. Ginseng: it has a very strong trait to boost adaptability. It increases the resistance and adaptability of our body as it fights various types of stress. Ginseng's medical effect usually boosts the workings of adrenal, and the effects include antioxidant, anti-hepatotoxic, and hypoglycemic traits. There are also reports that it strengthens immunity and lowers cholesterol levels. However, we should always remember that side effects such headaches and skin problems can occur when abused.

12. Goldenseal: it is the most frequently used herb in the USA. It boosts immune response and has antibiotic effects. The bitter taste of goldenseal and its digestion fluid secretion boosting effect make it popular in curing peptic ulcer and colitis.

13. Hawthorn: it is a natural product that has been used for hundreds of years both in the East and the Europe as folklore therapy. It is known to increase cardiac functions as cardiant. Research shows that it also has sedative and hypotensive effects, and countries such as Germany are using it with digoxin, a well-known cardiac medicine.

14. Hops: as an herb that adds a bitter taste to beer and acts as preservative in its fermenting process, hops have been used for several hundred years. It also has calming effect and sleep-inducing effect and is often used to cure anxiety and insomnia.

15. Licorice: just like the saying that someone is "like a licorice in the pharmacy," it has been one of the most widely used herbs for a long time. It is known to have effects that boost the endocrine system and liver functions, strengthening various organs. Licorice has a similar trait as adrenocortical hormones have, so

it can boost anti-inflammation activities and strengthen the liver as it can prevent the damaging of liver cells. Licorice is also used in liver symptoms such as hepatitis and liver cirrhosis and simple herpes, peptic ulcer, gastritis, cough, or lung-related diseases such as bronchitis. However, when large amounts are used for a long time, it can induce imbalance of electrolyte or high blood pressure. Therefore, high blood pressure and renal disease patients and pregnant women should abstain from using licorice.

16. Milk thistle: milk thistle has been used as liver tonic. Recent study shows that it is effective in inflammation and cirrhosis. It also cures liver damages by toxic agents and minimizes the sequel of inflammation. It is also reported to minimize the sequel following liver operations.

17. Nettle: it is one of the most popular natural herbs in the West. It has detoxification functions, is an immune-modulating tonic, and is facilitating the production of lymphocytes and therefore used to cure rheumatic disease, arthritis, allergic coryza, and infantile eczema. It is also used as diuretic.

18. Passion flower: it has been traditionally used as sedative in the West. According to recent study, it has anticonvulsant effects on the digestion system to cure conditions such as gastritis and enteritis. It also has sedative and anxiolytic effects and can lower blood pressure.

19. Peppermint: for hundreds of years, peppermint was widely used in the folklore therapy, known to help digestion. It gets rid of gas in the stomach, promotes secretion of bile, and has antibiotic effects. Clinically, it is used to cure stomach cramps, spasm of bile duct, gallstone, catarrh, pruritus, and urticaria.

20. St. John's wort: it has various effects such as anti-inflammation, wound-healing nervine, relieving the nervous system, and diminishing pain. It is used in treating neuralgia, anxiety, tension derived from stress, fibrositis, pain resulting from rheumatism, changes of physical condition in the menopause, depression, inflammation resulting from virus, influenza, and AIDS.

21. Saw palmetto: it is a natural herb that is in the palm family. Generally, it is known to increase the fertility of men. It is used to facilitate the secretion of male hormones, and clinical tests show that it is effective in curing benign prostatic hypertrophy and prostatics.

22. Senna: it is a natural product that is in the bean group. As a relic of the traditional medicine of ancient Arab world, senna has relieving effects and is used to cure constipation. As other stool looseners, patients may develop dependency when they overconsume senna, and it can result an imbalance in electrolyte.

23. Eleuthero: it is one of the best adaptogens, and it can strengthen stress coming from outer environments. According to a study, those who took eleuthero had lower incidence rates of chronic gastritis, diabetes, and atherosclerosis. They were able to recover relatively faster and had lower metastasis rates and more power to overcome the side effects of chemotherapy.

24. Valerian: it is a natural product that is in the valerian family and has been used as sedative. It soothes a "state of excitement" and gives sleep to those who suffer from insomnia. It has little side effect than from other sleeping pills, and

even taking it while drinking doesn't induce any synergy effects. The reason it's a good sedative to use during the day is because it doesn't make you feel blank like other sleeping pills.

25. Witch hazel: it is a kind of *Hamamelis virginiana* and is regarded as astringent. Witch hazel works as styptic that stops bleeding and is a cure for hemorrhoids, bruises, inflamed swelling, and varicose vein. It is also used as obstruent to stop diarrhea.

Diet

The mainstream idea is that "everything that is not Western medicine is alternative therapy." Therefore, any food or diet that is not generally prescribed in the Western medicine is regarded as complementary, alternative therapy. There are six types of complementary, alternative therapies related to eating habit and attitude.

Six Types of People Looking at Food

1. Survivors: these people eat to sustain their lives. They only eat the minimum portion needed to survive and only eat when they're in a situation to do so. Even in those necessary times, these people eat a little bit from the table. They don't like to give much thought to food and have little interest in eating.
2. Vaudevillers: this type of people are like the plump clowns who appear on vaudeville shows. Eating is like a performance to these people, and mealtime is very precious to them. They wake up feeling happy to eat breakfast and wonder what the lunch menu is right after having breakfast. A grand dinner is the best part of their day, and night snack is a must for them.
3. Disease avoiders: this type of people has a certain phobia for disease. They are the products of the so-called health experts. They stick to health books and experts only. With their fear of disease, they have restrictions on the food they consume. They consider only a number of foods that are right for them.
4. Fat fighters: this is a very unfortunate type of people whose daily life is focused on the fight against fat. They think that all food consumed will be stored up in their body as fat, and this is usually what happens. They eat a lot like the vaudevillers but don't enjoy food like they do. Fat fighters are filled with a kind of guilty conscience, an embarrassment, and a concern for obesity. They tend to spend a great deal of time at the supermarket, at a restaurant, or at the gym or hospital.
5. Faddists: they have all the concerns on their shoulders. They worry too much about the pollution of air, water, or food. This type of people only consumes food that is said to be good. All food is considered as poisonous material other than natural food without agricultural pesticides, vegetables grown by organic farming, or food bought at a healthy food store.
6. Health enhancers: this type of people are the real healthy ones. They enjoy the quality and the taste of food and the mood as well. They don't have a guilty

feeling when eating and aren't so picky when eating and don't necessarily follow the trend of what people call healthy food. Gym or hospitals are not frequently visited as well. They control their diet and enjoy eating, based on their experiences on what healthy foods are.

Types of Diet

There are numerous diets around the world, but let me introduce a few importance ones:

1. Atkins diet: it started to become popular from the 1970s, after when the book by Dr. Atkins, *New Diet Revolution*, became the bestseller. The biggest characteristic of the book is the recommendation to significantly reduce the amount of carbohydrate you intake. Generally, the food we consume has about 50–60 % of carbohydrate and Dr. Atkins recommends reducing it to one-third to a half.

   Carbohydrate is the major source of energy we need in order to move. As the diet makes you take less amount of carbohydrate, our body uses fat stored in our body instead. Therefore, it's good for weight control and promoting health. There is a report that a patient who used to get 140 units of insulin could stop it through the Atkin's diet.

   There is ample medical evidence that losing weight is good for treating high blood pressure, cardiac disease, diabetes, hyperlipidemia, and osteoarthritis. It can be indirect evidence that the diet is good for curing such conditions. However, some experts warn that taking high-protein, high-fat food for a long time can be a cause for adult disease.

2. Ornish diet: Dr. Ornish came up with a special diet that can decrease the risk factors for kidney disease, and it is to cut down on the intake of fat lipid to a large amount. According to his diet, intake of fat should be lowered to the level of 10 % in proportion to the overall calorie intake. In the Ornish diet program, mind-body medicine, relaxation therapy, yoga, exercise, and psychology therapy should be used together. Dr. Ornish takes an angiography as an example to show how coronary artery stenosis' patients regained their normal levels.

3. DASH (Dietary Approaches to Stopping Hypertension) diet: "DASH" is a short form of "Dietary Approaches to Stopping Hypertension." This diet emphasizes whole-food diet (eating vegetables and fruits) and taking low-fat dairy products. The diet focuses on lowering the level of fat to 27 % level and to increase the intake of fruits and vegetables. It's not a vegetarian diet, but the 11-week-long diet program reports that there was a significant effect of lowering blood pressure. Small portions of dairy products and meat are allowed in this diet, so people who are against the vegetarian diet can make themselves at ease.

4. Mediterranean diet: the diet consists of food generally consumed in the Mediterranean area, such as fresh vegetables, olive oil, fish, and poultry. It has a small amount of salt, and the olive oil decreases the level of harmful LDL cholesterol while maintaining the level of useful HDL cholesterol.

The diet includes grapes, wine, and artichoke, and they provide much anti-oxidants that prevent cardiac and liver diseases. The Mediterranean diet isn't singled out as a diet therapy, but it's tasty and easy to get the ingredients. It consists of food that is good for promoting health.

5. Macrobiotic diet: this diet mainly takes the vegetable diet from the East. The food contains rice, soy, and seaside and pickled vegetables. It was spread from the 1980s from a Japanese-American named Michio Kushi, and it is a diet for cancer prevention and treatment. It received great interest when a prominent doctor Sattilaro in the USA was reported to cure his prostate cancer with the macrobiotic diet.

   However, some experts who study the diet strongly recommend that other ways necessary for curing cancer, such as chemical therapy, surgical operation, chemotherapy, stress management, holistic fitness program, mind-body medicine, and spiritual treatment, be used together.

6. Gerson diet: it was established by a German doctor named Max Gerson in the 1930s. It is the original form of more than 20 types of metabolic diets that are popular these days. It is used as a way to treatment of cancer. It is argued that the detox process and the exacerbation of the immune system can be produced through the diet, which helps cancer treatment both directly and indirectly. Preparing food and the special containers to put in the food are difficult, so there are criticisms that patients can't do this alone.

   In the Gerson diet, vegetable and fruit juice with a lot of potassium is used. Vegetables, fruits, and grain that are used should be grown by organic farming. The diet used to have cattle liver juice but was eliminated when some patients gained disease through infected liver. The diet refuses animal protein intake, and quite a large amount of vegetable food is restricted as well.

7. Pyramid diet: this diet uses the nutrition distribution chart provided from the Human Nutrition Information Service of the Department of Agriculture in the USA. Foods that have to be taken much are shown in the bottom of the pyramid, and the little you need, the higher up it is shown in the pyramid. It is very easy to see the graph visually.

   The pyramid is divided into four parts. In the bottom, the flour-based food group is located where rice, bread, and cereal are included. Just above are fruits and vegetables. Above are dairy products such as milk, yogurt, cheese, meat including poultry and fish, and nuts including beans and eggs. At the top, fat, oils, and sweets take the place. It is a diet graph suggesting that taking the nutrients in the portion shown in the pyramid is helpful for promoting health.

8. Zone diet (according to nutrition distribution): it uses a strict set menu and it is composed of 40 % carbohydrate, 30 % protein, and 30 % fat. There is a certain zone or a belt according to which nutrients are contained in their ratios. Each person is prescribed with the best food for them according to zones. It decreases secretion of insulin, which is stimulated by carbohydrate, and seeks weight loss. The diet stresses that regular exercise and control of the overall calorie intake should follow.

9. Sugar Busters diet: each food is given a "glycemic index" according to the insulin secretion function. Foods are categorized according to their indexes, and it becomes the barometer for each person. This diet also stresses that regular exercise and control of the overall calorie intake should be followed.

10. Food according to blood type: blood type B comes from the nomads, so they should eat dairy products and small portions of meat, and chicken is not recommended. Blood type A can't digest meat well, so they are recommended to become vegetarians. Blood type AB shouldn't eat wheat such as barley, but soy, dairy products, seafood, and meat are fine. Blood type O has blood evolved from hunters, so they are advised to take meat-based low-plant food.

11. Diet using soy products: beans and soy have phytoestrogen, so it's good for preventing breast cancer. The fact that Eastern women have a lower incidence rate of breast cancer than the Western women is closely related to the daily habits such as breastfeeding and low-fat diet. Experts argue that their high intake of bean and soy is one of the contributors as well.

Recommendations for Diet

1. You should have motives and determination. A strong motivation is the most important. Even if you have a very good diet program, it's no use when there isn't a strong will to stick to it. Many people are attracted to the programs that are easy to follow and understand.

2. It is without doubt that vegetable diet is good for promoting health. According to the accumulated experiences and clinical studies, high-fiber content, low-fat content, and physiological protective substances such as flavonoids, carotenoids, lignin, and the antioxidants included in the vegetable diet are useful to decrease health problems such as adult disease.

3. Weight control is very important. Losing weight through diet is important, but efforts to maintain a healthy level of weight are the most important. Therefore, a regular exercise program should be kept up.

4. Have self-esteem. Having self-esteem is the most important for maintaining health. There is ample evidence that those who have self-acceptance and self-love are healthier than their none counterparts, such as having a relatively lower incidence rate of adult disease. In short, the same obese person with a high self-esteem is less likely to contract a disease.

Fasting

People eat to maintain health. However, there are traditionally handed-down methods where we can promote health by "fasting" (skipping meals). Fasting has been used as a therapy in the traditional medicine and was used by ascetics who cultivate themselves religiously. It has continuously been performed as a religious ritual as well. The following is the results of studies that explored what impacts fasting have on our body.

First, it gives rest to our organs. By fasting, the organs that receive food and decompose, digest, and absorb the nutrients from food can take a rest. Of course, the organs may become weak if not used often just like the muscles, but giving them a short rest will help them recover their functions.

Second, it increases the functions of the digestive system and internal organs. Through fasting, harmful elements such as uric acid or metal can be emitted out of our body. The emission process can be more useful when you drink fruit juice during the fasting period, rather than just taking water. The juice provides your body with vitamins, minerals, and enzymes that are essential for maintaining vitality.

Third is the cleansing of organs. Organs involved in the digestion process can take a rest while fasting. However, the organs that eliminate wastes work actively. Therefore, the liver, lung, kidney, and colon that get rid of the toxic elements can be cleansed as the wastes are driven out of the body. When fasting, you have a bad smell and the color of the urine changes to blackish. It is related to the toxic agents' emission.

Fourth, chemical elements in the blood can regain their balance. Irregular diet, eating fast, monophobia, overeating, repletion, and binge eating all make up irregular diet. The blood elements can regain peace and harmony through fasting. Blood tends to turn acid when we fast, so it is advised to drink fruit juice rather than just water. The fruit juice (tomato) that has alkaline is effective to regain the balance between chemical elements in our blood.

Fifth, our mind is cleared. After overeating, our energy is concentrated in the digestive system, and our body gets too relaxed and sleepy. However, our head clears off when our digestive system takes a rest. It is the main reason why monks or religious people go on fasting.

Sixth, it is good for weight management. Our bodyneeds protein to sustain. When the supply is cut during the fasting period, the accumulated fat goes into a transition process to become energy, to make up for the loss of the intake. Therefore, fasting gets rid of unnecessary fat and helps to fight off obesity. Other than that, fasting has the following benefits. It trains your mental ability, increases the self-sustainability of your body, decreases dependency on drugs, and induces comfortable sleep.

However, you should avoid fasting in the following cases: a malignant cancer, diabetes in process, active tuberculosis, pregnant women or those on breastfeeding, in a bad health suffering from heavy stress, an acute condition in process such as inflammation, an expendable condition in process, and on a particular drug treatment, such as insulin, digitalis, steroids, and penicillin. You should never go on fasting if you're suffering from one of these conditions. Many people ask whether it's okay to exercise when fasting. The answer is, "if you've been working out steadily, it's okay to exercise according to your ability."

If you've been fasting for a long time, it's very important how you end it. The period from the end of fasting to where you go back to your normal diet is called "supplementary eating period." The following are effective ways of going through the supplementary eating period.

Start with light meals, no overeating, and steadily move onto your normal diet. On the first day, start with food you can digest easily, such as fruits, vegetables, and yogurt. On the second day, add soup, porridge, and some vegetables to the first day. On the third day, start eating porridge and soft rice with small side dish. One day of supplementary eating period should be followed with 3–4 days of fasting. Therefore, 3–4 days of the period is suitable if you went on fasting for 10 days. Everything needs to be done in order to promote health. We should eat correctly, but correctly fasting is also important for promoting health.

Homeopathy

Since the old days, air was called "air" or "Gong-ki," referring to the "ki" (energy, spirit) that is in the empty place (Gong). Science found out later that in such an empty place, there is "ki" which is colorless, invisible, and untouchable and doesn't have any smell but that which is essential for maintaining life.

How would people believe if certain water has a healing effect, when it doesn't have any color or taste? Homeopathy therapists believe that it does have a healing effect. It is the mysterious and amazing trait of homeopathy and has been controversial among medical experts. In fact, the water used in homeopathy is similar to ordinary water when its components are analyzed chemically. That's why some people who don't have any understanding of the field say that "How can you cure people with ordinary water?," "It's nonsense," or that it's an exaggeration.

Homeopathy is a relatively new therapy developed by the German doctor Samuel Hahnemann back in 1810. He surprised the then medical field with his discovery. He argued that to cure some disease, drugs that give similar symptoms as the disease should be used. As an example, he took quinine. He said, "to treat malaria, which produces severe fever, we should use quinine that can produce fever in healthy people." The word "homeopathy" was used to imply that the "same type" (homeo) is used in this therapy.

In the West, it is called, "homeopathy." It is the word "homeo" (meaning "harmony") and "pathy" (meaning "disease or treatment") combined, and it can be translated into "a treatment that restores the harmony of the body." Those who experienced or are followers of homeopathy believe in the therapy as religion. However, those cynical about the therapy keep their view, and the difference of perspective rise from the "manufacturing process of drug."

According to the theory of homeopathy, the healing power of medicine becomes greater the more it is diluted. For instance, when 1 cc of medicine is diluted in 100 cc water, it would become 1/100. When the diluted 1 cc is once again mixed with 100 cc, it will be 1/10,000. When 1 cc of it is once more diluted in the 100 cc, it would become 1/1 million. It is argued that 1/10,000 content is stronger than 1/100 and that 1/1 million is stronger than the 1/10,000. In fact, the 1/1 million content is very similar to ordinary water, not containing much drug substances. Therefore, it goes against the conventional wisdom that higher concentration is stronger than lower one, whether it's medicine or poison.

However, if you look more closely into homeopathy, you would see that it also has a point. The diluting method used in the homeopathy is called, "succussion." It is a special way to mix two things by strongly shaking them. Every component has the materialistic side and the dynamic energy within them. Homeopathy believes that the innate dynamic energy is made more pure and its activation stronger through the "mixing and shaking" process. The 1/1 million content would be containing little medicine content in terms of materialistic aspect. However, through the "succussion" process, the dynamic energy is strengthened to several hundred times.

Homeopathy is used in various internal medicine and pediatrics. It is reported to have great effects on allergic conditions. In addition, it's more effective in acute conditions than in chronic ones.

India is where homeopathy is widely practiced. In India alone, there are about 70,000 licensed homeopathy experts. In France, the number is about 6000. Countries such as England, the Netherlands, and Russia have homeopathy experts as well. In South America, homeopathy is practiced widely in Brazil, Argentine, and Mexico. In the USA some 1000 experts are estimated to be in practice.

In Korea, homeopathy experts started to work 10 years ago. Nowadays, the number of experts and clinical researchers are on a rapid increase. In Oriental medicine, a therapy similar to homeopathy has been traditionally used, based on the odor theory. The recent boom of homeopathy is due to the Oriental medicine boom in the USA, which increased peoples' attention on complementary alternative medicine.

Homeopathy has both the traits of Western and Eastern medicine. The fact that it extracts components and atoms of materials and uses them by purification process is similar to Western medicine. Its emphasis on the dynamic energy and the concept of harmony is akin to Eastern medicine. Homeopathy has ample potential to combine the ideas of both Western and Eastern medicine to be a driving force to take the status of medicine to another level.

Light Therapy

Light therapy refers to inducing the physiological changes of the human body through natural sunlight or artificial rays. Dr. Charaka, who is known as the original expert of the Indian Ayurveda medicine, suggested early on in sixth century BC to use sunlight to cure disease. Since the 1970s, it has been accepted in the medical field that human behavior is related to the exposed time out in the sunlight.

Some people feel ungrounded happiness and a comfortable mind in spring and summer where there is longer daylight. They are also more satisfied with their life and encouraged to do more work. However, when fall and winter come, when there are longer nighttimes, these people tend to get sensitive and emotionally unstable. They tend to feel gloomy and sometimes suffer from a severe depression, sleepless nights, and eating disorder, such as loss of appetite or overeating. When spring comes again, these people tend to experience an uplifting of spirits. Such a seasonal cycle of emotional ups and downs is experienced by a lot of people. Therefore, exposing the patients suffering from seasonal emotional anxiety to sunlight can be a treatment.

There are several rhythms in our body, and all of them are controlled by hormones and other chemical substances. The "sleep-wake cycle" in which you feel sleepy at some time and wake up belongs to one of the rhythms. Light is a very strong awakening stimulant, and the "sleep-wake cycle" is controlled by the amount of sunlight that comes through our retina. The receptor in our retina transfers the sunlight stimulus to various parts of our brain, so that information on when to go to sleep and when to get up can be delivered. When there is lack of sunlight, however, we tend to feel drowsy and tired even in the daytime.

A hormone called melatonin induces drowsiness and depression, and sunlight tends to repress the production of the hormone. Some people say that they have trouble going back to sleep when they awake up in between sleeping to go to the bathroom. Being exposed to the bright bathroom light is related to the trouble.

Natural sunlight, which has all wavelengths of the ray, is the most ideal for treatment, and that is why artificial lights that have the full spectrum of the sunlight is regarded as the best. The barometer of brightness is called "lux," and the sunlight has 50,000 lux. Ten thousand lux is needed to cure seasonal emotional disorder. If the patient sits under the sunlight or even under the artificial light from 15 min to 3 h a day for treatment, he can benefit from the effects in just a couple of days. However, as ultraviolet ray is included in the general ray, which can cause severe damage to our body, too much exposal in the light should be avoided, and it is useful to use gadgets that block ultraviolet rays.

Conditions that can be helped through the sunlight therapy include seasonal emotional disorder, jaundice of infants, premenstrual syndrome, rashes or stimulant spots of the skin, migraine, high blood pressure, various stress-related symptoms, insomnia, and simple herpes.

Hydrotherapy

Hydrotherapy refers to using various forms of water to cure disease and maintain health. Since the ancient times, almost every culture around the world used hydrotherapy, and the various programs that were used in spas in the 1800s are the origins of hydrotherapy. Scholars accept that the Austrian farmer named Vincent Preissnitzs is the creator of hydrotherapy.

The most popular therapy in Eastern Europe is lying in a small bathtub for 30 min and ending it with a shower. The water in the tub contains much sodium, calcium, magnesium, carbon, and sulfur components. The carbon water is good for curing small injuries, burns and hardening of the skin, digestion problems, and allergies. Sulfur is known to be good for arthritis, chronic toxic symptoms, diabetes, skin problems, and urinary diseases.

Hydrotherapy is often used in traditional medicine, and in particular, in the field of rehabilitative medicine. Hydrotherapy is included in the complementary alternative medicine as the scope of using water and the treating patient has been broadened from the traditional medicine. Hydrotherapy can be conducted in hospitals, at home, and in spas. Hot, cold, and warm water can be used, and they can be used in various forms, ranging from liquid to steam to ice. It can be put into our body through our mouth or anus or can be administered outside of our body, such as sauna, shower, bathing, whirlpool, or a sitz bath. Spray or hose can be used or even hot moist pack.

The effects of hydrotherapy are as follows: the heat and coldness effect, massaging effect, minerals effect, and buoyancy effect. The cold massage, which is usually conducted through hot moist pack, contracts our blood vessels and diminishes blood flow. It soothes edema or inflammation and works as local anesthetic and relieves the conditions such as headache, toothache, nosebleed, sprain, bruise, abrasion, and cramps in the muscle. On the other hand, heat expands blood vessels and increases blood flow to decrease pain. In particular, the heat in the hot bath adds the massaging effect and the buoyancy effect, thereby decreasing the pain in the joints and relaxing tension in the muscle. Moreover, there are arguments that heat therapy increases immunity and is effective to curing chronic fatigue syndrome.

Whirlpool relaxes tension in the muscles and joints and is helpful to curing traumatosepsis on the skin and edema and for light chilblain treatment. Hydrotherapy accompanied with heat is known to be useful for curing insomnia, sore throat, cold, menstrual pain, cramps in the legs, neuralgia, and headache. A steady research should be conducted to identify the exact effects of the therapy, but hydrotherapy is forecast to be loved by the public.

Sense Therapy

Adapting to the surroundings is important to sustain life, and continuously taking in information is essential in the process. Tools in our body that are used to take in information are called sensory organs, and the most important ones are called the five senses. The five senses are vision, hearing, taste, smell, and tactile.

The vision of humans is not so dull compared to animals, but it's not so sensitive, either. Eagles can see little chicks that are several meters away in the broad daylight, and owls can see things clearly in the night, the things humans can't see in the pitch darkness. The eyes of horses are big and bulging, so they can see 360° without even turning their heads, whereas we don't have such a wide vision even with our eyes wide open.

Hearing is highly related to emotions. According to the types of sounds, we tend to be surprised, sad, and happy. There are reports that men tend to focus more on vision but women more on hearing. Bats that live in dark caves don't see with their eyes but prey on flying bugs by detecting the ultrasonic waves that humans can't hear.

The smelling sense we have is relatively dull. We have high adaptability in smelling, so we tend to easily lose the stimulus of smells. Even perfumes with rich fragrance tend to be lost on us when we smell it often. Dogs have highly developed nose and can smell 500 times better than us. Dogs can even smell scents that come several meters away.

Unlike other senses, the tactile sense can only work when the subject touches our tongue. Moreover, tastes can be distinguished with the aid of smelling sense. When you eat an apple with your nose pinched, it's hard to tell whether it's an apple or a raw potato.

The tactile or touching sense works in all parts of our body, but the most sensitive one among them is tongue and then comes the fingertips. Our back is the dullest when it comes to telling big or small things apart or the number of things that touch our back.

Recently, the interest and passion for complementary alternative medicine increased, and various therapies using the five senses are rising. In therapies that use vision to treat disease, various colors or lights are used, and sometimes pictures, sculptures, and porcelains are used. Red is related to increase instinctive passion, orange to reality, yellow to wisdom, green to peace, blue to a clear mind, navy (dark blue) to intuition, and purple to sacredness. Patients can be prescribed to each color according to their symptoms. Just like in sculpture, the functions of the brain can be stimulated by looking at a certain form. Sometimes natural lights like sunlight and artificial lights like laser are used.

As for therapies that stimulate our hearing sense, "music therapy" that helps cure anxiety and language disability and "nature sound therapy" that uses bird, wave, and stream sounds to promote health can be cited.

In the therapy that uses smell, aromatherapy is included. Dissolving fragrant oil, extracted and manufactured in a special way in the bath water when you take a bath, is one way. Mixing it with cream to do a skin massage and dropping a few drops in the towel to smell it several times are all ways used to cure stress and other conditions.

As for tactile, the odor theory of Oriental medicine, where you harmonize the five tastes (sweetness, bitterness, saltiness, sourness, and hot) to promote health, is the most popular.

Electric, magnetic, and ultrasonic waves, rays, laser, and ice are used alongside the traditional therapies such as acupuncture, moxa cautery, acupressure, and buhwang. Massage, manipulation, and touching therapy can be included here as well. The five-sense therapy will see a great breakthrough as a field in future medicine, if the experts from both the Western and Eastern medicine come together in research.

Colon Therapy

While a Pharaoh, the ruler of ancient Egypt, was having a picnic on the banks of the Nile River, Thoth the God of Medicine appeared before him in the form of a sacred bird, ibis. Thoth filled up its large beak with water and stuck the tip of its beak to its anus and put in all water into its anus. The monk doctors took it as a message from God and did an enema on Pharaoh.

The colon therapy, also known as colon irrigation therapy, is to strike a balance in the body chemistry through maintaining the functions of the colon. It also effectively gets rid of wastes in our body and restores the damaged functions of our tissues and organs. A healthy colon plays the most important role in absorbing and eliminating the wastes of essential nutrients. Colon therapy includes not only the irrigation of colon but also analyzing the structure and chemical components of feces and looking into the environmental, immunological factors, and psychosomatic effects.

Our body needs energy to sustain life, and we need to eat, drink, breathe, excrete, and emit carbon dioxide to get the living energy. In most Western cultures, the "input" aspect, where you put something into the body, is stressed. However, generally in Eastern culture, "output" is emphasized. This means that "how to eat good food and think good things" is important in the West, whereas "how to get rid of the toxic agents out of the body and how to empty our minds off of bad thoughts" is stressed in the East. That's why fasting (fasting or abstaining from food) and excreting are very important in the East, and there is an emphasis on expiration, rather than inspiration, in breathing exercises such as hypogastric breathing.

Food that enters our stomach through the gullet go through the small intestine that is 6–7 m long with a diameter of 2–3 cm. It goes into the colon, which is about 1.5 m long with 6 cm of diameter, and stays there for some time before coming out of the anus as feces. The colon is not just storage for useless wastes, but it is a very important organ. Most of the moisture and nutrients from the wastes that entered colon are bound to be reabsorbed. There is most moisture in the colon in morning time, so just after you wake up is the best time to excrete. Moisture in the colon disappears as time goes by, so you may suffer from constipation if you develop a habit of going to bathroom in the evening.

About 500 types of normal flora live in our colon. They decompose the wastes to make vitamins B and K and amino acids that our body needs. In the process, about 500–800 cc of gas composed of indole, skatole, and methane are produced, which become gas. About 33 % of the feces are made up of dead flora, another 33 % is the dead cells from the epithelial cell of the intestine, and the rest 34 % is composed of food wastes.

According to a study, the animals which have long colons have relatively short life span. Enema is often used in Western medicine as well. Enema is used when constipation continues or when a colon checkup or operation is planned or when excreting by oneself is impossible due to stroke or damaged spine. Recently, those who are for enema is on the rise, using it not only in terms of sickness but also to promote health and to supply nutrition or drugs through the anus.

From the past, Koreans also believed that eliminating coprostasis from the colon is helpful to our health, calling coprostasis the waste that sticks to the walls of large intestines. The oldest records about stomach cleansing go back 90 years, written by Dr. John Karvey Kellogg from Michigan, USA, who pioneered the field of natural medicine. To avoid an operation as much as possible, he conducted the colon irrigation on 40,000 of his patients who were suffering from digestion problems. In the 1920s and 1930s in the USA, the colon irrigation therapy was very popular. About

60 years ago, Dr. Max Gerson developed "coffee enema" and it is still frequently used in many countries to cure cancer.

The following conditions are known to be prerequisites for our large intestine to function ideally:

1. "Whole-food diet" is recommended. A balanced diet consisting of high-fiber foods such as grain, bean food (legumes), vegetables, and fruits is needed.
2. There should a balance in the distribution of symbiotic bacteria. There are about 500 types of flora in our body. In the digestive system, some 60 types of flora help out with digestion, synthesize the necessary nutrients, and maintain the pH level (acid-base balance). They also repress harmful flora in our body.
3. Mucosa of the colon should be healthy. Mucosa or surface cell layer lining the intestine should make the essential nutrients to be absorbed well into the blood, should secrete various hormones and lubricants, and should prevent the absorption of harmful toxic agents.
4. Tension of the muscle in the wall of the large intestine should be maintained at an appropriate level. The peristalsis should be done about 15 times a minute.
5. Feces should be emitted out of the body in suitable time. There are arguments that "Bowel movement should be thorough and frequent. To effectively emit toxic residue, about 2–3 times of bowel movement is desirable."

Colon therapy experts argue that cleansing of the colon facilitates the normal function of the colon and prevents toxic agents to settle or leaky gut syndrome and cures the conditions. A typical colon cleansing therapy goes like this: First, you put in a tool such as speculum into the anus. Filtered water or water mixed with herbs and oxygen is slowly put into the colon, before taking them out. The process is repeated for 30–45 min, and about 2–6 l of water is consumed. Generally, enema cleanses the 30 cm of the sigmoid, which is the lower part of the colon. Irrigation, however, can cleanse off the entire colon, which is about 1.5 m long. The following are the conditions that can benefit from irrigation: backache, bad breath, coated tongue, indigestion, sinus congestion, loss of concentration, headache, gas, bloating, constipation, skin problems, and fatigue.

Irrigation can also facilitate intestine muscle exercise and help production of bile in the liver, and indirectly, it is beneficial to curing high blood pressure, arthritis, depression, helminthiasis, and lung disease. Treatment effects can be increased when other alternative therapies such as acupuncture, homeotherapy, or special exercise therapies are conducted together. However, irrigation shouldn't be applied when there is ulcer, inflammation, or tumor in the colon or when you suffer from a severe hemorrhoids or when your body is in a weak condition.

IMS, Intramuscular Stimulation

IMS, or intramuscular stimulation, is to stimulate the muscle by injecting a relatively thick and long needle into the skin. It was developed and spread by Dr. Chen Gunn in Canada in the mid-1970s. In the beginning, the goal of the therapy was to put the needle deep into the skin to give a physical stimulus to the muscle so that pain can be relieved. Later, it included stimulating the nerve root related to the painful local part, not only the local part itself. Sometimes monitors that can observe the needle that goes deeper in to stimulate the nerve root parts are used as well.

The difference of IMS from other acupuncture is that its diagnosis and treatment are not dependent on meridian massage and its points. It's also distinguished from MPS, or myofascial pain syndrome, in that it doesn't entirely depend on trigger points in terms of diagnosis and treatment. IMS usually stresses the symptoms related to the radiculopathy, and the basis of its theory lies in is the supersensitivity of receptor. In short, IMS is about dulling the supersensitivity of the receptor, which is caused by the nerve root lesion, by the strong stimulus of the needle.

Hyperthermia

Our body is programmed to let out heat naturally and to fight infection or inflammation. Every method that is to make heat artificially to treat local parts or bodily conditions is called hyperthermia. Heat is one of the powerful tools that can fight diseases.

Quantum Medicine

Quantum medicine is a treatment that goes beyond molecular biology to include the concept of atom. Quantum energy is divided into the energy from the electrons and the energy from the subtle particles, which surround the electrons. By analyzing the energy, the normal and abnormal condition of our body is revealed. In the therapy, the source of the sick energy is stimulated with the subtle electromagnetic waves to be restored to its healthy state.

Instruments are used in the quantum medicine, which is called "magnetic resonance analyzer" in the USA and "quantum resonance analyzer" in Japan. The instrument is used in research and operation. It was introduced in Korea recently and is in use.

Juice Therapy

Juice therapy is to use the fresh juice taken from fruits and vegetables to nourish and restore our body. When you're suffering from stress or a disease, the therapy can be used as a way to maintain health by giving nourishment. Practitioners of juice therapy argue that it is good for stimulating the immune system, lowering blood pressure, and eliminating toxic agents. It is also known to be effective in treating diseases resulting from environmental factors, food allergies, and indigestion problems.

Urine Therapy

Urine therapy is to drink urine as a way to keeping health. Usually, the practitioners drink their own urine. Urine has information that reflects various physiological conditions of our body. This therapy is based on the theory that the information of the urine stimulates the physiological mechanism of our body so that the unhealthy factors can be corrected and complemented. More study is needed to back up the therapy.

Taping Therapy

Taping therapy was created and distributed through a Japanese Dr. Kase Kenzo in the 1970s. First, it was used to relieve pain but is now expanded to treat secondary diseases related to muscle pain and other conditions apart from pain. Taping therapy is putting on elastic tapes on the muscle part where pain can be felt due to tension and damage. When the skin is uplifted through the tape, the space between the skin and the muscle is enlarged, and the circulation of blood and lymph fluid is increased through the space to ease off the pain. Other explanations of the theory include gate control theory and cutaneo-vascular reflex.

References

Amiel H (1985) Journal intime. Macmillan, London (Vaillant EG, trans: Lee Deok-Nam. Conditions of happiness. Frontier (Seoul), 2012, p 36)
Brooks G (1986a) Lactate production under fully aerobic conditions: the lactate shuttle during rest and exercise. Fed Proc 45:2924–2929
Brooks G (1986b) The lactate shuttle during exercise and recovery. Med Sci Sports Exerc 18:360–368
Byun Kwang-Ho, Chang Hyun-Gap (2012) Stress and mind-body medicine. Hakjisa, Seoul, pp 39–42
Gong In-Duk, Ye Byung-Il (2012a) Body saving prescription for exercise. Thinksmart Press, Seoul, pp 62–63
Gong In-Duk, Ye Byung-Il (2012b) ibid., pp 185–186
Gong In-Duk, Ye Byung-Il (2012c) ibid., pp 87–88
Gong In-Duk, Ye Byung-Il (2012d) ibid., pp 121–127
Gong In-Duk, Ye Byung-Il (2012e) ibid., pp 241–242
Gong In-Duk, Ye Byung-Il (2012f) ibid., pp 114–116
Hargreaves M (1995) Skeletal muscle carbohydrate metabolism during exercise. In: Hargreaves M (ed) Exercise metabolism. Human Kinetics, Champaign, pp 41–72
Hwang Nong-Moon (2007) Think hard! Random House, Seoul
Jeon Se-Il (2004) Complementary alternative medicine. Gyechukmoonwhasa, Seoul, pp 160–258
Junger A (trans: Cho Jin-Kyung) (2013a) Clean, Sam and Parkers, Seoul, p 175
Junger A (trans: Cho Jin-Kyung) (2013b) ibid., pp 59–60
Junger A (trans: Cho Jin-Kyung) (2013c) ibid., p 69
Junger A (trans: Cho Jin-Kyung) (2013d) ibid., pp 310–312
Junger A (trans: Cho Jin-Kyung) (2013e) ibid., pp 191–195

Kim Hye-Yun, Lee Yung-Keun (2013a) 100 year living in a city. Goodbook, Seoul, pp 174–201
Kim Hye-Yun, Lee Yung-Keun (2013b) ibid., pp 202–222
Kim Hye-Yun, Lee Yung-Keun (2013c) ibid., pp 207–210
Kim Hye-Yun, Lee Yung-Keun (2013d) ibid., p 213
Kim Jae-Ho, Park In-Tae, Son Rak-Sung, Jeon Yong-Kyun, Kim Yong-An, Han Dong-Yup (2004a) Exercise and health. DanKook University Press (Cheon An), pp 171–178
Kim Jae-Ho et al (2004b) ibid., pp 219–236
Kwon Yong-Wook (2004) How to keep healthy well-being with fearless ageing. Chosun Ilbo Sa, Seoul, pp 42–48
Lee Yung-Keun, Choi Joon-Yung (2011a) Doctor detox. Sogeumnamoo, Seoul, pp 196–218
Lee Yung-Keun, Choi Joon-Yung (2011b) ibid., pp 136–145
Lee Yung-Keun, Choi Joon-Yung (2011c) ibid., pp 186–187
Lee Yung-Keun, Choi Joon-Yung (2011d) ibid., p 174
Morley J, Colberg S (2008a) Science of youth (trans: Jung Joo-Yon). Migibooks Press, Seoul, p 68
Morley J, Colberg S (trans: Jung Joo-Yon) (2008b) ibid., pp 80–82
Oh Hong-Keun (2004) Medicine of natural therapy. Jeonghan Health Books, Seoul, p 19
Powers S, Howley E (2008) Power physiology of exercise, 6th edn (trans: Choi Dae-Hyuk, Choi Hee-Nam, Jeon Tae-Won). Lifescience, Seoul, pp 62–63
Rath T, Harter J (2010a) Wellbeing finder (trans: Sung Ki-Hong). Winners Book, Seoul, pp 12–13
Rath T, Harter J (trans: Sung Ki-Hong) (2010b) ibid., p 205
Shrand J, Devine LM (2013a) Use insert paper of stress (trans: Kim Han-Kyu, Kim Moo-Kyum). Joong Ang Books, Seoul, pp 133–134
Shrand J, Devine LM (trans: Kim Han-Kyu, Kim Moo-Kyum) (2013b) ibid., pp 128–130
Shrand J, Devine LM (trans: Kim Han-Kyu, Kim Moo-Kyum) (2013c) ibid., pp 140–141
Shrand J, Devine LM (trans: Kim Han-Kyu and Kim Moo-Kyum) (2013d) ibid., pp 143–145
Shrand J, Devine LM (trans: Kim Han-Kyu, Kim Moo-Kyum) (2013e) ibid., pp 145–148
Shrand J, Devine LM (trans: Kim Han-Kyu, Kim Moo-Kyum) (2013f) ibid., pp 148–149
Shrand, J, Devine LM (trans: Kim Han-Kyu, Kim Moo-Kyum) (2013g) ibid., pp 134–136
Shrand J, Devine LM (trans: Kim Han-Kyu, Kim Moo-Kyum) (2013h) ibid., pp 136–138
Shrand J, Devine LM (trans: Kim Han-Kyu, Kim Moo-Kyum) (2013i) ibid., pp 130–131
Song Yung-Kyu (2011a) The science of staying young. Wisdom House, Seoul, pp 155–156
Song Yung-Kyu (2011b) ibid., pp 156–157
Song Yung-Kyu (2011c) ibid., pp 165–167
Song Yung-Kyu (2011d) ibid., pp 170–171
Song Yung-Kyu (2011e) ibid., p 187
Song Yung-Kyu (2011f) ibid., pp 196–210
Song Yung-Kyu (2011g) ibid., p 134
Song Yung-Kyu (2011h) ibid., pp 240–241
Sul Joon-Hee (2012) Physical remodeling. CNB Media, Seoul, pp 60–63
Vaillant EG (2012) Conditions of happiness (trans: Lee Deok-Nam). Frontier, Seoul, p 18
Willett WC (2009) Eat, drink, and be healthy (trans: Son Soo-Mi). DongA Ilbo Sa, Seoul, p 41

Chapter 4
Pharmaco-gelotology

4.1 Introduction

Humans are made up of mind and body. Nowadays, laughter is held in high esteem as more indicators are revealed that show laughter is useful to promoting health. One example would be the rapid spread of laughter therapy around the world. Pharmaco-gelotology, one of the tools of social medicine (SM), is generally related to improving a person's complexion or facial expressions.

Why is improving one's complexion so important? As I mentioned earlier, I believe that facial image control is one of the crucial aspects of SM therapy, including diet, physical condition improvement, and stress management. Face is one of the defining points of impression in first encounters. Some even go further to say that one's life can be determined on how one looks. In this sense, face doesn't only mean outlooks or features; it is a broad concept which gives off a person's aura that includes one's heart and inner feelings.

In the words of a man who is renowned for his physiognomy studies, facial image is not about destinies or how one's life is bound to flow. Facial image or impression can be changed by a person's will or how he thinks. He also tells us that good impression can brighten our society, going beyond giving advantages to each person involved. We know from experience that when we face the world with good facial image in our daily lives, good energy comes from within us and ultimately the "vital force" is shown through our face:

> There are more than 60 muscles on our face. Using 44 muscles among the 60 can brighten our facial image or expressions. Facial expression, in fact, can be easily changed depending on our efforts. … Just like the saying, "Laughter brings good luck," bright facial expression can bring good luck. (Ju Seon-Hee and Jin Se-Hun 2013a)

As is already proven by "health exercise," muscular strength can be gained with regular exercise. Just like muscles, laughter is a part of a good facial image that can be achieved by using your facial muscles. Laughter is vitalizing energy, and you should laugh often. This is the mechanism of how the vitalizing energy, known as the laughter, works to change ourselves and those around us in a positive way:

© Springer Science+Business Media Singapore 2016   193
B.-H. Han, *Therapy of Social Medicine*, DOI 10.1007/978-981-287-748-2_4

First, the brain gives out serotonin and endorphin when we laugh, and it results in happiness and an elevation of feelings (Lee Im-Seon et al. 2009).

Second, it has been revealed recently that laughter changes the status of 23 genes in our body as the genetic "switch" is turned on, prompted by the increase of messenger RNA. It has also been revealed that NK cells, the simple cells which attack cancer cells head on when they are found among immune cells, are activated and grow in number. The result is the increased NHS that seeks to maintain homeostasis (Park Soon-Ok and Kim Soon-Ja 2013). With this, laughter therapy has been given greater importance in curing "almost incurable diseases."

Third, each individual's vital energy shown in their faces has NHP. In particular, SHS based on reciprocity takes effect and lights up the atmosphere, and it acts as a "social catalyst" that not only makes it easier to build new relationships but also to solidify existing relationships. It has been revealed that laughter plays an essential role in developing personal relationships and forming friendliness, which is necessary to maintain human network (McAdams and Powers 1981; McAdams et al. 1984).

According to art researchers, minor differences based on aesthetic standards can be overcome by unique expressions and constructed images. It means that simply having a smiley face can boost one's beauty and amiability. A research that compared an expressionless face and a smiling face showed that the latter had the eyebrows in the part of the middle of the forehead go up a little bit, followed by the uplifting of the eyes (the part where there are hairs under the eyes) by 1.5 mm. It also accompanied a 6-mm widened mouth and the upward crooks of its corners by 3 mm (Ju Seon-Hee and Jin Se-Hun 2013b).

People laugh when there are funny things, and the laughing itself can brighten our hearts and please others. If laughter is a type of muscle exercise that we can choose of our own will and if our hearts (the inside) and laughter (the outside) can be reversible, we have ample reason to study "beautiful laughter (BL)" among other ordinary laughter. This is because natural laughter, born out of a pure heart, is beautiful to look at. In turn, artificial laughter, made on purpose to boost health, is also beautiful to see, because it can change our negative hearts to a positive one which can be healing.

Laughter is translated into "gelos" in Greek, and it originates from the word "hele," which means "health." Therefore, beautiful laughter, or BL, can be regarded as one of the representative social medicines (SMs) that go beyond boosting one's personal health to cure societies. Pharmaco-gelotology will firmly establish itself to a branch of SM therapy. So here, I would like to name the studies of BL as one tool of SM as "pharmaco-gelotology." The studies will look deeper into BL, which will be the number one step in improving facial expressions, the ultimate goal of which is a healthy life and happiness.

People living in modern society suffer from various stresses as they are exposed to infinite competition with the rapid advancement of science technology. Laughter has been regarded as important since the days of ancient medicine, as it was known to have positive impacts on pneuma/anima, the core of life. The body fluid theory of the days believed that the balance of four body fluids (black bile, yellow bile, mucus, and blood) was fundamental to health.

In Korea, the saying "when you yell with anger, you gain a year, and when you laugh with joy, you become a year younger" shows how good laughter is. Laughter is an act of expressing one's joyful mood. Laughter is made up of a loud and unique sound added with facial expression, as it a communicating tool of arousing similar feelings in others. Laughter intrinsically has social traits and it is contagious; laughing sounds infuse listeners with good feelings, and it prompts to make them laugh in return, solidifying our social community.

For the last 2000 years, laughter was regarded as one of the essential elements of humanity, and it has been analyzed and discussed in traditional methods in various fields such as theology, philosophy, archeology, sociology, psychology, physiology, and linguistics (Martin 1998; Fry 2002). Can only humans laugh? Aristotle (384–322 BC) was the first to announce that only humans are animals that can laugh. The definition was enlarged by Conrad-Martius (1957) who said that humans are beings that can laugh. Rabelais (2002) emphasized that laughter is a unique trait of humans, and his statement argued that laughter is one of the specialties of humans that set them apart from animals.

But studies show that humans are not the only animals who can laugh. Zoologists researched the forms of laughter by the young chimpanzee, known by Darwin, and they found out that similar forms of laughter can be found in other anthropoids such as bonobos, orangutans, or gorillas (Preuschoft and van Hooff 1997; van Hooff and Preuschoft 2003). There is also evidence that even anthropoids have basic sense of humor. Chimpanzees and gorillas that were taught to use language as a form of communication use language in a humorous way, such as replying with rhymes and humorous reactions. They also did funny actions using words that don't connect with each other (Gamble 2001).

The evidence show that the humor and laughter of humans are productions of natural selection and that laughter originated from social play. We can presume that they are a part of the gesture-call system that was formed before the development of language and that they evolved from play signals of primates. Intelligence, the evolved linguistic ability, and the play activities of ancient people that make people laugh are thought of as mental adaptation of what we call "humor" nowadays (Caron 2002). Laughter, made up of play activities, has been playing a very important role in our society, going beyond the biological and cultural evolutionary stages of people.

Emotional theorists nowadays have been finding out objective grounds that laughter has various positive functions both in personal and social life. Laughter relieves excessive nervous energy (Freud 1928), increases solidarity in a society (Coser 1959), relieves stress (Martin and Lefcourt 1983), washes away negative feelings (Levenson 1988), and diminishes anger (Tomkins 1984). It has also been revealed that even fake smiles can uplift one's mood (Foley et al. 2002). Unconditional, fake laugh lets the cold air in the outside into the brain and decreases the brain temperature. Nerves of muscles that are related to our eyes, nose, and mouth are connected to the brain and stimulate it (Michel and Roberta 2003).

The study results show that beautiful laughter (BL), emphasized in my book, is a precious SM that can restore both NHS and SHS that are lost to humans. In terms of SM therapy, BL is a health exercise that can catch all three birds, which are disease prevention, antiaging, and longevity. BL is also a health stressor that can relieve stress. All these good sides of BL have been effectively backed up by the study results mentioned above. It has been proven by many people throughout a long period of time. The bottomline is that humans are prone to laugh.

As long as people live among people in a society, it is important for us to leave our mark. Even if one doesn't have stunning humor and wit, he can make a good impression of himself by breaking the ice among new people. Laughter acts as a supplementary tool that can bring back the memories of something else. If two people met in the past and laughed together, it can make them remember the past situation well in the future. Ultimately, when they meet again, it can boost their friendliness. As such, laughter acts as a social catalyst whenever and wherever.

Apart from pathologic laughter, there are many feelings that arouse laughter. There are feelings such as pleasure, joy, happiness, and satisfaction, but there are also arrogance, mockery, humiliation, contempt, the dark pleasure of seeing someone's failure, sarcasm, rebellion, trick, craftiness, nastiness, dejection, a sad laughter, and a bitter laughter, which are natural and artificial. This means that laughter can be either a beautiful laughter out of a pure heart or a pretense from a false heart. For instance, "I'm not laughing because I feel happy" is a phrase often used by people, and it is an expression to describe the sadness one feels in the inside even if his face may be smiling. Fake smiles and laughs may look artificial and insincere, but that is also good because it can overturn negative feelings to positive ones.

In his book about the theological analysis of laughter, the German theologian Karl-Josef Kuschel praised the beauty of laughter, saying, "laughter is not only a cure to the heart, but it also makes our body beautiful. There is no one beautiful than a laughing person." Recently, there are some patients at hospitals who actively laugh with a definite resolution. Considering the harsh condition of the patients, the laughs are beautiful gifts that give them health.

Everyone wants to live a healthy and cheerful life. We are living in the twenty-first century where "Healthy 100 Years Old" is nothing out of the ordinary. As we find answers to the profound question of "how should we live?" I guess one solution would be to "keep laughing as we are born crying." Charlie Chaplin left a famous phrase, "Life is a tragedy when seen in close-up, but a comedy in a long shot." This is why we desperately need BL, which is of the people, from the people, and for the people:

Life is heavy, laugh is light.

4.1.1 Definition of Laughter

Laughter is a phenomenon of the shaking of the diaphragm, hysterical exercise of the uvula and the soft palate, and certain twists of facial muscles. It can occur from various reasons such as itchiness, joy, madness, ridicule, and nervous gas (Morris

2000). It is also a motion reflection that happens when 15 facial muscles on the surface of the face contract simultaneously. Laughter doesn't occur without the change of breathing, and although it is a reflex action, it doesn't have a biological aim as other behaviors. The only function of laughter is freeing someone from nervousness (Korean Britannica 2001).

According to Darwin, how laughter can be induced and what its function may be depend on the social and biological situation the laughing person is in. This means that laughter can't be entirely described by the relative position the laughing person is in, in regard to the other person or the basic intention of the person making the other one laugh or any traits of the people involved. Rather, laughter can be best described by analyzing each case and the social, biological situation that it takes place in (Darwin 1998).

As you can see, laughter is not only a biological reaction but also a social behavior. That is why the mechanism of laughter is complex as well. Laughter is sometimes used to hide other feelings such as shyness, humiliation, or anger. As Freud said, whether it is based on the outside stimulus or an inside cause, laughter lets off extra nerve energy and it develops into sociopsychological aspect (Lim Hyo-Soo 2000a).

The definition of laughter is summarized well in Ryoo Jong-Hoon's book about laughter therapy and health, and the following is taken from his book (Ryoo Jong-Hoon 2007).

4.1.1.1   Lexical Definition

1. Expression of satisfaction
   Laughter is an expression or a sound that is made when a person is satisfied. It reveals one's instincts which are shown when one is satisfied, as things go as planned. However, laughter is also an artificial act that gets rid of conflicts to smooth out relationships. In this case, the aim is to have a control over the situation to make it as he planned. Therefore, laughter has two faces.
2. Expression of momentous joy
   Laughter is a product of a happy heart, and it shows that the laughing person has peace in his heart. People who don't have inner peace find it hard to laugh even when he is surrounded by happy things. His heart is filled with desires and he just can't laugh from the bottom of his heart. Laughter washes away conflicts and awkwardness, and it is the key to a successful life. Laughter is shaped by good character, such as the mind to look after others. Laughter itself is a blissful journey.

4.1.1.2   Broader Definition

1. Expression of imagery feelings
   Laughter and heart communicate with each other. Laughter stems from the heart, but when you keep laughing, you can change your heart. Laughter can come out

spontaneously from a satisfied and peaceful heart, and it can also be artificially made. In this case, laughter can change your perspective on life. Laughter comes out from a pure heart. Therefore, laughing is a vital activity mingled with feelings and psychological aspects. However, an embarrassing laugh can be made when you are in a subtle and complex situation.

Heartfelt laughter is produced when you are satisfied with a certain result or when your wishes are fulfilled. However, manipulated laughter can come out in a totally different situation. When there is a specific goal in your mind, you can lie to yourself and make fake laughs. But as I mentioned, even the fake laughs can promote health.

Laughter is a message from the resolute heart. Laughter is a basic signal that expresses a pure heart, whether it is a humble laughter that makes other people to smile or a smart laughter that is brought out after hours of painstaking efforts or a fake one to make someone happy. In the end, laughter is the reflection of our heart.

2. Change of perspectives

The heart decides how we should act and the result determines a successful life. We don't necessarily laugh because we are happy, but rather, we are happy because we laugh. When you smile, it changes your attitude, and it also changes your perspective on life to be more positive and proactive. Laughter gives you room to put yourself in someone else's shoes.

Laughter infuses living energy in the boring and frustrating everyday life and provides our mind with healthy spirit. It serves as a barometer to relieving stress.

4.1.1.3 Smaller Definition

Laughter is a simple combination of facial muscles that is derived from pleasure and happiness. Our face can stage various laughs: natural laugh, a bright laugh that makes others to smile along, a big laugh that comes from satisfaction, a "smoke-screen" laugh that is produced to put a halt to fights, a political laugh that have specific goals, and lastly, a laugh of realization that accepts the finite traits of human life.

4.1.1.4 Philosophical Definition

Humans are born incomplete. People should try to improve good character and restore the smile on their faces. Laughter is a representation which shows that he is ready to accept himself and others as they are, and that is why we need to laugh more to have a successful life. Laughter itself is a vital activity which shows that we exist. It is also the result of our thoughts. Even fake laughs can be a barometer of vitality and passion, a sure evidence of vitality. It is very hard for the sick to laugh out loud. Patients suffering from illness find it hard to smile, as in many cases both their body and heart are wounded. Therefore, laughing is evidence that the patient is on his way to a healthy life.

4.1.1.5 Physiological Definition

In physiological terms, laughter is the result of brain activity. Back in March 1989, Doctor Iszak Fried at UCLA University Hospital discovered a part in our brain. It was where it made people laugh when there is a stimulus. While he was treating an epilepsy patient, he found a 4-cm^2-large part that controlled our laughter. It was in the fore of the nervous system, which controls our arms and legs in the left cerebrum. He also found out that when there is any stimulus in the part, patients laugh even when it's not humorous. It was discovered that the 4-cm^2-large part that controlled our laughter can also move muscles in our cheeks. It induced the patient to think of happy memories which ultimately caused the patient to laugh.

The 4-cm^2-large part (which controls our laughter) is located in the overlapping area between the lower part of the frontal lobe (beside the left forehead) and the upper part of the middle of the brain (limbic system). The part where the two overlap is called the "A10 section," which controls reasonable judgment and feelings. The part is composed of dopamine, a neurotransmitter that controls good feelings, and a mass of high protein.

What is the definition of laughter? It is a voluntary expression of feelings caused by the laugh inducer. It is the product of a pleasing mental activity shown with our body and face, as they react to stimulus, happiness, and funny situations. To sum up, laughter is induced by an outside stimulus, and the stimulus is recognized in the brain to be expressed through our body and face.

4.1.2 Conditions of Laughter

People nowadays have a hectic life. It isn't easy to make these people laugh, who are burdened with stress and nervousness. However, if you know the essence of laughter, it is easier to trigger laughs. Generally, you need the following three conditions to make someone laugh (Kim Kyung-Tae 1991).

4.1.2.1 Laughter Should Be Humane

Human beings are not perfect. So the word "humane" is equal to being incomplete, imperfect with many faults and shortcomings. Being imperfect is the best condition to trigger laughs. For imperfect people like us, laughter is granted as a privilege. Humans can laugh at something and make others laugh as well. For instance, "Mickey Mouse," along with many animal characters in Disney, makes people laugh not because the character itself is funny but because they mimic people. They have love triangles like people, and they sing and dance and fight just like us. That is what makes people laugh by looking at those characters. The key here is the personification of animal characters. People laugh and smile at the "humanity" of the characters, not at the animals themselves. Similarly, comedians who can mimic gun, train, car, and plane sounds make people laugh, and it's because they can mimic machinery sounds with their human mouths.

According to the philosopher Bergson, no laugh can be made without humane traits. People tend to laugh at characters who have faults and shortcomings, and he says that those characters were created to ridicule rules and authorities that oppress us. In this sense, "humane" can be related to the laughs produced by humans as a group. Our laugh tends to be a group activity in many cases. Bergson says that people who feel isolated can't laugh and that laughter is contagious. He says mob psychology induces laughter, and the examples are shown well in the groups of people laughing on public transportations and the effect of laughing audience in studios. Thinking that laughter has a definite, useful social role to play, it can be defined as a "group laugh." By laughing, it is certain that people are responding to a demand or oppression from the society, which is why a laugh can be said to have a social meaning. In this context, "social" means getting rid of social rigidness and ways to improving it.

4.1.2.2   Laughter Should Be Free from Feelings

Feelings turn away laughs. Being incomplete, cynical, and shy are not such positive traits at first glance. In order for these traits to induce laughter, we need pureness, which is an absence of feelings. Incompleteness without pureness would be mere foolishness, and cynicism and shyness would become nothing less than annoyance. However, when pureness and other traits can be shown together, it can move other people's hearts. "Pureness" is a loving trait.

Bergson said that there is no bigger enemy than feelings in terms of laughter. This shows how carelessness can be dangerous to laughs. Laughter is produced naturally when our heart is at peace and when there is pureness in it. For instance, when a movie star acts with an exaggerated air, onlookers tend to stop laughing at the awkwardness. Similarly, when people openly talk too much about sex, listeners tend not to laugh as there is a stronger feeling of shame or awkwardness. Both cases are where strong feelings got in the way of laughter.

It may be hard to believe this, but laughter is produced much in logical, reasonable people than in emotional people. Goethe said that sensual people tend to laugh even at things that aren't funny, the intelligent at everything, and the logical not even at laughable matters. People with strong feelings tend to look at their surroundings with a hint of their own feelings, so they can't laugh at things that generally trigger people to laugh. Logical people are cold ones that normally don't find life so funny, and they tend to laugh less. Sensual people laugh at even the smallest things because they are carried away with their own funny ideas and associations. Intelligent people find joy in petty little things in life due to their highly functional brain. However, that doesn't mean their laugh is meaningless.

As for Korea, the following make up the social atmosphere: the ideological conflict of the two Koreas and the military tension arising from it, the polarization from the high-speed compact economic growth, and feelings of anger and deep sorrow resulting from the society. As a result, the Korean society is lacking of composure with its innate culture of "hurry up and get going." Therefore, the Korean society has to restore laughter to make it a healthier and brighter place. It should also break free from too much feeling misleading us to misinterpreting social phenomena.

4.1.2.3 Laughter Should Have Intellectual Connections

In some cases, laughter in one society isn't contagious to other societies. This is due to the lack of intellectual or intelligent connection between the two, which is made up of language, culture, and habit. Humor in Korea may not be funny in the USA and vice versa. Every subgroup in the society also has their own code that triggers laughter. Girl students and soldiers serving in the military all have their own points of laughter and culture. It will be hard to make them laugh without intelligent connections.

4.1.3 Categorization and Types of Laughter

4.1.3.1 Categorization of Laughter

Then why do humans laugh? Supposing that the cause of laughter is something comical, it is impossible to explain causeless laughter. Generally, scholars see that comical assets, humor (joke), and laughter are all the same. This is what Kim Jin-Ak said, who analyzed theories and researches at home and abroad to establish the definition of humor:

> Humor is intrinsic and natural (...) Humor is expressed with a laughter that has a positive link toward the subject, such as love, compassion and pity for people. Satire is a type of humorous criticism. It is a form of literature that is linked to words and sentences that are used to accuse, expose and ridicule wrong deeds, foolish acts and bad customs. Humor has a positive attitude towards its surroundings, while satire poses a negative stand. The subject of satire has to be worthy to talk about, and it shouldn't be a mere lampoon. Irony stems from the suspense between words and their meanings. It is a type of conversation that shows the double meaning between the expressed word and its real meaning. Irony is divided into word-related irony and situation-related irony. In terms of how delicate it is, it can be divided into a simple or a sophisticated one. Wit is made complete by language. Wit is composed of words that can connect seemingly unrelated ideas with the twisting of words. Humor is natural; wit, a product of education or sophistication which is cultivated. Intelligence, wisdom, reason make up wit, and it is an intelligent behavior induced from a reasonable mind, and it is the technical humor created in the human brain. (Bae Hyun-Ja 2001)

Generally speaking, humor is equal to comic, and comic is divided into an objective and subjective one. Satire, joke, wit, and irony all fall into the category of subjective comic. Humor, on the other hand, is expressed by laughter, induced by the disharmony of jokes. It is an emotional response to happiness in various social settings. It is a mental process that creates or recognizes something funny, and it is mentioned as a component of intelligent perception (Martin 2007).

4.1.3.2   Types of Laughter

Based on health, laughter can be categorized into two: one that promotes health and the other that hinders health. The following are the types of laughs that are good for health:

1. Pokso: a sudden laughter
2. Hongso: a loud laughter
3. Huiso(a): a pleasing laughter
4. Huiso(b): a meaningless laughter or a pretty smile
5. Gyoso(a): a seductive laughter
6. Daeso: a loud laughter with big sound
7. Gyoso(b): a seductive, flattering laughter
8. Miso(a): a soundless laughter
9. Miso(b): a flattering laughter
10. Bangso: a tough laughter
11. Chiso: a foolish laughter

As you can see, BL is a health-promoting laughter that is based on the love for humanity. There are also health-deteriorating laughs, such as gallows humor, harmful humor, caustic humor, and demeaning humor. They induce laughter that is poisonous to our body, and they are as follows (Ra Won-Ki 2004):

1. Gaso(a): a fake laughter
2. Gaso(b): a demeaning laughter
3. Ganso: a cunning laughter
4. Gyeongso: a looking-down-on laughter
5. Gumso: a sharp, knifelike laughter
6. Goso: a bitter laughter
7. Giso(1): a ridiculing laughter
8. Giso(2): a joking laughter
9. Naengso: a cold laughter
10. Biso: a nasal laughter
11. Joso: a sneer-like laughter
12. Chiso: a cynical laughter

4.2 Laughter Theory

Humans laugh. We laugh because we are born that way.

Plato (Plato, 428 BC–348 BC) talked about foolish humor in his book *Philebos*. The dialogue between Socrates and Protagoras is valued as one of the longest-surviving examples of comic theories.

In the book, Plato defines foolish humor in the mouth of his teacher, Socrates. First, not knowing yourself is a foolish humor (this is where the famous quote "Know yourself" comes from). In particular, it is foolish to not know exactly how wealthy, beautiful, and competent you are. Second, not every ignorance or lack of discretion is foolish. The people with those traits trigger foolish humor only when they are powerless. Therefore, his laughter theory is about the foolish humor of ignorance (Ryoo Jong-Yung 2005a). In other words, the so-called weak, who have no power to revenge for themselves or act out when they are ridiculed, can be seen as foolish. As they can't ridicule the strong, their weak ignorance puts them in a position where they are ridiculed.

One of the glaring examples of such ignorance is "Don Quixote" in Cervantes' novel, Don Quixote. He is depicted as a foolish man who can't tell a windmill from a giant. Laughing at a weak person such as Don Quixote, as he does foolish things or unrealistic behavior, is common among people of all times and places (Lee Kang-Yup 1998). We don't have to look far. In our daily lives, we tend to meet people who like to say this and that about matters they don't know well, and those people make us laugh. It is the point where we feel that it is comical. This is a good example of foolish humor which makes us laugh.

We can't leave out Aristotle (384 BC–322 BC) when we talk about laughter. His remarks on laughter are the most classic explanation which has been criticized and corrected for so many times. His laughter theory is a revised version of Plato's and it is written in *Poetik*. Aristotle believed that foolish humor is related to ugliness, and he captured the characteristic that sets comedy apart from tragedy as "an imitation of lower type":

Comedy, as I mentioned, is an imitation of a lower type compared to ordinary things. A lower type than ordinary things here isn't related to all types of evil. Rather, it is only so when it is about something funny, which can be considered a part of ugliness. Funniness is, so to say, both a mistake and a fault. However, as a "funny, crushed mask" doesn't cause pain, it is just a fault that doesn't inflict pain or hurt feelings. (Aristoteles 1961)

Therefore, comedy depicts people that are inferior to us, and it tells us that these types of people make us laugh because it makes us recognize "hamartema" or "hamartia" that is not painful or destructive. Here, "ugliness" isn't about physical beauty, but it is an evil that can be perceived instinctively, and "faults" are simple mistakes that are related to weakness or shortcoming that are relatively unimportant (Horn 1988a). Aristotle generalizes "no harm" by citing "a funny mask" as an example. His words "a funny mask that is crushed in a funny way doesn't inflict harm" isn't about the pain of a third person (bystander). It refers to the pain itself, which may be felt by the person who is ridiculed. We have to see that the laughing theory of Aristotle went one step further than the one promoted by Plato. For in order for laughter to be developed into social medicine, "safety" must be secured firsthand, and this was first established by Aristotle for the first time.

Funniness arising from mistakes can be found often nowadays. For example, there is Chaplin in the Charlie Chaplin movies, clowns in circuses, and comedians who appear on funny TV shows. All of these people are recognized by the public as people whose job is to make people laugh, so their intentional mistakes always have an element of "no harm" in them. They are different from mistakes found in our everyday lives. Based on the "no harm" trait, we can laugh at the foolishness, clumsiness, and other mistakes and shortcomings, in the boundary that these faults are not harmful to us or to the people around us or pose severe danger in the society (Kagan 1989).

Funny language, behavior, and comical figures in the *Rhetoric* of Aristotle are used in comedies and in our everyday lives, and a few examples are as follows (Ryoo Jong-Yung 2005b):

1. Comical language: Homonymie, synonymie that confuses people; schwatzhaftigkeit, which refers to repeating words; paronymie, used often in playing of words; diminutivform, abbreviating nouns as babies; wortveränderung, which is changing words with incorrect pronunciation; and wortform, word forms that are expressed with faulty grammar, are a few of the examples.
2. Comical behavior: Comical behavior includes the following: creating good or bad characters by makeup or change of roles, fraud, expressing the impossible by using fantasy-like traits, incorrect description of cause and effect, inappropriate expressions by using useless methods, unpredictable or alarming behavior by making comical reunion, depicting characters in an ugly way by using caricature, cheap-looking dance by a choir, selection of something worse than expected, and unrelated words among the dialogues of characters.
3. Comical characteristics: Comical characteristics include der alazon; der eiron who are puzzling, humble people where it is hard to know who they really are; and der bomalochos, who are funny men.

For example, the word "pun" derived from the concept refers to playing with words. It includes funny language, punning, jokes, fresh talk and funniness created by using two words that have the same pronunciation but different meanings, and dual language. It is using humorous words, making fun with words that have different meanings but have similar or the same pronunciations which can confuse people, or using words that have various meanings. Words are flexible ingredients that can create everything. There are words that still hold their original meanings in some special contexts even though it lost all of its original meanings. Humor actively makes use of these traits of language, and it includes using words that have various meanings or double meanings or pun and emphasizing one aspect than the other with the same word (Kim Hwon-Hwan 2006a). In short, humor can maximize comical behavior or situation by paradoxically changing general ideas or by using cliché expressions and changing quotes and sayings in a funny way. As you can see, all of these are possible using language as the medium, so the importance of language in laughter theory should be given credit.

Aristotle defined that humans are "animals that can laugh," and he believed that laughter is made in diaphragm. In our body, diaphragm acts as a bridge between the upper and the lower part of the body. Therefore, laughter, produced from the diaphragm, also has two origins. The upper part refers to sophisticated, mental sphere and the lower part symbolizes impulsive and cheaper sphere. People tend to laugh by mental motives such as witty language but also by tickling or sexual stimulus (dirty jokes) (Ryoo Jong-Yung 2005c).

Aristotle also believed that laughter is related to age. Young people tend to react with great energy. They tend to love or hate with more force than aged people and have a sense of wit as they like laugh. Here, wit is a tamed arrogance. However, aged people tend to think their future is limited and grieves much from small things. They don't have the heart to laugh or have witty senses, as sorrow can't be combined with the pleasures, which are derived from laughter. Furthermore, Aristotle argued that pleasure-giving laughter is good and is same as virtue. He also argued the need of fellowship among people in the society and emphasized the necessity of laughter (clown) and evaluated the importance of laughter (Ryoo Jong-Yung 2005d).

As an answer to the question "What makes people laugh?," Aristotle only referred to the relationship between certain characteristics of the subject that make people laugh and the people who laugh. That is why his description was regarded as superficial and lacking. Therefore, many critics tried to reform or add to his laughter theory. However, various theories and discussions that follow Aristotle's only focused on describing and categorizing separate examples, and they all fall into his concept of comedy, in which all people tend to laugh at the "foolishness" of people (Lim Hyo-Soo 2000a). Later, research on laughter and comical aspects was dealt in physiological, philosophical, and aesthetic point of view, and psychological and social aspects were added in the eighteenth century. However, steady research is yet to find out a general answer to what makes people laugh.

Now let's look at the three theories, starting with the "superioritytheory" to "incongruity theory" and "relief theory." In each theory, the cause of laughter is by superior feelings, disharmony of recognition, and settlement of psychological tension, respectively. The three theories can cover a general explain of the laughter theory and, therefore, are practical.

4.2.1   Superiority Theory

From the sixteenth century (14th in Italy) to the seventeenth century, with the Renaissance in Europe, the laughter theory underwent great changes. It broke free from a spiritual afterlife, which was taken as the norm for several centuries in the Middle Ages. Instead, the laughter theory was discussed and researched considering humans and their current life just like in the ancient Greek and Roman times.

Thomas Hobbes (1588–1679) tried to systematically categorize the descriptions and the differing opinions on laughter.

Hobbes (1840) categorized laughter in the following three aspects. First is the "superiority theory" where laughter is induced through superior feelings and contempt. Second is the "contrast theory" or "incongruity theory," which is about the contrast between expectations and reality. Lastly, there is the "combination explanation theory" which is a mix of the two theories.

According to the "superiority theory," laughter is produced when people compare others' faults with their own or their past faults, as is expressed in his book, *Human Nature*:

> The passion of laughter is the same as sudden glory. It is made from a sudden thought about superior feelings that is produced when we compare others' faults with our old self's. Many people tend to laugh at such sudden reminders of their past faulty behaviors, as long as they dishonor their current selves. (Hobbes 1840)

As you can see, the laughter described by Hobbes is similar to a cynical laugh that is produced when you see someone's unfortunate situation. It makes his definition of superiority effective only in limited situations. According to Hobbes, laughter-inducing behaviors are fundamentally rooted in others' faults and shortcomings, which make people get a superior feeling. The feeling turns into "sudden glory" that is the source of pleasure. For example, when people laugh at a person who slipped on ice, it can be a physical "fault" or weakness on the part of the slipped, and the other laughing bystanders may feel a sense of superiority that they don't have such a physical defect. Or they can be reminded of a similar occurrence of their own in the past and feel a sense of superiority or "sudden glory." The principle also applies to comedians, where the popular comedians tend to have "below than average" physical traits. Their characteristics make ordinary people laugh, because most people feel superior to their comedian counterparts.

Henri-Louis Bergson (1859–1941) is a household philosopher of the twentieth-century French living philosophy, and his 1900 essay book about laughter and its meaning of humor caused a stir back then. Bergson recognized the limitations of the existing "good deed theory" and promoted a dichotomous theory (form of life and structure) which saw laughter as mechanical that is added to the vital aspect. He said, "Life constantly evolves in time and life itself never goes back or repeats itself. In spatial aspect, life has coexisting elements, and they exist together, and not one element can belong to two different lives as they are complementary. Every being or life is a representation of an exclusive system that can't be copied. The outside characteristics that distinguish life from simply being mechanical are continuous changes of forms, and the perfect individuality in a series of sequence that is embed in the fact that it is impossible to reverse phenomena" (Bergson 1994a).

The opposing mechanical aspect refers to things that aren't natural, and they go against the flexibility, mobility, and time aspect of life. There are times when human beings are regarded as without life. It's when their mechanical traits that go against the natural aspects of life show up because of inertia, oblivion, habit, stubbornness, and bluffing. At these moments, people tend to laugh at them. In situations where adaptability and agile flexibility are needed as people's traits, certain "mechanical stiffening" makes us laugh. The "mechanical stiffening" means that life with flexibility is hardened. Flexibility is a natural state of life, and stiffening is lacking life and is the destruction of mentality, that is, when unmaterialistic aspect of life is altered as materialistic. As you can see, Bergson's laughter is based on pure intelligence and therefore isn't compatible with feelings. That is why he said that however small someone's fault may be, it can't produce laughter from the bystanders when it makes people think about their own fears and compassion. If there is a hunchback person in front of you, it will be something tragic when you see with compassionate eyes. However, seen with an objective point, it can produce laughter from the bystander as the body seems unnatural. Often times, deformity or abnormality in cartoons tends to produce pleasure and a light feeling rather than fear or shock. This is because humorous cartoons usually have powerful tools that suppress compassion.

Now we know that in order for laughter to be produced, we need to be in a state of "insensibility," that is, to be a "careless person." Being "careless" is a psychological stand on the part of the laughing person but is needed on the laughing person as well. Why? Because "carelessness" is a mechanical trait and it is the only condition that enables you to recognize comedy. In other words, carelessness is a temporary state of insensibility, which needs pure intelligence. Indifference is a "distance" that a self has toward himself or his counterpart. It is both an inside and outside distance, and being comical ultimately means that one has a "distance" against his own self, with which he can reflect on himself.

Therefore, when there is a greater feeling of carelessness and when it is systemized as in the case of Don Quixote, it becomes even more comical. Let's look at an example. Korean men would remember having embarrassing moments when words about "communication security" slipped when they picked up the receiver, right after they finish military service. Such experiences that are in our unconsciousness produce laughter with untimely behavior and language. This is why Bergson said that "comical things rise from unconsciousness" (Lim Hyo-Soo 2000b).

Based on the state of "insensibility," Bergson saw the characteristics of laughter as being collective and the social role of laughter as a "punishment that relieves defects that hinder social life." In other words, Bergson argued that laughter is like a punishment that is given to the stubborn individuals in the society. Some people think laughter is frank, but whether it exists in real life or is the result of imagination, Bergson believed that it acts as a tool to hide certain agreement among people, thereby hiding a type of complicity conscious. What society hates is the "rigidity" in this sense. When people laugh, thinking that they are like the others, they are given the silent right to laugh at the person who acts differently or makes mistakes. Therefore, Bergson said that laughter itself is a "cold" one, meaning it is a sneer or a cynical laugh.

Bergson also believed that humor is strengthened when we have cold indifference and go deeper down to see the behavior that is conducted in the lower part (i.e., evil deeds, mechanical movements), rather than turning to the upper part (i.e., goodwill), such as irony (Bergson 1994b).

In short, comedy is the representation of inadaptability in a society, and comedy can't exist apart from people, who are life themselves. Bergson believed that the function of such laughter is in "correction." He argued that as the objective of laughter is the behavior of correction itself, the role of laughter is to emphasize and correct rigid things that are contrary to being alive and that are stuck, mechanical, and careless that is in contrast to paying attention and automatismé that goes against free activities. Bergson also argued that the role of laughter is to replace rigidity with flexibility, to harmonize individuals with others by readaptation, and ultimately, metaphorically speaking, to make round the sharp edges (Bergson 1994c). In this sense, laughter is both the judge of evil but can also erase the real value of the utmost holiness and honest truth. In conclusion, Bergson's laugh is an insight which is to maximize the "distance" between the self and the object that is laughed at, so that the self can critically see himself or the object (Go Hyun-Kyung 2006).

In contrast, the laughter theory promoted by M. M. Bakhtin reports that the absence of the distance between the self and the object is what produces laughter. According to his words, "it is produced from the people, and specifically, it is a destructive laugh that demolishes descriptive and hierarchical distance that tries to fixate things. Laughter makes the self and object to narrow the distance and it has a powerful force to attract them to an area where artificial contact is impossible. There, we can touch every aspect of the object, turn them upside down, and strip them naked. We can even avoid, expose, look at and experiment with it freely. Laughter discards the fear and a sense of sacredness of the object and the world. (…) Laughter is the most important asset of 'looking down upon something' that is needed to get rid of fear. If this aspect is not considered, the world can't be beheld as it is, or 'realistically,' he says" (Bakhtin 1982).

This is different from the "reflective distance" promoted by Bergson. Bakhtin's "distance" is subjective and aesthetic, which doesn't allow access to the object, as the subject sees the object to be an absolute one. In this respect, the subject creates tradition and an aura around the object, and hierarchy is established between the two in the process, where one can't bridge the distance to get to another. The hierarchical distance hinders laughter to be produced. Bakhtin focused on laughter that can be made when absolute, hierarchical distances such as authority or seriousness are destroyed. In short, every being loses all authority in laughter, and there is no distance or authority in laughter, and the world exists in the same time frame as the laughing subject or self. Precious being can't be the object of laughter, so laughter itself means that the object is upgraded to the surface from the bottom. Even the self is spitted, rising from the surface of the representation. The distance in Bakhtin's laughter theory is both something to be destroyed as well as something that has hierarchy, which stems from the subjectivity and mysterious feeling that the self feels toward the object. Bergson saw that the self held a superior position than the object, and it was reversed in Bakhtin's case. As a result, the two talked about "distance" in the laughter theory but had opposing views on the self and object that were located on the both ends of the "distance."

Another person who talked about laughter is Bernard Shaw, who said that laughing without compassion is a form of feeling sadistic satisfaction that is hard to be felt in our everyday lives. Shaw thought that it is the most animallike element of human nature that enjoys low comedy (Shaw 1998). The critical positions on laughter can be found often in Aristophanes, Shakespeare, and German romantics' comedies.

4.2.2 *Incongruity Theory*

After the eighteenth century, the so-called incongruity theory or contrast theory, developed in Germany, looked at laughter to be produced from irrational conflicts between expectations and reality. The first person to argue the "incongruity theory" of laughter was James Beattie (1735–1803). As a writer and a philosopher, he summarized the laughter theories of the era in his "Essay on laughter and ludicrous composition" (1764):

> Laughter seems to rise from looking at the combination of conflicting elements in the same group. (…) I don't agree with the Hutcheson's view of laughter, who said that the cause or the object of laughter is "a cheapness that is contrary to dignity." Rather, I want to use more ordinary words to describe the cause and object of laughter. It is "the contrast between something appropriate or inappropriate. Or the contrast between a unified, or seemingly unified relationship in the same group and the absence of that relationship." (…) Some people may ask what the characteristics are that bring pleasant feelings to produce or arouse laughter. I would say that it is the rare combinations and incongruity that is made in a group, which is thought to be made up with a certain correlation or combination. Then when does such combination arouse laughter? I believe that the recognition of this, except for the case when a more authoritative feeling is aroused, can always, or at least, in many cases, produce feelings that can make us laugh. (Beatti 1975)

Beatti did well to set apart laughter and sneer by accepting Aristotle's argument (in England) and criticizing the "superiority theory" of Thomas Hobbes. Beatti also accepted the arguments of Francis Hutcheson (1694–1746), who expanded the concept of laughter to go beyond ethical traits to reach historical and cultural sphere. By developing Hutcheson's theory further, Beatti cast a good arguing point in the laughter theory. His works later sparked Immanuel Kant (1724–1804) and Arthur Schopenhauer (1788–1860) to cast their version of the "incongruity theory," which is a step further from his.

This is how Schopenhauer explains laughter in his well-known book, *Die Welt als Wille und Vorstellung*:

> Laughter isn't produced from different things every time. Rather, it is produced from incongruity that is suddenly recognized between one concept and the real objects. The objects have been thought of as in correlation to the concept, and laughter is nothing more than the expression of the incongruity. The incongruity is produced often times when two or more real objects are thought from a concept and when the oneness of the concept is transferred to the objects. Next, it is significantly revealed that the perfect distinction between the objects and the concept is the same as the objects in a unilateral way. Nevertheless, there are some real objects that make us feel the sudden incongruity between the concepts, which encompasses objects. However, it is useful to note that the more right it is to include the real objects to the concept, and the bigger and starker the incompatibility between the objects

and the concept, the humor rising from the disparity becomes stronger. To put it another way, every laugh is paradoxical, and that is why unexpected encompassing is produced as a motive. The encompassing takes place whether it is expressed via language or behavior. This is the correct explanation of something "humorous (funny)" put in a simple way. (Schopenhauer 2003)

Schopenhauer saw that the disparity is what produces laughter. He thought laughter and funny things are the same. His "incongruity theory" took a knowledge-based perspective, so it is often called as the "intellectual incongruity theory." Schopenhauer paid attention to the good aspects of laughter as well. For instance, he argued when a person slips, laughter is produced from the recognition of the bystander that the slipped person did something that is out of the ordinary. This shed new light on people's awareness and turned hostile laughter into a favorable one.

Similar idea can be found in Kant as well. In his book *Critique of Judgment* (1790), Kant focused on the inner thug that lives within us. "In everything that makes us think about impressive, lively laughter, there is something corrupt that can't be satisfied with our knowledge. Laughter is a type of a feeling that can be felt when strained expectation turns into a feeling of emptiness" (Hartmann 1995a). In Kant's words, laughter didn't come from superior feelings but highlighted "strained expectations." However, it then is recognized as an objective, strange "object" that becomes nothing more than emptiness. His argument follows like this. "We should know that expectations don't change into the active opposition of the expectant party, but into emptiness. Think about it. When someone talks about history, we listen with expectant hearts. The expectant feeling will be turned into utter bitterness when we find out that is not true" (Hartmann 1995b). As you can see, the comical cause that was expressed both as "a mistake and fault" by Aristotle was understood as "disparity" by Kant. Kant also pointed out that life can be comical without human weaknesses. Therefore, Kant's laughter encompassed broader and generous emotions. According to Kant, laughter is like a generous pleasure that you feel in a situation like this. You see someone being embarrassed, when he later realizes that he prepared food that is unsuitable for the occasion (Kant 1998). In short, in Kant's point of view, laughter refers to a feeling of generosity in which "laughing with ourselves who laugh at our neighbors" or "laughing with our neighbors who laugh at us." When we have a more generous attitude toward human foolishness, we can earnestly enjoy being funny. However, it doesn't mean that we can always say okay to the foolishness of ourselves. It's just that our lowliness, sense of failure, and the hidden contempt we have for ourselves are diminished and healed by our laughter.

Taking Kant's theory one step further, Freud stressed "situational comicalness," which revealed even the complex traits of laughter. Freud didn't agree that the antagonistic distance between the self and the other induced comical situations. Though a person may laugh at the faults and weaknesses of the other, the laughter stems from the situation itself, as the person could be in a similar situation next time. It has nothing to do with feelings of superiority. It puts the comical situation on the center rather than the superior feelings. The realization that the comical situation could happen to any one of us is what makes the person laugh, so the laughter is not an antagonistic one but a favorable one. Freud's laughter theory isn't such a simple one. He points out that laughter produces some type of "illusion" about the reality and has the power to deny reality itself. This shows that it is hard to describe the function of laughter in a simple way.

Spencer argued that laughter is a "signal of an effort when you are hit by a sense of sudden emptiness." T. Lipps also described that laughter is produced when something that had seemed meaningful, valuable, and somber reveals to be petty. In this sense, the end results are about emptiness as well (Kim Hwon-Hwan 2006b).

In every society, there are common rules which dominate our consciousness. When something goes against such common rules, people tend to think that it is paradoxical and irrational. This also produces laughter. According to the incongruity theory, presumption and result always have some differences, and the difference produces laughter. G. E. Lessing said the following: "Irrationally, the contrast between the reality and one's thoughts are always comical. The contrast between promise or expectation, and the execution of it is comical and funny" (Lessing 1991).

The everyday mundane life can seem very fresh when seen by a new perspective. In a dry situation, the act of laughing itself can be energy in our life. People feel not only pleasure but also a sense of sheer joy when the social leaders' "gross dignity" (be it those in power or who have money) is quickly turned into a joke. The longer the distance (gap) between the two objects that are being contrasted, the more laughter is produced from irony. After the new government came to power in Korea, the chief secretary of the president was known to have sexually harassed an intern who was similar to his daughter's age, in the new president's first visit to the USA. His actions became an international laughingstock, and it is one of the big disparity examples that I mentioned.

As you can see, the laughter that is shown in the "incongruity theory" includes "satire" about the society. The disparities, irrational customs of the era or the foolishness, hypocrisy, and defections are pointed out and ridiculed in satire, which is one of the forms to express comical feelings. Satire is always made up of negative and critical attitudes of the reality. Satire is about contradicting someone in a higher level and attacks the counterpart with ridicule and cynicism. Furthermore, it has an educational meaning, which is the reforming negativity of the object. Therefore, satire is a "beautiful laughter" where the negative motives are improved as a positive one, based on passionate emotions and pure knowledge. Essentially, satire is grounded in "humanism." It protects human values, which are the attitude of protecting what is right, the pursuit of moral goodness, and the respect for aesthetic things (Kim Ji-Won 1983a).

As seen from above, many people regarded that the irrational contrast between the presumption and the result and the incongruity stemming from comparison were at the center of laughter. When paradox and irrationality prolong, confusion and complaint arise, and the feeling of tension is only washed away when they are hit and dispersed by the paradox ones. It is precisely when the tension is relieved when we feel comical feelings. Therefore, solving the paradox is the same as recognizing that it is nothing and that it is emptiness and incongruity.

Karl Marx's (1818–1883) opinion on the comical things is directly related to the disparity or paradox. About the comical aspect of the history, which is revealed throughout the development of history, he says this in *Der Achtzehnte Brumaire des Louis Bonaparte* and *Zur Kritik der Hegelschen Rechtsphilosophie* (Ryoo Jong-Yung 2005e):

> Hegel described somewhere that every great historical facts and figures arise twice in history. But he forgot to add that they happen once as a tragedy, and once as a farce. (Marx 1946)

> [...] it is mistaking the era, and it is a stark contrast to the public goods that are recognized generally. The current German identity, an unfruitful result of the ancien regime, which had been revealed all around the world, proudly believes that it is still given a trust, and is demanding the world to believe this illusion. [...] The ancien regime of today is nothing more than a comic actor in the world order, where the real actors have all died out. When history gives up the past form, the history experiences various steps that are strict. The last step of the global form is comedy. By the handcuffed Prometheus, the Greek gods have suffered a huge blow. In the dialogue of Lucianos, the gods had to suffer another comical blow. Why does history move on like this? It is to say goodbye to the past in a pleasant way. We demand those in power in Germany to give us the pleasant historical tradition. (Marx 1957)

The sayings of Marx lay a fundamental ground as we understand the historical and social characteristics of comical things. He revealed that historical incidents and famous figures that had tragic traits in particular circumstances can be given a comical trait in the change of history. In other words, in his interpretation of something being comical in history, he revealed the paradox that is in the comical things. Marx saw that the reality of the individuals (Louis Bonaparte) and the reality that has historical grounds (the identity of Germany/ancien regime) are types of disparities, that is, paradox. Later, the paradox was accepted as an essential part of comical history. And the comical history continues today.

4.2.3   Relief Theory

Laughter was an issue that couldn't be ignored by the philosophers and thinkers. To those people who pondered on the existence of human being day after day, laughter, which is one of the essential parts of humanity, was something that stuck with them for some time. The serious attitudes of them are a sheer irony, as the characteristics of laughter are to hate and destroy seriousness.

The "relief theory," which is also called as the "arousal theory," reports that laughter is produced when stimulus is resolved in a stressful situation. Basically, it saw that relief from strained feelings is what produces laughter. Before that, Descartes saw that we laugh when we first become angry at evil and then realize that the evil can't do us any harm. Hartley also viewed that laughter is a signal of joy when something painful or surprising is removed (Kim Hwon-Hwan 2006c).

Freud argued for the political aspect of laughter, saying that "Reason, critical judgment and oppression are the things that joke fight their way through." He persisted that laughter is the great force which fights against the beliefs of reason-centered and individual-oriented Western custom. The subject that is dissolved by laughter is the one which believes that it can exist in a single form. However, that is an illusion. Humans live not only in thoughts but also in body. They live in the mind and emotions as well. They need material things as well as sexual life. Therefore, the subject dissolving itself with laughter is a good way to make its living joyful.

The psychological social theory of Freud is as follows. First, certain traits and responses of psychology are inherent, permanent, and general. Second, every human being has a common psychological mechanism, ability, and symbolism. Third, in our moral selves, there is a general, unconscious force, and the "id" refers to the oppressed impulse or instinctive needs of the unconscious self. "Superego" oppresses "id," as it is a value system that is learned from a culture or is a personal conscience. In other words, "superego" is an "internalized society," which is a force that commands individuals' actions according to moral judgment, just like the conscience. It is also a moral (social) self that continuously strives to aim for perfection. Lastly, "ego" is a conscious self that connects the "id" and the "superego." As you can see, his theory argues that psychological devices such as oppression, reflection, and resolution are general (Garbarino 1995).

So according to Freud, laughter is an active expression of the "ego" which aims to fight against the pains of the reality with "pleasure principle." He said that it is about responding more flexibly to the oppressions arising from the reality, so that the ego can be protected and healed from pain. He also said that the essence of laughter is to free the ego from stress and oppression felt in painful situations (Freud 1997a).

In this context, Freud defined laughter in this way: "When the things that we thought meaningful are laid bare as things that are totally meaningless, therein lies the essence of comical process. When we give meaning to a description with a psychological inevitability and then is taken away that meaning at an instant, the description seems comical to us. In this situation, meanings can be understood in various ways." He believed that "the contrast between sens and non-sens" are the foundations of comical feelings, that is, laughter (Freud 2003b).

The words "sens" and "non-sens" are same as the terms meaningful and meaningless that we use in our everyday lives. Let's look deeper into the words for clear understanding. "Sens" has three meanings in French. First, it is about "direction." The word "meaning" that we generally use means direction. Second, it is about sense, which refers to the sensory organs in our body. Third, it is about "meaning" and bears a certain "systematization" in itself. When the first and the third meanings of "sens" are combined, it is related to the "doxa," which is a social meaning. "Doxa" has two aspects, "bon sens" and "sens commun." "Bon sens" is about a "right direction or work." "Sens commun" is about "common direction" or "common sense." "Doxa" contradicts with "para-doxa." "Doxa" is about values and beliefs that are generally accepted in an era or in a society. "Non-sens" and "para-doxa" go against the common rules and therefore refer to the conversion of conventional beliefs (Deleuze 1999a).

In every era and society, there is conventional wisdom that is accepted in usual situations. The conventional wisdom that is made before can be referred to as common sense, ideology, or code. However, there is a kind of a desire beyond the conventional wisdom, which has the force to converge it anytime. The force becomes stronger when the conventional wisdom can't speak up for the society where it is shared, and that is the power of non-sens and paradox. "Bon sens" drives everything and value to one way, that is, to work. However, "non-sens" and "paradox" agree to both directions at the same time. Furthermore, "paradox" and "non-sens" can be interpreted into various directions and meanings according to systematization (Kim Hwon-Hwan 2006d).

More important is that the comical effect of "non-sens" is that it makes us strive to know the hidden meaning of the "non-sens." However, we can't find any meaning in it and they are meaningless in real terms. In that moment of deception, we can let off pleasure freely, in the "non-sens" context. This is the essence of meaning that is in the "non-sens," and it is the pleasure of "non-sens." Therefore, the paradoxical thinking and the downward direction to the "non-sens" produce humor and laughter. For instance, the disharmony, breaking free from forms, exaggeration, distortion, deformation, and omission are major devices that transform (in a downward form) traditional, ideal regulations and laws, which are used in cartoons and caricature. It is the point where laughter is produced.

Many paradoxical opinions found in these arguments on laughter tell us that laughter doesn't exist in pure forms in most cases but in various combinations. To put it another way, the festive atmosphere made by laughter has to be pleasant to begin with. However, in order for it to be something more than a simple escape from the reality, the freedom from stress and the recognition of the reality of the laughing person should be reconsidered. As for laughter based on satire, it has to have a critical view on the subject. However, it can break free from "cynicism" only when it has a community that can look at it and laugh at the subject together.

As a result, we can say that at the both ends of the spectrum, we have a blind laughter that only chases after the simplest pleasure and cynicism (cold laughter). In between the two, there are various levels of laughter, which have satire and humor in different ratios mingled together. When we recognize how the insides of human-minds are dynamically combined with reason and emotion and how we are faced with disparities and paradoxes, we will know that humans are not just "beings that can laugh" but are "beings that are bound to laugh":

First, are there people who can say they know themselves? Just like the words of the great Monk Soong San (the mentor of Monk Hyun Kak who graduated from Harvard University), "Only I don't know." So we have no choice but to laugh at our fundamental ignorance.

Second, are there people without faults or defects? There is no perfect human being, so we laugh at the fundamental foolishness of ourselves.

Third, are there people who don't feel pain and stress in reality? There is no one without stress, so it also makes us laugh.

Fourth, are there people who can escape death? Life itself is full of emptiness, so we can't help but laugh.

4.2.4 From Laughter to Humor: A Paradigm Shift

In the early seventeenth century, Thomas Hobbs regarded laughter and cynicism as the same. However, starting from the mid-seventeenth century, laughter was given a new role in the UK, as it was seen as an expression of pure human feelings. The emotional experience was regarded as pleasing as well. In the eighteenth-century sentimentalism coupled with enlightenment, humans were thought of as being born with "good intentions" and "ethical sense." Against this backdrop, the concept of laughter underwent a paradigm shift as related to humor. With the rise of humor concept, the characteristics of humans and their subjective motives and situations began to be recognized. Some individuals who became financially successful put great emphasis on "sociality," and it was regarded as one of the essentials of harmony and reconciliation in the upper society. Laughing and crying together were used as a propaganda, a gesture of social reconciliation (Ryoo Jong-Yung 2005f).

Laughter, which used to be assimilated with cynicism, took on a new meaning of "humor." And the process was conducted with a change of viewpoint on humans. It is shown well in the book by Shaftesbury (1671–1713), where he criticized the role of selfish laughter of Hobbs (superior theory of laughter) and used cynicism as a tool of sense:

> I believe that truth can take every perspective. One of the important perspectives and natural medium to give light to the things to aid people to have a perfect recognition is cynicism itself. And that cynicism is a way of proving weaknesses in some subjects. By way of proving this, we discern whether the subject has the right value to be laughed at. All people who use this as evidence would allow for this much sometime. (Shaftesbury 1711)

The word "humor" originated from the word "humor" that refers to the bodily fluid and disposition of humans. H.M. Koelbing, medical historian, describes it in detail with body fluid theory (Ryoo Jong-Yung 2005g):

1. The Greek doctor Alkmaion (born in 520 BC) said that humans have four bodily fluids and that each has warm, cold, humid, or dry traits.
2. The Greek philosopher Empedokles (born in 483/482 BC) argued that the world is made up of four fundamental elements, which are air, water, fire, and earth. Aristotle combined the four bodily fluids of Alkmaion and the four fundamental elements of Empedokles. He said that air is warm and humid; water, humid and cold; earth, cold and dry; and fire, dry and warm.
3. The Greek doctor Hippocrates (460–370 BC) and his students believed that the four fundamental elements exist in human's bodily fluids as well. They argued

that the following groups of two are the same: air and blood, water and mucus, earth and black bile, and fire and yellow bile.

4. Galen (129–199 AD), a Roman doctor from Greece, said that the dominant bodily fluids of each person are related to the disposition of each person. Blood (Lat. sanguis) refers to a pleasant (or hot-tempered) person, mucus (Gr. phlegma) a mucus person (dull and slow person), bile (Gr. chole) a person of bilious (person who is quick to anger), and black bile (Gr. melas chole) a melancholy person (a gloomy person).

5. The body fluid theory or the study of dispositions has been maintained until the eighteenth and even to the nineteenth century in medicine. In psychology, the study of dispositions still is the foundation for the study of characteristics to date.

Later, the concept of humor was established in late sixteenth century in the UK. In the forward of Ben Jonson (1572–1637)'s play Every Man out of His Humour, the then meaning of bodily fluid was described with the critic Asper's words:

> Every human body has bile, black bile, mucus and blood. These continue ceaselessly and don't stop, and hence their name "bodily fluid." As long as they have these traits, the word can be transferred to disposition in a general sense. If someone is occupied with a particular characteristic and when it is combined together to make the flow of his passion, mental and physical force go in one direction, it is natural to call it characteristic humor. (Schmidt-Hidding 1963)

According to Schmidt-Hidding, the bodily fluid of humans is not set permanently, but they are flexible in each individual. It means it has had great volatility in its combination since the fifteenth century. Therefore, the characteristics of the emotion, mood, and even whim are all changeable. Despite the changeable traits, pleasant people were called as "people with good bodily fluids (humor)," which can be translated into someone being in a good mood or someone who is kind. If someone is in a good mood or is kind every time, he was regarded as the one having a "good sense of humor" or having a "sense of humor." The word "humor" here developed into "disposition," "mood," "atmosphere," and "taste." Since the late nineteenth century, people without a sense of humor wasn't regarded as a whole being in the UK (Ryoo Jong-Yung 2005h). In this respect, we can see that humor has a lot of subjective aspects to it. In short, the expression that someone "has a sense of humor" includes the meaning that he is self-centered or is ethnic centered, and the expression can be used in both individuals and groups.

Now let's look at the definition of humor in the dictionary: (1) characteristics that are shown in accidental incident, action situations, or expressions of ideas which induce laughter, disharmony, or awkwardness (laughter or pleasure); (2) the ability to discover, express, and evaluate ideas, situations, accidental incidents, or disharmony (mimicking or expressing something funny); and (3) the action or effort to make something seem funny (Webster's Dictionary, 1984).

A. Horn distinguished "humor" and "satire" in a simple way, by the level of harmlessness of the foolishness. That is, when something foolish is "not at all dangerous, and has absolutely no harm," it is distinguished as "humoristisch," "humorvoll," and "humorig." When the foolishness is at a dangerous level, it is called "satirisch" (Horn 2, 1988b).

In Korea, the concept of humor has so many synonyms, ranging from irony, wit, ridicule, pun, jokes, and meaningless pranks. Scholars have various opinions on humor, and they are not well categorized. For instance, Kim Sa-Yup used the term "pun" to mean "comic" and "comical" and "joke" to replace the meaning "humor" (Kim Sa-Yup 1957). However, Jeong Dong-Hwa used "joke" as the same word as comic and "pun" meaning fun. In a wider sense, humor in Korea can include concepts such as fun and joke (Goo Hyun-Jeong 2000), but the content is about the contrast between comical things or an indirect explanation of the "incongruity theory" or "superiority theory" (Son 1999).

Comparing humor with other types of information, humor usually sets the relationship (meaning) between disharmonies, and by suddenly showing them to us, it tends to make us laugh. Now, let's look at the essential concept of humor, which has become a critical point in "social skills" as it makes us pleasant and makes us smile with beautiful laughter. Let's look at it from the following three perspectives, entirety, subjectivity, and observation (Dosio 1989):

1. Entirety: Humor doesn't focus on the foolish individuals or their particular behaviors. It only jokes about the foolishness of life in general. It doesn't sit still on lowering the higher people, just as in parodies, and neither does it focus on giving power to the lower people like irony. Humor relates the individual finite people with infinity by comparing it with ideology. In the perspective that everything great and small are nothing in the face of infinity, it denies both at the same time.
2. Subjectivity: Humor stems from wit. However, when wit only goes so far as to relate two things that are different and lacks a sense of self, humor is added with a reason for irony that is self-conscious. In this way, subjectivity is equal to wit that makes subject out of which that does witty actions. The subjectivity of humor is mixed with a pure feeling that is extremely sensitive to its faults with a strict sense of criticism. It makes it unstable but never gives up a compassionate stance toward the subject.
3. Observation: Humor is based on deep insights in various realities that we face in life. When the secrets of the world are revealed based on the insights, they become humor, which is the highest form of subjective jokes. Humor has the powerto highlight the paradoxes in life in a witty sense, which are as follows: greatness that always comes with beautiful laughter based on the cognitive impulse that wants to reveal the outsides of life, the healthiness that hides and makes the illness not seen, and heroism based on self-deceit. Humor makes all tools of jokes fall on knees to this cause. Therefore, humor is an aesthetic form that has the intentions of recognition and observation.

As you can see, the essence of humor is not on the subject or the expression of it but rather on subjective attitude. It is also closely related to the outlook on life and how you view the world. Therefore, it seems that humor has the highest aesthetic value among the forms of subjective jokes. Humor, on the aspect of laughing motives, falls into the category of wit, satire, or irony, which is under the boundary of comedy that nullifies things that are noble and resolute. However, it's unique in that it doesn't show antagonistic feelings toward the subject by contradicting it but embraces it with love and compassion. In short, humor looks at the subject as it is and tries to dismiss the unpleasant feelings that arise from disharmony by embracing and assimilation (Kim Ji-Won 1983b).

People tend not to be satisfied with experiencing comical things that occur in life but have tried to produce comical things intentionally. Humor is totally a subjective comedy, so it is related to our actions and efforts to make it. That is, humor, whether it is an observatory comedy or a situational comedy, is something that is produced intentionally. There might be slight differences on whether the humor is pleasant or the satire makes one angry, but in the perspective of "comical" spectrum, it is hard for us to define whether a story is related to humor or satire.

4.2.4.1   Freud's Humor: Superego Humor

Freud distinguished the processof humor in two ways. His arguments can be explained as in the perspective of the so-called scaffold humor:

> Let's say there is a prisoner who is destined to die on a scaffold on Monday. When he says, "The week is starting off so smoothly," the prisoner himself and the people who are unrelated to the humor can feel a sense of pleasure, which is the first kind. The second kind is a humor writer, in which case the characters that are the focus of humor, don't have to be humorous themselves. People who have to pose humorous attitudes are people who make subjects out of these people. In this case, readers and the audience share the joy of humor just as in the first case. (Freud 1998a)

To Freud, humor comes to the person in question, or to someone outside, despite its characteristics. In short, humorous attitudes are regarded to pose pleasure not only to the people who pose the attitude but also to the people who are unrelated to it. As you can see from the "scaffold humor," the prisoner is faced with a desperate situation, being in the face of death, and it can give rise to a strong sense of compassion on our part. However, when we realize that the prisoner is not so much concerned with the situation, our compassion is oppressed. From the positive attitude of the prisoner, who doesn't stop to let himself feel miserable in the face of death, Freud discovers a certain mental attitude that is noble and transcendent. As in the words of Charlie Chaplin, "Life is a tragedy when seen in close-up, but a comedy in a long shot."

Transcendent is a type of a mental attitude and it is "self-dualization." When someone takes humor from another person, the person puts himself in the position of elder, assimilating himself with a father figure. He gains superior feelings by treating others as young people. This person can laugh because he knows that the relationship, conflicts of interest, or pains that have significant meaning on young people are trivial things. However, we can't help but ask what it is that allows the person taking humor from others to do this. This is by the "superego," an instance.

According to Freud, humor is like the superego (parent) consoling the self (child) with its pains, saying, "It's nothing." Just as in the humor spoken by the prisoner, it is looking down at oneself from a "meta-level" (Garatani Gojin 2002). However, this is similar but different from irony, which can sometimes have contempt at oneself which is in pain or in the troubles of reality, even risking death. By doing so, irony shows itself proudly, the high-ranking self which can risk those. Irony makes people unpleasant; however, humor emancipates others who hear it. The humor of Freud comes from the "reconciliation of superego," so that the self don't have to succumb to or be intruded by various difficulties that the self confronts in reality:

> Humor is a simple tool that aims to gain pleasure despite the uncomfortable feelings that hinder pleasure. Humor replaces it, and shows itself instead of the expression of the feelings. Maybe this is what humor wants to say; "Look, it is a dangerously-looking world. But it is a mere joke of children. A little prank from children!" It is superego that consoles the much-afraid self with humor. If the superego consoles the self and protects it from pain, it doesn't go against the opinion that the superego stems from the "instance" where parents used to take its place in the child's mind. (Freud 1998b)

In the end, Freud's humor is a mental attitude where the superego transcends the finite human conditions and situations. According to Freud, the task of humor is to "eliminate the development of excitement" which gets in the way of pleasure that exists in a situation. That is why humor discovered by Freud is the power of superego, which regards all pain and troubles of this world as "nothing" in an instant. If joke is made to make oneself superior than the other, humor is a skill to become superior by lowering oneself than the world. Therefore, even when the world gives us any sorrow or disappointment, when we can laugh at us, we can become superior to the world. Nothing can claim victory against humor, which appears at the last moment. By looking into the inner world of humans, Freud woke up the self which oppresses animal instincts and one-dimensional desire and adapts to the reality. He showed the world of morally mature superego by teleporting to a higher new world. Freud says that "humor is a rare and noble quality." The essence of the quality lies in "distancing." According to Freud, in humor, there is "authority that doesn't exist in wit," and humor writers are people who "change the stressing points of psychology into superego, being free from his self" (Freud 1963).

As you can see, Freud starkly shows that people can always experience, beyond the objective situation ("to distance or to look at something from another perspective"), the subjective and positive humor. Beautiful laughter has the power to overcome and look beyond the current situation at an instant, thereby making people taste the "beautiful, noble victory of the mentality." Based on the fact, beautiful laughter always secured the superego, and we have to take note of this fact. Therefore, as there was a paradigm shift from cynicism to humor, by taking one step further, we can reinterpret humor in a modern sense:

> Humor gives birth to beautiful laughter. In short, humor is the mother of beautiful laughter.

4.2.4.2 Deleuze's Humor: Non-sens (Meaningless) Humor

Gilles Deleuze (1925–1995) wrote in his book *The Logic ofSense* that humor is a Socrates style of irony, a technique of depth and length, and a technique of downward expression that is against the upward expression (Deleuze 1999b). To him, humor is a downward direction to the "surface," which is not to the higher level or to the deeper level, and he says that it is a deeper "surface" and "skin" than other grounds where uniqueness, paradox, non-sens, and sens exist:

> The adventures of jokes, the double destruction of deeper level and higher level for the surface are all adventures of stoic wise men. However, it is also adventures of Taoist hermit. Taoist hermit, which goes against the stoic's Brahmanism, and the Buddha's height, famous issues, Zen riddle and public documents all prove the disparities of signals semiotic process, and refers to the meaningless (non-sens) of signal process. Sticks are general tools, the teacher of questions and the mime and food are answers. The wise focus on the surface is to discern subject and incidents. In the emptiness which composes their realities, they communicate in the Aion which can never be filled by them but which is used as their stage. (Deleuze 1999c)

In linguistic sense, humor is a description that reveals the disparities of the semiotic process and the infinite repetitive traits of the signal process to Deleuz. For instance, the disparities of the semiotic process are shown as a "Buddhist revelation" in Zen Buddhism, which means that realization in Buddhism is transferred from heart to heart, and so it doesn't rely on language or characters. The meaninglessness (non-sens) of the signal process is shown in "ilchegegong," which means that everything is empty. It doesn't refer to a complete nothingness but that something is trivial (Kim Hwon-Hwan 2006e). In short, it means that "you can be free from everything (situations or problems) when you set your heart on the right way." The difference is that the direction of the heart can be different. In the case of Freud, he emphasized that humans can "teleport" by using humor, to the fabulous, high level of new world (superego) that is allowed to humans. However, as for Deleuze, the direction is not upward but downward. Deleuze feels that the ultimate goal of good is a world of meaning (natural order) where it can be directly accessed without going through direction, revelation, or semiotic process. The thing that descends from the history of good is not a sacred book but stories that depict the everyday lives of monks (stories of realization) and Zen riddles. Therefore, all stories that appear in Zen Buddhism are not ironies of Socrates or Freud-like humor but are more akin to stoic humor which puts the utmost value on "mental values" and jokes that are cutting.

In addition, Deleuze describes the attitude difference between irony and humor in relation to the law and good in his book *Masochism*. According to Deleuze, irony is a way that looks good as a ground for higher principles and law. However, humor is a downward movement from the law and its result. In short, irony is understood as a process of thinking that makes us depend on the concept of good that is superior to law. Humor is a more just good than law is and that humor is a trial that seeks to authorize law:

According to the concept of classical law that is driven from Plato, law can be seen from two perspectives; a principle that makes up the foundation or the result of it. Seen by the first perspective, the law itself is not one-dimensional, but it is a secondary or alternative force that depends on the utmost high principle that is good. From the second perspective, abiding by the law becomes the "best" policy that has the image of good. Righteous people abide by the law of the nation that he is born into or living in, and thereby does the best action that he could. (Deleuze 1996a)

Deleuze said that the classic concept of law had been turned upside down by Kant that law no longer depends on good but that the good itself is made to rely on law. This means that the foundations of law isn't grounded by a higher principle or that the rights of law is driven from the principle but that law takes its root on the principle itself and gains meaning in the form:

Now law becomes an absolute law itself, not in need of any specification or grounds. The concept of law in Plato's perspective only dealt with laws that were about various fields of good or about various situations regarding the best. However, Kant talked about the moral law, and was able to apply it to the things that could have been left untended by the moral law. The moral law of Kant is a revelation in a pure form, and it is irrespective of contents, subjects, the fields of action or situation. Moral law is the form of law itself, and it is the law. Therefore, it doesn't need a higher principle. (Deleuze 1996b)

Let's presume that law no longer can take its root from good as an existing, higher principle. If the law that is defined in the pure form has its content in an indefinite form and has no ingredient, subject, or limits and therefore has no one to claim it as their own, then the content of the law is indefinite. Because of the trait, it cannot but be defined as a sin in the perspective of the person who obeys it. Therefore, the only way left to overturn the law is to accurately obey the law.

Humor is in contrast with the upward movement of irony that aims for the transcendent principle in the higher level. Humor is a downward movement from the law to its results. Law, in this case, is not overturned by the upward movement of the irony that seeks a higher principle. It is overturned by the downward movement of humor which contracts law to its detailed results.

Metaphorically speaking, Deleuze saw that irony, the way toward good as a ground of higher principle and law, was sadism (an abnormal way of fulfilling one's sexual desire by sexually abusing the other or feeling pleasure by attacking or giving pain to the other). Humor, in contrast, which overturns law and everything related to Plato, was regarded as masochism (a mental state where one feels sexual pleasure by being mentally and physically abused by the other). Deleuze saw that just as a sadist with an inclination toward irony is a logician of principles, masochist is a humorist and a logician of results.

In this way, Deleuze criticizes Freud, who said that the superego is related to sadism and realistic self to masochism and that humor stems from the "mediation of the superego." He also said that just as the law, which took its roots on the higher principles, is dead, superego is also dead. Deleuze thought that humor is a victory of realistic self over the superego, and he didn't think that humor is an expression of a strong superego as Freud argued. Freud believed that humor inevitably gives additional benefits to the self and shows a resistance, firmness, and coldness toward the self which wants to form a partnership with the superego. He thought that humor shows the victory of narcissism. However, Deleuze argued that the benefits of the self are not "additional" as Freud believed but are a main and essential one. Humor, despite being the results of masochism, is an action of self which is the victor, and it is a skill that escapes and denies the intention of the superego (Deleuze 1996c).

Now, tragedy and nastiness/irony give its place to a new value, which is joke/humor. If irony is a similar outside trait between an existence and object or between I and representation, humor is a "similar outside trait between sens and non-sens" (Deleuze 1996d). Therefore, Deleuze's humor itself is the criticism of the revival and organism mindset of Plato which traps all meanings in oneness and similarity. To him, humor is a process that shows the world of paradox and non-sens, which makes it impossible for a one-directional fixation of all semiotic process and signal process in language. It is also regarded as a tool that directs it to the potential or sensitive reality of "incidents" and "surface" regarding what's happening. At the same time, the peculiarity and surface trait of the incident change its face in pure terms, forming a "flat surface of the inner world." The "flat surface of the inner world" is like an "organless body" where all objects and unmaterialistic things are regarded the same. It is also the destination of all things that move downward, and it can also be referred to as a "flat surface of unconsciousness" (Kim Hwon-Hwan 2006f).

Paradox is same as overturning, in that it goes against the rules and the common sense that dominates our lives. It is deviation from situations and expectations. Paradox is a resistance toward the world and, at the same time, a basic form of opening a world of thinking toward variety and multiple by going beyond the limitations. That is why it nullifies conventions and common sense meanings to let us stand alone on the horizon of non-sens. Therefore, as a systematization of paradox, the production of humor challenges to nullify all dichotomies. However, it is required to do the following: cross-sectional systematization of substance, form, reality, and real objects and subjective ridiculing such as a detailed "standing alone on the part of non-sens" on the various, multiple alignments. For instance, in the concept of classical beauty, order, proportion, and harmony are all elements of beauty. The things that are on the contrast, that is, inharmonious body, breaking free from regulations, exaggeration, distortion, reformation, and omission are all traits that arouse humor. They are the tools that can change traditionally handed-down, ideal rules into nonsense, and that is when laughter is aroused. The wider the gap is, the bigger laughter is produced. Generally, abnormality in cartoons and caricatures gives pleasure and laughter, rather than feelings of ugliness or shock.

The language we use is made up of two aspects. One is "vocabulary," which refers to a variety of words. The other is "grammar," a combination rule of these words. If one is left out, sentences will be awkward. For instance, "mother is doing the laundry" is a complete sentence. However, if there is no grammar, then it will be a strange sentence, "mother the laundry is doing." If there are no words, then only the structure "noun+subject postposition+noun+object postposition+verb" will be left out. Therefore, two new aspects are needed to make a sentence. The aspect of "selection" that chooses the words and "combination," where the words are connected, are the aspects (Chin Jung-Kwon 1994a). The "selection aspect" is "metaphor," which is a way to think A as B, and the important role is understanding. The "combination aspect" is "metonymy," which is a way to express an object by referring to the objects' characteristics or things that are near them in space and time, rather than directly referring to the object itself.

When explaining the basic rule of language formation, R. Jacobson refers to the two aspects. Metaphor is the basic rhetoric for poems, which is the combination of languages that is based on similarity. Metonymy is the combination of languages based on proximity, which is a basic rhetoric for prose. The selection of words is based on similarity, and it is presumed to be interchangeable. Therefore, the process of selection is similar to the thinking process of metaphor. However, the combination of words is based on proximity. The fact that the combination of words is based on proximity means that the process is similar to a metonymic thinking (Lee Seung-Hoon 1995). Jacobson argues that the response of the person who has a similarity disorder is metonymic, and those with proximity disorder show metaphor-related responses (Chin Jung-Kwon 1994b).

Let's say humor is defined as "fall" or a skill of going downward just as in Deleuze's way, rather than excluding a surpassing mindset of Freud's as a thinking or mental activity. In this way, the dichotomy that divides the object of thinking and the subject of thinking, object and non-object, culture and nature, good and evil, and expression and content loses its exclusive effect. In order for the "nonsense humor" by Deleuze to be established, the organic conspirator relationship among substances form, reality, and realities that lies in the dichotomy should be broken down.

4.3   Laughter Therapy

4.3.1   The History of Laughter Therapy

4.3.1.1   The Birth of Laughter Therapy

The renowned journalist Norman Cousins (1979), who also worked as the editor for *Saturday Review*, said at a medical group that "Laughter has the potential to cure." In August of 1964, Cousins was diagnosed with a rare disease called "ankylosing spondylitis," and his doctor said that he wasn't likely to recover from it. About 1 out of 500 patients recover from the disease, and it is a critical condition where inflammation is produced in every knuckle of joints. It comes with a severe pain where the patient is impossible to bend his fingers. The doctor told Cousins that he contracted the disease by heavy metal contamination (pollution). He presumed that Cousins had the condition due to an excessive intake of smoke from his diesel car, which he used when he visited Russia on behalf of the US government.

Cousins knew that there was no special cure for the disease. On the verge of giving up all hope, he thought of the thesis "The stress of life by Hans Selye" (1956), which he read some time ago. In the thesis, it was said that "Our body reacts to

stress" and "negative feelings bring out chemical changes in our body, and ultimately wastes adrenal." Based on the two presumptions, Cousins believed that positive thinking and feeling can cure his disease. Several years ago, he also heard from
Doctor Albert Schweitzer, whom he meet in Lambarene of Africa, that laughter has
mysterious healing powers. Remembering this, Cousins made up his mind that he
would live. He believed that courage, which is used to overcome the pains in reality,
and hope not despairing in any circumstance are important elements that promote
our mental and physical health. Cousins also strongly believed that laughter and
humor erase negative thoughts and give energy in our lives. William Hitzig, his
long-time friend and doctor, also agreed with him that laughter and pleasant feelings
would aid in overcoming the disease. Hitzig encouraged Cousins to go on.

Cousins asked his nurse to read him humor books. He watched Hidden Camera
and Marx Brothers, the two most hilarious movies in the era, giggling immensely.
Laughter took immediate effect. Cousins wasn't able to sleep without painkillers
and sleeping pills, but after 10 min of laughter, he was able to sleep peacefully for
about 2 h. When the laughter medicine had done its effect, he would watch the movies again and make his nurse read the humor comic books to him, even in the middle
of the night. But hospital wasn't an ideal place to laugh. Laughing to his heart's
content at a saddening "prison" wasn't an option, as it was rude to other patients,
and he was frequently labeled as a lunatic.

Cousins had no reason to stay at the hospital. Hospitalization guaranteed no cure,
and it wasn't the doctor who gave him hope of survival. As mentioned, hospital
wasn't a good place for him to laugh out loud. He only had to pay a third of the
hospital room for a cozy, quiet hotel room near the hospital. So Cousins got out of
the hospital, conducted laughter therapy, and took vitamin C as well. The doctor
prescribed 26 pills of aspirin and 12 pills of phenylbutazone. The medicine, painkillers and antiphlogistics, had much side effect. When taken, the two brought out
rashes in his entire body, and it felt like hundreds of red ants were biting him. So in
order to solve the severe problem of inflammation, Cousins took a large amount of
vitamin C as his cure. By conducting the laughter therapy, he was able to move his
thumb without pain in 8 days, and his blood precipitation rate steadily went down,
after hitting 80.

When Cousins was hospitalized, his blood precipitation rate was 88. Before the
week passed, it skyrocketed to 115. Blood precipitation rate is a general way to see
the speed of red blood cells (millimeters in hours) as they precipitate in the test
tubes. The speed of precipitation shows how severe inflammation or infection is.
For instance, blood precipitation rate of flu is from 30 to 40. When the rate goes over
60 or 70, doctors see that it is a very serious disease.

It took him several more years to fully recover, but Cousins was able to become
healthy again from the status of suffering from a rare disease that was to become his
deathbed. He was able to play golf and tennis without pain again, to enjoy horseback riding, and to push the buttons on his camera. Based on his experience, he
published his book titled *Anatomy of Illness* in 1968. It became a bestseller in the
USA and gained much popularity among the public. It remained in the bestseller
chart for 40 weeks in the *New York Times* (Kim Yong-Un 1997a).

Cousins lived a healthy life of 75 years. For the last 12 years of his life, he worked as the visiting professor at the medicine department at UCLA, where he promoted positive feelings such as laughter, hope, faith, love, the will to live, goal of life, and delight. He tried to come up with scientific evidence that these can be helpful to patients who are fighting against severe diseases. His efforts are shown in his book *The Biology of Hope*, which was published in 1989, 1 year before his death. The following is quoted from the book:

1. Human body is stronger than people think. Public education related to health issues trick people into thinking that humans are much weaker and less strong than they really are. As a result, we as a nation seem as though are filled with weak people and hypochondria patients. Franz Ingelfinger estimated that 85 % of all diseases are self-limited. The fact should be highlighted in the reeducation of the American people. Furthermore, therapies, especially drug-related therapies, should be limited in use.

2. Patients are prone to be captured by fear. The ability of the doctor to calm the patients down is a major component that activates the body's innate curing ability. Giving the patients a peace of mind and boosting their confidence can be a great help to making the best of the treatment.

3. Considerate doctors have great interest in the treatment environment. The surrounding environment related to treatment can have an effect on the treatment.

4. A strong will to live and other positive feelings such as belief, love, goals in life, determination and humor are all biochemical realities that affect the treatment environment. If negative feelings are physiological elements that worsen the condition, positive feelings are physiological elements that overturn the disease.

5. Depression has a negative effect on the immune system, and is a critical cause that worsens our physical health. When depression is overcome, almost automatically, the number of immune cells that fight against the disease increases, and they become more active. The most effect way to prevent depression is to have a strong will, a firm determination, and to engage in interesting and useful activities, which all point to a firm goal to live. The role of the doctor is also very important. Good treatment depends on how much emotionally the doctor can react to the patient's needs.

6. There is no guarantee that active attitudes of the patients turn directly into treatment tools. However, it can make a useful environment that can aid the treatment process. It will also help both the patient and the doctor to aim for the best, and to achieve the best of what they can.

7. Patients' condition tend to shift depending on their expectations, whether it is positive or a negative.

8. As there are some cases where the condition gets better, without expected, published books related to the medical field is in a good place to discover such evidence. It is only natural that both the doctors and the patients want the best and try their best to attain it.

9. It is more useful for the doctor to tell his patients to take on the challenge, rather than giving obscure opinions. When the doctor treats severe disease, he has to make sure the patient puts in special effort, and make him understand that the effort is worthwhile.

10. Family members, friends and social groups can help the patient as he fights against the negative feelings that are bound to follow the diagnosis of a severe disease. Our brains arouse feelings of fear and helplessness when we hear bad news. Therefore, strong support from the family members and friends can help to achieve a balanced emotional status or to recover from pain.

11. Medical therapies are not the ultimate judges. Patients' emotions when they undergo diagnosis can have an effect on the test results. This holds especially true when heart-related diagnosis is made. The environment of the test and patients' feelings can have an impact on the test results. We should also remember that modern techniques can't entirely be an alternative for the doctor's diagnosis.

12. The ability of the doctor to listen carefully to the patients' stories is more important than the answering questions about the diagnosis. Understanding all elements that produce disease is as important as checking the sick parts.
13. Lastly, I want to say that the general public's interest on the patients, who have given themselves to the doctors, has increased throughout the last ten years. To tell the truth, I felt somewhat downhearted by some medical education and realities. It would have saddened me all the more if I had to give up the most important result that I had gained from the ten years I spent in college of medicineby observation. Most medical experts (students, professors, nurses and doctors) can take pride on themselves that they are working in this rewarding field and that they understand the philosophical aspect of their occupation (Cousins 1992a).

4.3.1.2 Development Period

After Cousin's anecdotes were reported in the medical world, many doctors had second thoughts about laughter therapy, which had been regarded as nontraditional, peripheral, and alternative therapy. It received wide interest from the medical experts. Some professors in the prestigious medical universities, such as Stanford and Harvard, have started clinical tests on laughter. Theses that say laughter helps relieve stress and cure disease have appeared, as well. With the changing trend, laughter therapy became widespread in North American countries. In particular, Doctor William Fry at Stanford University researched on the relationship between laughter and health for 40 years. The following is quoted from his book *Advances in the Clinical Use ofHumor*, where he reported on the physiological effects of laughter:

- Natural painkillers such as endorphin and encephalin are produced from pituitary glands.
- Mysterious chemical substances are produced in adrenal, which cures inflammation that causes pain and neuralgia.
- As artery is relaxed, the circulation of blood and blood pressure is lowered.
- Laughter helps ease stimulus on all organs of the body.
- Laughter diminishes the amount of cortisol in the blood.
- Heart attacks can be prevented by easing stress, anger and stimulus.
- Laughter increases the pulse of heartbeats, thereby stimulating the circulation of blood and affecting body muscles.
- It prevents diseases in the circulatory system, which can be the cause for stroke.
- It relieves the pains on the part of the cancer patients.
- Three to four minutes of laughter doubles the heartbeat, and supplies more oxygen to blood.
- It can produce effects on the chest, stomach and the upper muscles of the shoulders as if you exercised (Kim Yong-Un 1997b).

Vera Robinson, a nurse and a professor of the college of nursing at the California Fullerton State University, received her doctor's degree on her thesis on why the use of laughter is important on the medical experts. She published the first textbook of laughter therapy, *Humor and the Health Professions*. In 1986, Canadian psychologist Herbert Lefcourt and Rod Martin wrote in the book *Humor and Life Stress* the results of stress and emotional response by their research on laughter and humor. They said that humor and laughter are the most efficient ways to relieve stress.

4.3.1.3 Transformation Period

Laughter therapy underwent transformation period when professors Lee Burke and Stanley Tan at the college of medicine at Loma Linda, California, gave medical proof. Norman Cousins, who was at the UCLA in those days, gave a part of his research fund to the two professors (Cousins 1992b). Doctor Burke's theory was that laughter strengthened immune system. He did a research with ten healthy men and made them watch a hilarious, 60-min movie. He checked the men's immune body changes in the blood before, during, and after the men watched the funny movie. As his expectation, it was revealed that the interferon-gamma hormone, which is an antibody that prevents pathogenic bacterium in the body, is secreted much when people laugh. In his later studies, it was revealed that there was a significant decrease of cortisol, which is a hormone which has the repressive power on immunity. Naturally produced blastogenesis was discovered to increase greatly. Dr. Burke argued that laughter is the "real medicine," not a complementary alternative medicine. The phrase symbolizes the healing power of laughter by an expert who has conducted long-term studies on the physiological effects of laughter.

The "laughter festival" first began at a Jewish hospital in New York in 1995. After supported by Toyota, the Japanese motor company, the festival spread to nine more hospitals in New York. It developed into a very popular program to be broadcast in 600 hospitals across the USA.

Patty Wooten made a textbook on laughter especially for nurses (Wooten 2002) and formed a nurse laughter group. In more than 570 hospitals in the USA, nurses in clown costumes make rounds in the wards and make the patients happy. Wooten runs this program where laughter is used as one of the medicine to cure patients. She was also the chair of a global body that promotes laughter therapy and said that "laughter isn't taught as a cure in traditional medical schools, but the situation is rapidly changing." Wooten prospected that laughter therapy will be taken as a regular subject at medical and nursing schools and her forecast become a reality before long.

4.3.1.4 Activation Period

Laughter therapy is not only for the patients who are sick, and it is becoming widely known among the general public. Doctor Madan Kataria at the Department of Surgery from Mumbai, India, who established "Laughter Club International," contributed to the popularization of laughter.

In March of 1995, the "Laughter Club International" kicked off with five members. In just 1 month, the number of members increased to thousands. He once said,

"The sun gives sunlight to the ground without a special reason, and the wind comes and goes. Only people try to laugh with a reason. That is why we lost how to laugh." Members follow him and start with a simple exercise. Then artificial laughter is produced, followed by a natural laughter with sounds, which is to be replaced with a hard laugh when the mood goes up. As you can see, the club uses laughter yoga to give health, pleasure, happiness, and peace to the general public, including patients. Doctor Madan Kataria argues that the body, mind, and spirit can be integrated through the laughter yoga. Madan Kataria visited Korea in March of 2008, contributing to the spread of laughter therapy movement in Korea.

In 1999, "Patch Adams" produced and distributed a movie on laughter therapy. The movie had the message that we should meet people, not patients, and stressed that patients are humans as well. "Patch" plays the main character in the movie and is taken from a real-life person. His real name is Hunter Adams. The movie contributed to the production of comedy movies on laughter therapy.

Another person who contributed to the widespread of laughter therapy is Steve Wilson, a humorist and clinical psychologist. After he met with Madan Kataria in 1998, he developed laughter yoga with more psychological and scientific clinical tests. Wilson founded and runs the "World Laughter Tour," and related clubs have been made in various countries. There were 300 in the USA in 2006 and 480 all around the world. As of late 2009, more than 5000 leaders in the USA who engage in laughter therapies have trained in the seminars from the club. Wilson continues to actively promote laughter movements in and out of the country (Wilson 2004).

Recently, laughter-diet academies that make people exercise while laughing is gaining popularity in the USA, numbering up to 1000. When we laugh and exercise at the same time, various muscles can be moved. To put it into perspective, 80 facial muscles, 650 body muscles, and 206 bones can be moved. Furthermore, all organs in our body can be moved as well, according to the strength and method of laughing. Therefore, laughter can become a health exercise. Laughing out loud for 15 s can burn 12 cal, and laughing for 3 min produces the same effect as doing sit-ups 25 times. If you want to use laughing skills to exercise, various stages ranging from laughter breath to laughter stretching should be learned professionally (Han Gwang-Il 2006).

4.3.2 The Definition of Laughter Therapy and Laughter Therapist

All around the world, activities related to laughter therapy is being widely promoted. BL, or beautiful laughter, is used in various fields, such as facial image control, preventing cold and other severe conditions like cancer. Beautiful laughter promotes level of immunity and at the same time improves mental and physical health. It is one of the representative social medicines (SMs) of the twenty-first century that elevates individuals, families, and the society.

There is a phrase that "Even artificial laughter helps health." From this, we can presume that laughter needs training and exercise. The relationship between emotion and expression is not one way, so when our emotion changes, our facial expression shifts and vice versa. It is because the part that controls emotion in the cerebrum is near the part that controls exercise. The latter part controls our facial expressions, and the two interact with each other. Therefore, putting on a sulky face will make you feel dissatisfied at the things around you. However, even putting on an artificial smile will elevate your feelings. The theory that our facial expression has an impact on our inner mind is called the "facial feedback theory" (Lee Min-Kyu 2008). Laughter therapy, as described above, is a therapy that depends on the various natural healing power of laughter and on its sociopsychological effects.

The American Association for Therapeutic Humor, AATH, states that laughter therapy uses funny episodes and expressions in our daily lives to promote health and comfort (AATH, 2004). Ultimately, laughter therapy is a behavior-cognitive therapy that seeks to increase people's quality of life and find happiness (Seo Hye-Yung 2012).

In Korea, laughter therapy emphasizes that it differs from medical treatments in the sense that it has to go beyond physical treatment to change our psychological status to promote both physical and mental health. In other words, voluntary or involuntary laughter can be used to maintain, recover, or prevent physical, psychological, social, mental, and spiritual functions. The goal is to make people live a desirable life and maintain a healthy relationship with people. Therefore, it means using laughter to express his physical and emotional status to find happiness. And by maximizing the physical and mental functions that remains in the body, laughter therapy is to bring out positive changes. Laughter therapy produces good experiences of voluntary and involuntary laughter. In the case of laughing sounds, there are just silent smiles that appear on the face, laughter with small sounds, and big laughs that shake your body and hilarious laughter where you feel stomachache. Laughing sounds shouldn't be a burden on the larynx, and a good laugh is a strong one which can be produced by people who don't have severe complications of lung and heart-related diseases. When we hear others' laughter, it stimulates us and makes our laughter all the more joyous.

Laughter exercise makes an intentional laughter that is guided by the laughter therapist, which is produced for more than 10 s. Through laughter movement, heartbeat is increased, and the number of breaths taken changes, which are ways to strengthen our heart functions. When you first start the laughter movement, 40–60 % of the maximum exercise potential should be conducted. Big laughter exercise time should be gradually increased until it reaches 20 min. The frequency of the big laughs such as hilarious ones and the ones that give you a stomachache should begin at two times to be increased to three to four in the middle period and five to six in the later times. It should be repeated until you reach the five to six limit. Laughter therapy as a group treatment program is the significant element that produces immediate response of pleasure and comfort at the same time. It induces the gathered people to interact with immediate laughter and can give feelings of joy and positive emotional and physical changes, ultimately promoting health.

The following is the role of the laughter therapist, which is an occupation that is gaining popularity nowadays. As for individuals, laughter therapist treats the negative functions of the body, mind, spirit, and environment with laughter. In social sense, laughter therapist seeks to solve social pathologic phenomena. Laughter therapist gives happiness and peace to families and religious communities and promotes attention span of students and fun education at schools. In companies, a laughter therapist boosts the morale of the employees with fun management and passes down the principle that productivity can be increased through this. In hospitals and welfare facilities, a laughter therapist takes on various roles. Therefore, laughter therapists should be equipped with intelligence, morality, and flexibility. Furthermore, they should fully be prepared for the program and also have flexibility in running the program in each situation. In short, results produced in the programs are important for laughter therapists, but they should also consider the following: "How does the laughter therapist manage the program? In what way, content, and skill?" and they should know "if the participants are working in the program with passion and an active attitude." They should always keep in mind "whether the program is managed according to the goal of the group."

As you can see, laughter therapy provides various humormechanisms that can produce laughter, such as taste, sound, picture, written materials, humor, performance, exhibition, imagination, experiential activities, dance, tours, leisure sports, recreation, quiz, artificial laughter, and so on. It is not only a mediator that provides information on laughter but also gives behavioral and psychological treatments about laughter. Therefore, it should be sustainable and inclusive service to people from all walks of life, regardless of age, gender, or condition. The most important is that the state of happiness should be felt through laughter.

Lastly, in order for systemized treatment recreation such as laughter therapy to be a success, an organic and effective communication between the professional experts and the treatment team is needed. The following are the major roles each should assume (KAAHS 2006):

1. Doctors and nurses – focus on medical problems
2. Psychology counselors – focuses emotional problems
3. Physical therapist – recovers physical skills and functions
4. Occupational therapist – instructs skills for self-sustainability
5. Occupational therapist – instructs occupational skills and ways to land jobs
6. Language therapist – focuses on language and communication
7. Social worker – provides resource information through counseling and help people to adapt to new surroundings
8. Laughter therapist – manages and runs laughter treatment programs
9. Recreation leader – manages and runs recreational programs

4.3.3   The Effects of Laughter Therapy

Recently, interest on laughter therapy is increasing both home and abroad. Therefore, various clinical researchers are trying to identify the treatment effects of laughter. Results differ according to the treatment subject and mediating methods. Reports show that laughter therapy has various physical and mental effects.

4.3.3.1   Physical Effects of Laughter Therapy

According to Berk and others, the test results of adults who were shown 60 min of humor video showed a decrease in stress hormones, such as cortisol (Berk et al. 1989). It was also revealed that laughter had a significant effect on diet and weight loss (Jang Kyung-Soo and Lee Dong-Kyu 2004).

At first, laughter increases heart rate, blood pressure, tension of the muscle, and breathing rate. However, a relatively short relaxation period replaces the laughter, and the blood pressure decreases, whereas the circulation of the body, the digestion, and the saturation of oxygen in the body are activated. This leads to the decreased bodily reactions related to stress. In particular, a loud laughter stimulates 231 muscles out of the 650 in our body, affecting the cardiovascular, respiratory, and musculoskeletal system. It has the same effect as doing a whole body exercise. When a person laughs, it is the same as doing aerobics for 5 min. Laughing for 1 min is similar to exercising 10 min and laughing for 20 min is as same as rowing with all might for 3 min. It is even argued that laughing 45 min a day can cure all diseases for people living in the modern (Fry 1992). In short, laughter relieves the tension in the muscles and decreases any abnormal bodily reactions by strengthening the cardiopulmonary functions. With an effect similar to that of exercise, laughter also has a positive impact on the coping skills of stress.

4.3.3.2   Psychological Effect of Laughter Therapy

One of the most researched areas of laughter therapy in Korea is related to anxiety and depression. For instance, Kim and Jun did a singular laughter therapy that lasted 60 min on the elderly. The result showed that the experimental group had a significant increase of good feelings than the control group, in terms of their reaction to psychological stress. However, depression and anxiety levels showed no meaningful changes. In the physiological stress reaction, contraction period blood pressure and the amount of cortisol decreased statistically significantly. However, the blood pressure of relaxation period and pulse showed little changes. In immunologic stress reaction, the ratio of natural killer cells and the amount of immunoglobulin G had no significance statistically (Kim and Jun 2009). Kim also provided the type 2 diabetes mellitus patients who are hospitalized with a 60-min laughter therapy a day for three consecutive days. Their state anxiety and depression scores all showed a decrease at the time of termination. Lee and Sohn gave the local people who underwent petroleum damage four laughter therapy classes. The class lasted for 4 weeks, 60 min at a time, once a week. The result showed that the anger (disposition) significantly decreased in the ways the anger was expressed in the experimental group. However, anger (status) didn't show a statistically meaningful decrease, although it did decrease later in the experimental group. In terms of mentalhealth, experimental group showed a statistically meaningful decrease in physical tendency compared with the control group (Lee and Sohn 2010).

The anxiety of the following patients was lowered by laughter therapy: soldiers, cancer patients, backache patients, and inflammatory bowel disease patients. As you can see, it has been revealed that laughter therapy resulted in the decreased feelings of depression, the elevation of feelings, and the decreased of contraction period blood pressure in the following patients: elders, women in middle ages, cancer patients, blood dialysis patients (Heo 2007), backache patients, and stroke hemiparesis patients.

4.3.3.3   Physiological Effects of Laughter Therapy

After the research of Dr. Fry, laughter has been known not only to stimulate muscle-exercise, pulse rate, and exchange of oxygen in the relationship between laughter and health but also to promote sympathetic nervous system and cardiovascular system. When we laugh, the movements of heart muscles and blood pressure rise, and we breathe more rapidly. As a result, the circulation of blood in the artery and vein is increased, and the flow of oxygen and nutrients to the tissues is activated. Endorphin, which is secreted when laughing, gets rid of pain and increases sleep. It not only controls feelings of depression and anxiety (Lebowitz 2002) but also stimulates catecholamine, the neurotransmitter of the sympathetic nervous system, and the production of immunoglobulin. It also activates natural killer cell (NK cell) (Bennet and Lengacher 2006; Hajime 2004; Berk et al. 2001; Burns 1996). Moreover, laughter increases the flow of blood circulation and strengthens heart functions, thereby increasing bodily circulation and cardiopulmonary function. It is clinically confirmed again and again that it also prevents heart attack and numerous diseases related to the cardiovascular system (Fry 1994).

Recently, Jeong Jong-Soon summarized the physiological effects of laughter therapy by looking into the research:

1. When we laugh, natural painkillers such as endorphin and encephalin are produced from pituitary gland.
2. Mysterious hormones that cure inflammation such as pain and neuralgia are secreted from adrenal when we laugh.
3. Laughter relaxes artery, and the circulation of blood is activated and the blood pressure is lowered.
4. Laughter relaxes all organs throughout the body.
5. Laughter diminishes the amount of cortisol in the blood.
6. Laughter prevents heart attack by decreasing stress, anger, and anxiety.

7. Laughter increases heart rate (pulse), helping the circulation of blood and affecting the muscles.
8. Laughter prevents disease in the circulatory system that causes stroke.
9. Laughter relieves cancer patients of pain.
10. Three to four minutes of laughter doubles the pulse rate and provides more oxygen in the blood.
11. Laughter produces a similar effect on the chest, stomach and shoulder muscles as exercise (Jeong Jong-Soon 2007).

4.3.3.4 Emotional Effects of Laughter Therapy

After laughter was known to act as an antidote to relieve stress (Wooten 1996), laughter was also reported to increase self-esteem, to promote positive thinking and confidence, and to decrease pain (Bennet and Lengacher 2006). Laughter is a natural response to humor and controls stress, anxiety, depression, and feelings and also promotes learning abilities (Bennet et al. 2003). In Korea, there are also studies that report the effect of laughter therapy on stress. Let's look at the process up to the laughter response. First, there has to be a stimulus of humor, and the emotional reaction is produced, varying from pleasure and delight to happiness. As a result, laughter is produced (Heo Eun-Hwa 2007). Laughter gets rid of feelings of tension between people, elevates positive atmosphere, makes our minds and body healthy, and becomes a useful alternative to make us get out of unfortunate situations. Laughter is a self-tool that can produce such good results and is a good stress reliever. There are also studies on laughter, cognitive behavior, and emotions. In particular, laughter is a helper that lets us get rid of unfortunate situations and painful moments. Moreover, laughter is reported to have positive impacts on the women after they recover from childbirth and on the breast cancer survivors' quality of life.

Laughter exposes people to various possibilities where they can restore confidence, self-esteem, recovery from fatigue, quality of life, and well-being. It also makes people to be more relaxed as they go about their daily lives. As you can see, research on the effects of laughter therapy on self-esteem and emotional peace and the altogether result of health promotion is increasing.

4.3.4 Laughter Therapy of Korean University Hospitals

[Seoul National University Hospital]

Laughter therapy: It is a therapy that uses laughter to relieve bodily and emotional pain and stress. Medicine of mental health is in charge of laughter therapy.

1. Definition: It is a therapy that uses laughter to relieve bodily and emotional pain and stress. It is used as an alternative way to promote health and recover from disease.

Since the historic times, laughter has been steadily used in medicine. In the early thirteenth century, some surgeons used laughter to relieve patients from the pains from operation. In the sixteenth century, Robert Burton used laughter therapy as a way to cure melancholy, and Richard Mulcaster used it as a way of exercise. In the seventeenth century, Herbert Spencer used laughter to get rid of excessive tension, and Gottlieb Hufeland used it to help digestion in the nineteenth century. In the twentieth century, Doctor James Walsh in the USA used laughter to stimulate the intestines. In the field of medicine, laughter has always been a subject of research.

Laughter therapy in the modern society started from Norman Cousins, who was the editor of *Saturday Review* in the USA. He once suffered from ankylosing myelitis and endured great pain due to the stiffening bone and muscle. One day, he realized that pain was reduced after he watched a comedy show. He found out that 15 min of laughter took away 2 h of pain. Later, laughter therapy aided much in curing his disease. In a university hospital in California, he set out to study the medical effects of laughter. Since then, research on laughter therapy has been conducted.

2. Types: There are various kinds of laughter. Passive humor is laughing as you watch funny movies, comedies, books, and any materials that are prepared. Spontaneous or unplanned humor is finding something to laugh at in your daily life. The ability to find laughter in ordinary things can be helpful when curing cancer. Laughter therapy can be applied in the following cases:

   - Relieving patients' pain
   - Stress management and emotion control of ordinary people
   - A way of treating anger, depression, and feelings
   - Promoting doctor-patient relationship
   - Increasing mutual communication

   Laughter therapy is broadly applied to many other areas.

3. Preparation: Before patients are prescribed with laughter therapy, they should be thoroughly evaluated whether laughter therapy is right for them. Burton Leiber said that the following three aspects should be taken into account:

   1. Time: For instance, laughter can't be understood when the patient is in the harshest conditions.
   2. Degree of acceptance: In some instances and in some people, the actions that drew laughter from other patients may not work.
   3. Content: The content that is made to produce laughter should be considered whether it is suitable for the patient, in terms of his character and cultural context.

4. How to administer laughter therapy: Laughter therapy can be provided alone or can be utilized as a part of treatment program such as mental therapy or stress relieving method. According to each situation, laughter therapy can be conducted in a group or individually. Movies, audio materials, books, games, and various materials can be used to induce laughter. As a way of exercise, continu-

ous laugh or smiling can be utilized. According to the purpose of the treatment and patients, various ways can be used.

5. Duration of time: It can vary according to each treatment.
6. Results and complications

   1. Immunesystem: Laughter brings about changes on the substances that are related to the immune system. The number of interferon-δ, white cells, and immunoglobulin increases, and cortisol that repress immunity and epinephrine decrease. There are also reports that NK cells, which kill cancer cells, are strongly activated through laughter.
   2. Neurohormone system: Laughter increases the secretion of neurotransmitters such as endorphin and enkephalin in the brain, which diminish pain. It physiologically supports that laughter increases the endogenous energy against pain. Furthermore, one of the representative stress hormones, cortisol, is lowered in its concentration in the blood.
   3. Cardiovascular system: Laughter eases blood vessels, lowering blood pressure and accelerating blood circulation. It also increases breathing and oxygen availability.

   There are other reports that say laughter improves allergic conditions and diabetes and has similar effects as exercising.
7. Side effects and aftermath: Laughter therapy can be safe when it is used with conventional medical treatment. Laughter therapy can be very important to the patient or his family, but if it is used to avoid certain problems, it can be harmful. In addition, laughter can cause temporary pain after specific kind of operations, but after recovery, it boosts condition and doesn't leave a permanent harm. Patients' values and cultural differences should be considered as well. Some patients can't accept laughter, and efforts to induce laughter by humiliating others should be taken seriously. When the condition calls for medical treatment such as cancer, patients shouldn't solely rely on laughter therapy. When conventional therapy conducted in hospitals are prohibited or delayed due to laughter therapy, serious results may arise.
8. Related therapies: Psychology therapy, music therapy, art therapy, cognitive therapy, behavior therapy, relaxation technique, and stress management.
9. Disease to be treated: Cancer or other specific diseases.

There aren't ample scientific evidence that laughter is an effective way of treating cancer or other specific conditions. However, laughter has many good sides. Laughter affects various systems in the body, and it brings about positive bodily changes and relieves pain. It also eases stress and negative emotions, at the same time improving satisfaction on life. Many hospitals utilize laughter therapy to ease patients' pain and fight over disease. To the patients at hospice hospitals, laughter therapy can be helpful in recovering their vitality and positive outlook on life, as they suffer from fatigue from a long fight over cancer (Source: Seoul National University Hospital/Naver 2014).

References

Association for Applied and Therapeutic Humor (2004) Essence. Retrieved 31 Jan 2005, from http://www.aath.org/home_1.html, p 1
Association for Applied and Therapeutic Humor (2004) Essence. Retrieved 31 Jan 2005, from http://www.aath.org/home_1.html
Bae Hyun-Ja (2001) Study on satire of Kim Seung-Ok's Novels. Master thesis, Ewha Womans University
Bakhtin, MM (1982) The dialogic imagination: four essays (trans: Emerson C, Holquist M). University of Texas Press, Austin
Beattie J (1975) An essay on laughter and ludicrous composition. In: Battie J, Essays. Hildesheim, pp 587–590. In Ryoo Jong-Yung, Aesthetics of laughter, Yuroseojuk, 2005, pp 180–181
Bennet MP, Lengacher CA (2006) Humor and laughter may influence health. I. History and background. Evid Based Complement Alternat Med 3(1):61–63
Bennet MP, Uanice MZ, Rosenberg L (2003) The effect of mirthful laughter on stress and natural killer cell activity. Altern Ther Health Med 9(2):38–39
Bergson H (1994a) Laughter: current view on the meaning of comic character (trans: Jung Yun-Bok). Segyesa, Seoul, p 79
Bergson H (1994b) ibid., pp 105
Bergson H (1994c) ibid., pp 23–25
Berk LS, Fry WF, Hubbard RW (1989) Neuroendocrine and stress hormone changes during mirthful laughter. Am J Med Sci 298(6):390–396
Berk LS, David L, Felton S, Tan SA, Bittman BB, Westengard J (2001) Modulation of neuroimmune parameters during the eustress of humor-associated mirthful laughter. Altern Ther 7(2):62–76
Burns C (1996) Comparative analysis of humor versus relaxation training for the enhancement of immunocompetence. Unpublished doctoral dissertation, Biola University, La Mirada, CA
Caron JE (2002) From ethology to aesthetics: evolution as a theoretical paradigm for research on laughter, humor, and other comic phenomena. Humor Int J Humor Res 15(3):245–281
Chin Jung-Kwon (1994a) Aesthetics Odyssey 2, Sae Gil, pp 196–197
Chin Jung-Kwon (1994b) ibid., pp 200–201
Conrad-Martius H (1957) Das Sein. Munchen, S. 23
Coser RL (1959) Some social functions of laughter. Hum Relat 12:171–182
Cousins N (trans: Lee Jung-Sik) (1992a) Hope, laugh, and therapy. Bumyang Press, Co. Ltd., pp 356–358
Cousins N (1992b) ibid., pp 188–189
Darwin C (trans: Choi Won-Jae) (1998) On the expression of emotion in human and animal. Seohaemunjip, pp 180–196
Deleuze G (trans: Lee Kang-Hoon) (1996a) Masochism. Ingansarang, p 92
Deleuze G (1996b) ibid., p 93
Deleuze G (1996c) ibid., p 142
Deleuze G (trans: Lee Jung-Woo) (1996d) ibid., p 249
Deleuze G (trans: Lee Jung-Woo) (1999a) Logics of meaning. Han Gil Sa, p 31
Deleuze G (1999b) ibid., p 58
Deleuze G (1999c) ibid., p 42
Dosio D (1989) Dictionary of aesthetics and art science. Mijinsa, Seoul, p. 280
Foley E, Matheis R, Schaefer C (2002) Effect of forced laughter on mood. Psychol Rep 90(1):184
Freud S (1928; 1959) Humor. In: Strachey J (ed) Collected papers of Sigmund Freud, vol 5. Basic Books, New York
Freud S (1963) Der Humor. In: Ders., Gesammelte Werke. Bd. 14, Frankfurt a. M, S. 386
Freud S (trans: Lim In-Joo) (1997a) Relationship between joke and non-consciousness. Open Books, p 181
Freud S (1997b) ibid., p 224

Freud S (trans: Jung Jang-Jin) (1998a) Creative writer and dreaming. Open Books, p 10
Freud S (1998b) ibid., p 17
Fry WF (1992) The physiological effects of humor, mirth, laughter. JAMA 267(13):1857–1858
Fry WF (1994) The biology of humor. Humor Int J Humor Res 7(2):111–126
Fry WF (2002) Humor and the brain: a selective review. Humor 15:305–333
Gamble J (2001) Humor in apes. Humor Int J Humor Res 14(2):163–179
Garatani Gojin (trans: Lee Kyung-Hoon) (2002) Materialism as humor. Munhwa Guahak Sa, p 127
Garbarino (1995) Sociocultural theory in anthropology: a short history (trans: Han Kyung-Goo, Lim Bong-Gil). Iljogak, Seoul, pp 103–104
Go Hyun-Kyung (2006) Study on humor expressions in object art. Master thesis. Korea National University of Education
Goo Hyun-Jeong (2000) Structure and production mechanism of humor story-telling. Hangul, No. 248, Academic Association of Hangul, p 162
Hajime K (2004) Reduction of plasma levels of neurotrophins by laughter in patients with atopic dermatitis. Pediatr Asthma Allergy Immunol 17(2):12–14
Han Gwang-Il (2006) Laughter therapy. Sam Ho Media, Seoul, p 48
Hartmann N (trans: Jun Won-Bae) (1995a) Aesthetics. Eul Yu Press, p 473
Hartmann N (1995b) ibid., p 474
Heo EH (2007) Effect of laughter on mood, stress response and health-related quality of life among hemodialysis patients. Unpublished master's thesis, CHA University, Pocheon
Hobbes T: Human nature, or the fundamental elements of policy. Being a discovery of the faculties, acts, and passions of the soul of man, from their original causes; according to such philosophical principles, as are not commonly known or asserted. In: The English works of Thomas Hobbes of Malmesbury; now first collected an edited by Sir William Molesworth, Bart., vol IV, Reprint of the edition 1840, Aalen 1962, ch. 8, pp 11–25. In Ryoo Jong-Yung, Aesthetics of laughter, Yuroseojuk, 2005, p 127
Horn, Andras 1: Das Komische im Spiegel der Literatur, Versuch einer systematischen Einführung. Würzburg 1988, S. 41. In Ryoo Jong-Yung, Aesthetics of laughter, Yuroseojuk, 2005, p 69
Horn, Andras 2: ibid., S. 194 In Ryoo Jong-Yung, Aesthetics of laughter, Yuroseojuk, 2005, pp 38–39
Jang Kyung-Soo, Lee Dong-Kyu (2004) A special report on laughter. Ran Dom House Korea, Seoul
Jeong Jong-Soon (2007) Study on effectiveness of laughter therapy programs. Master thesis, Cho Sun University
Ju Seon-Hee, Jin Se-Hun (2013a) Face reading woman and facial image changing man. Open House, p 4
Ju Seon-Hee, Jin Se-Hun (2013b) ibid., pp 71–72
Kagan MS (trans: Chin Jung-Kwon) (1989) Aesthetics lecture 1. Sae Gil, p 206
Kant I. Anthropologie in pragmatischer Hinsicht. Bd. VII. Kap. 76. In: Kant I. Gesammelte Schriften. Hrsg. von der Königlich Preussischen Akadmie der Wissenschaften, Berlin und Leipzig, 1900ff., S. 261f
Kim EH (2009) The effects of laughter therapy on the anxiety and depression of diabetic patients. Unpublished master's thesis, Sogang University, Seoul, p. 43
Kim Hwon-Hwan (2006a) Concerning the Visual Non-sense in Cartoons: Centered on the Humor. Master thesis. Kongju National University, p 52
Kim Hwon-Hwan (2006b) ibid., pp 9–10
Kim Hwon-Hwan (2006c) ibid., p 10
Kim Hwon-Hwan (2006d) ibid., p 5
Kim Hwon-Hwan (2006e) ibid., pp 23–24
Kim Hwon-Hwan (2006f) ibid., p 27
Kim Ji-Won (1983a) Literature of humor and irony. Moonjang Press, pp 33–35
Kim Ji-Won (1983b) ibid., p 31
Kim Kyung-Tae (1991) You can make others laugh. Jisiksanupsa Co. Ltd., pp 23–29

Kim Sa-Yup (1957) Essence of laugh and irony, literature and linguistics, No. 2, Academic Association of Literature and Linguistics, p 5

Kim Yong-Un (1997a) Healthcare theory of laughter. Yeyoung Communication, Seoul, pp 12–17

Kim Yong-Un (1997b) ibid., pp 60–63

Kim YS, Jun SS (2009) The influence of one-time laughter therapy on stress response in the elderly. J Korean Acad Psychiatr Ment Health Nurs 18(3):269–277

Korean Association of Aerobics Health Science (KAAHS) (2006) Education Guidelines for Leaders of Dementia Prevention Campaign. 21 Century Education, Seoul, pp 183–190

Korean Britannica Online (2001) Laughter. www.preview.britannica.co.kr. Retrieved in 2014/6/10.

Lebowitz KR (2002) The effects of humor on cardiopulmonary functioning, psychological well-being and health status among older adults with chronic obstructive pulmonary disease. Unpublished doctoral dissertation. The Ohio State University, Columbus

Lee Im-Seon, Bae Ki-Hyo, Paik Jung-Seon (2009) Introduction to laughter therapy. Changjisa, Seoul

Lee Kang-Yup (1998) A fool story: the real meaning of laughter. Pyungminsa, p 282

Lee Min-Kyu (2008) Psychology of affirmation destinating my life. One and One Books, Seoul

Lee Seung-Hoon (1995) Current view of modernism. Munye Press, Seoul, p 252

Lee YM, Sohn JN (2010) The effects of laughter therapy on anger, anger expressions and mental status after oil spill in victimized community residence. J Korean Acad Psychiatr Ment Health Nurs 19(2):186–195

Lefcourt HM, Martin RA (1986) Humor and life stress – antidote to adversity. Springer-Verlag, New York

Lessing GE (trans: Yoon Do-Joong) (1991) Lessing. Soongsil University Press, pp 186–187

Levenson RW (1988) Emotion and the autonomic nervous system: a prospectus for research on autonomic specificity. In: Wagner HL (ed) Social psychophysiology and emotion: theory and clinical application. Wiley, Hoboken, pp 17–42

Lim Hyo-Soo (2000a) Study on the comic characters and laughter induction of light comedy films in North Korea. Master thesis, Dong Gook University, pp 9–12

Lim Hyo-Soo (2000b) ibid., p 19

Martin RA (1998) Approaches to the sense of humor: a historical review. In: Ruch W (ed) The sense of humor. Mouton de Gruyter, Berlin, pp 16–60

Martin RA (2007) The psychology of humor: an integrative approach. Elsevier Academic Press, Burlington

Martin RA, Lefcourt HM (1983) Sense of humor as a moderator of the relation between stressors and moods. J Pers Soc Psychol 45:1313–1324

Marx K (1946) Der Achtzehnte Brumaire des Louis Bonaparte. Berlin 1946, S. 9, Anmerkung. In Ryoo Jong-Yung, Aesthetics of laughter, Yuroseojuk, 2005, pp 295–296

Marx K (1957) Einleitung. Zur Kritik der Hegelschen Rechtsphilosophie. In: Karl Marx, Friedrich Engels. Werke, Bd. 1, Berlin 1957, S. 382. In Ryoo Jong-Yung, Aesthetics of laughter, Yuroseojuk, 2005, p 296

McAdams DP, Powers J (1981) Themes of intimacy in behavior and thought. J Pers Soc Psychol 40:573–587

McAdams DP, Healy S, Krause S (1984) Social motives and patterns of friendship. J Pers Soc Psychol 47:828–838

Michel JB, Roberta L (2003) The role of laughter in traditional medicine its relevance to the clinical setting: healing with Ha! Altern Ther Health Med 9(4):88

Morris D (trans: Science Generation) (2000) Man watching. Ggachi, p 17

Park Soon-Ok, Kim Soon-Ja (2013) Immunology of laughter. Omunhaksa, pp 10–11

Preuschoft S, van Hooff JA (1997) The social function of "smile" and "laughter": variations across primate species and societies. In: Segerstrale UC, Molnar P (eds) Non-verbal communication: where nature meets culture. Lawrence Erlbaum Associates, Hillsdale, pp 171–190

Ra Won-Ki (2004) Study on laughter therapy in the Bible. Master thesis, Ho Nam Theological University and Seminary

Rabelais F (trans: Kwon Kook-Jin) (2002) Gargantua. Jung Press, p 7

Ryoo Jong-Yung (2005a) Aesthetics of laughter, Yuroseojuk, pp 57–60

Ryoo Jong-Yung (2005b) ibid., pp 73–74

Ryoo Jong-Yung (2005c) ibid., p 78

Ryoo Jong-Yung (2005d) ibid., p 79

Ryoo Jong-Yung (2005e) ibid., p 295

Ryoo Jong-Yung (2005f) ibid., p 160

Ryoo Jong-Yung (2005g) ibid., pp 36–37

Ryoo Jong-Yung (2005h) ibid., p 37

Ryoo Jong-Hoon (2007) Health theory of laughter therapy. Eunhye Press, Seoul, pp 59–63

Schmidt-Hidding W (1963) Humour and witz. München, S. 95f

Schopenhauer A (trans: Kwak Bok-Rok) (2003) The world as will and representation. Eul Yu Publishing Co. Ltd., p 106

Seo Hye-Yung (2012) Test for effectiveness of laughter therapy programs on self-esteem and creativeness in elementary schoolchildren. Master thesis. Myung Ji University

Seoul National University Hospital (2014) Laughter therapy. Retrieved from http://terms.naver.com/entry.nhn?docId=927817&cid=865&categoryId=1734, 2014/1/11

Shaftesbury AAC, Sensus communis. An essay on the freedom of wit and humor (1711). In: Shaftesbury. Sämtliche Werke, ausgewählte Briefe und nachgelassene Schriften. Herausgegeben, Übersetzt und kommentiert von Wolfram Benda, u.a. Bd. 1/3, frummann-holzboog 1992, p 18. In Ryoo Jong-Yung, Aesthetics of laughter, Yuroseojuk, 2005, p 162

Shaw GB (trans: Cho Yong-Jae) (1998) War and hero. Dongin, pp 30–35

Son Semodol (1999) Principles and methods for humor formation. Hanyangomun, No. 17, Han Yang University, p 159

Tomkins SS (1984) Affect theory. In: Ekman P, Scherer K (eds) Approaches to emotion. Erlbaum, Hillsdale, pp 163–196

Toshio D (1989) Dictionary of aesthetics and science of art. Mijinsa, p 280

van Hooff JA, Preuschoft S (2003) Laughter and smiling: the intertwining of nature and culture. In: de Waal FBM, Tyack PL (eds) Animal social complexity: intelligence, culture, and individualized societies. Harvard University Press, Cambridge, MA, pp 260–287

Webster's Third New International Dictionary (1984) USA Merriam-Webster Inc

Wilson S (2004) The world tour (DVD): makes good news! volume 1 – 2003 contains 5 videos! The World Laughter Tour, Columbus

Wooten P (1996) Humor: an antidote for stress. Holist Nurs Pract 10(2):49–59

Wooten P (2002) Compassionate laughter. Jest Press, New York

Chapter 5
Conclusion

5.1 Everybody Wants to Live 100 Years Old with Health

The substantial increase in life expectancy is one of the great human achievements of the past century. The rise in life expectancy over the last century has led to a huge increase in the diseases associated with later life – noncommunicable, often chronic diseases such as cancer, diabetes, and dementias. The risk factors for these diseases are predominately connected to people's lifestyles earlier in life, with major factors being smoking, poor diet, insufficient physical activity, and alcohol overuse. Such being the case, individuals are eager to take the responsibility to fight off these diseases by utilization of "something new and charismatic" rather than drug, since drug itself is not enough for man enable to live 100 years old with health.

This book starts from introspection on materialistic discourse ("new drug development"). Creative resignation and destruction originated from such a fundamental introspection on drug made it possible to go beyond the drug-full world. New drug development is only one little part of the world of medicine, which is only clinging to the infrastructure called productivity. In this sense, a new hope is necessary for man enable to live 100 years old with health. As motivation refers to forces coming from within a person that account for the willful direction, intensity, and persistence of the person's efforts toward achieving a specific goal or vision that is not due to ability or to environmental demands, this book was strongly motivated to reset the direction of the materialistic discourse by replacing productivity with imagination. As a result, the concept of social medicine (SM) is introduced in the world for the first time, based on the premise that "people are health prosumers."

Now, it is declared that the world of medicine is made up of two parts: one, social medicine of the superstructure and the other, visible drug of the infrastructure. Traditionally pharmaceutical scientists have focused on new drug discovery by the objective experiments in "wet laboratory" based on natural sciences ("nanoscience"), while the social and administrative pharmacists concentrate on the discovery of new social medicine by logical abstraction and imagination in "dry laboratory"

© Springer Science+Business Media Singapore 2016
B.-H. Han, *Therapy of Social Medicine*, DOI 10.1007/978-981-287-748-2_5

based on the "big science," convergence of multidisciplinary programs including social sciences, and humanities.

Finally, as it is expected that a paradigm shift should bring from drug to social medicine for the healthy 100-year age in this century, the current dominant discourse that the productivity-based infrastructure defines the imagination-based superstructure must be in vise versa:

Imagination is much greater than knowledge.
Health helps those who help themselves.
Mature life with healthy aging is everyone's self-actualization.

5.2 Social Medicine Is a New Hope for People

In this book, there is a dream of establishing the "social medicine of hope, drug-free world." Competent pharmacist is a professional for drug development and drug utilization, while supreme pharmacist is the expert of medicine who makes a newborn drug useless and helps people to give up drug use, just as supreme military strategist wins without fighting.

Social medicine is "everything that helps our health except drug products," which consists of two key elements originated from natural healing power (NHP) in vitology of Oriental medicine: homeostasis (natural healing strength, NHS) and reciprocity (social healing strength, SHS). Interestingly enough, the top secret of our life was revealed in 1953 by James Dewey Watson and Francis Crick: Genes are made of DNA, consisting of two strands of double helix. As such, social medicine simply consists of two strands of double healings. In other words, social medicine is regarded as remaining margin, while drug is a core part in the contemporarypharmacy.

Social medicine (symbol of superstructure) meets unmet needs of drug (symbol of infrastructure). According to Maslow's need hierarchy, five levels of needs are included: physiological, safety, social and belongingness, esteem, and self-actualization. And these needs are arranged in prepotent hierarchical order. Prepotency refers to the concept that a lower-order need, until satisfied, is dominant in motivating a person's behavior. Once a need for therapy is satisfied by drug in infrastructure, the next higher need for longevity, well-being, and happiness in superstructure becomes the active source of motivation. And this is a raison d'être of social medicine.

Since social medicine is a *charismatic*independent variable, each government in the world needs to develop "structures of social medicine" aiming to help local authorities to use their resources effectively to promote health, well-being, and happiness in later life and ensuring that people can live independently for longer and are engaged in civic life, and their potential is recognized so as to help address social issues of healing, without drug.

5.3   Therapy of Social Medicine

The new concept of social medicine creates opportunities for engaging with people to design and deliver their own healthcare services in the real world, which leads to therapy of social medicine. In short, therapy of social medicine is defined as all the intervening events or activities including health and illness behavior for health management and improvement or methodology derived from the theory of social medicine.

Therapy of social medicine is boundless via horizontal and vertical differentiation. In the case of literature, poem or reading therapy is being developed. In the artistic field, there is music and fine art therapy. In religion, spiritual therapy or temple stay is gaining popularity, and the same goes for play and laughter therapy in the cultural sector. In environmental field, natural therapies such as sunlight, stone, flower, forest, and fragrance have emerged, while talking, shopping, watching TV, sauna, traveling, and caring pets are practiced as new therapies in lifestyle and hobby sector. In this respect, therapy of social medicine is spreading and being distributed faster in many different ways. Therefore, it is nearly impossible to enumerate each horizontal differentiation for therapy of social medicine within this book.

On the other hand, as therapy of social medicine is practiced to the point of physician's prescribing according to each disease (e.g., diet and exercise for diabetes, enforced laughing for cancer, gum chewing for dementia, etc.), vertical differentiation occurs. It will become a niche buster. When the methodologies specialized from therapy of social medicine in various sectors are studied and completed horizontally and vertically, one picture of "The World of Social Medicine" will be revealed naturally.

Here, four major therapies of social medicine including health diet, health exercise, health stressor, and beautiful laughter as well as two methods originated from CAM including evacuation (−) and filling (+) were explored and developed for health and healing. In addition, CAM-derived SM therapies were introduced elaborately for the individuals and community concerned.

Understanding the important interaction between people's health and social and physical environments is only a very recent development. With this in mind, therapy of social medicine rather than drug therapy must be quite new and innovative. In addition, therapy of social medicine could benefit not only physical activity but also social links and spiritual/mental health and healing since it expands beyond all kinds of CAM.

If private and public health structures are to overcome the health-related challenges to addressing the issues surrounding this aging society, it is vital that people first make the most of health and healing opportunities therapy of social medicine creates, since there is no other way for the new challenges of responding to an aging population with long-term health planning.

Generally, local governments are seen as being the fount of innovation in governance. This is largely because local governments deal with smaller populations and because they operate closer and faster to the population they govern and further away from the center where a more bureaucratic approach such as drug therapy is needed in the healthcare system. The key health-related issues of each locality can be addressed by targeted initiatives, and innovative strategies can be developed that encourage more integrated working between departments. Such being the case, local governments are in a good position to use this experience and links with the local community to ensure that the voices of older residents are heard, and the issues effecting them are addressed in local health and healing strategies with a more liberal therapy of social medicine. Health officials, health professionals, and lay members in a small society can enhance this healthcare and healing process by collating resources and ideas from different departments, encouraging integrated working and avoiding doubling-up efforts on particular health issues with each therapy of social medicine.

By and large, the success of a public health and healing message lies in its ability to persuade and inform and that in turn depends on the trust, communication, and respect that the public give to the orator of the message. If local authorities – which do benefit from being democratically elected and close to their local communities – are deemed by the public to speak with authority on public health and healing issues, their message might have more penetrable value. This could be of significant value when initiating public health and healing campaigns such as "therapy of social medicine (no drug)" which can facilitate healthy aging.

While it is imperative that the current healthcare system takes a holistic approach to care, it will take some time for policy-makers to build up a rich bank of evidence and good-practice examples on how to deliver the better health program based on the theory of social medicine and therapy of social medicine addressing the health and healing needs of our aging society without drug that interacts with public transport, environmental policy, and so on.

5.4   Ending Remarks and Suggestions

The rise of social medicine and therapy of social medicine creates an opportunity to tackle the challenges presented by the rapidly aging population at a grassroots level all over the world, with long-term health and healing initiatives rather than short-term solutions.

Particularly, preventative social medicine will need to be developed which ensure older people are healthy and independent for as long as possible. This will involve taking a life course approach to public therapy of social medicine, as a good health and healing in old age requires early detection and intervention. In addition, such preventative policies focusing on therapy of social medicine by their very nature bring financial rewards and health improvements in the long term.

Further work in the health- and healing-related academic societies should be done on each therapy of social medicine, especially laughter therapy with cost-effectiveness. And each central government in the world needs to develop structures aiming to help local authorities make the most of the changes by supporting them to improve their health and healing services for older people. Developing outreach services in near future must be a target that each local government embraces by taking a life course approach to health and healing and by commissioning services that both encourage healthy aging and improve the health of the current old enable to enjoy the mature life with a new hope of establishing therapy of social medicine in the community level.

Index